Alfonso Baruffaldi, Andrea Baruffaldi
Martino Baruffaldi, Livio Yoshinaga

With the collaboration of Pasquale Romano

DIGITAL TECHNIQUES IN IMPLANT SURGERY AND PROSTHETICS

From chair-side to the DIGIT-Skyn concept technique

Forewords
Tiziano Testori
Pascal Valentini

edra
PUBLISHING

Original title

Alfonso Baruffaldi, Andrea Baruffaldi, Martino Baruffaldi, Livio Yoshinaga

TECNICHE DIGITALI IN CHIRURGIA E PROTESI IMPLANTARE. Dal chair-side alla tecnica DIGIT-Skyn concept

ISBN: 978-88-214-5216-1

Book Publishing Manager: **Costanza Smeraldi**, Edra S.p.A.

Paper, Printing and Binding Manager: **Paolo Ficicchia**, Edra S.p.A.

Cover: **Roberta Venturieri**, Edra S.p.A.

Layout: **Fulvio Martello**, Como, Italy

Copyediting: **ALTER EDOM s.r.l.**, Noventa Padovana (PD), Italy

ISBN: 978-1-957260-19-8

eISBN: 978-1-957260-27-3

Edra Publishing US LLC

3309 Northlake Boulevard, Suite 203

Palm Beach Gardens, FL, 33403

EIN: 844113980

info@edrapublishing.com

www.edrapublishing.com

Printed in Italy by Faenza Group S.p.A. Faenza (RA) – December 2022

Authors

Alfonso Baruffaldi, MD, DDS

Graduated in Medicine and Surgery from the University of Bologna, MSD in Odontostomatology from the University of Parma.
Professor of a number of master's degree Courses.
Lecturer at national and international courses and conferences.
Practitioner in Piacenza (Italy), where he specializes in implantology, oral surgery and digital techniques.

Martino Baruffaldi, DDS

Graduated in Dentistry and Dental Prosthetics from the State University of Milan.
Winner of the 2018 Riitano Award at the national AIE Congress (Italian Academy of Endodontics).
Tutor at the IRCCS Galeazzi Orthopedic Institute of Milan, in the Endodontics-ROC and Oral Surgery departments, 2019-2020.
Practitioner in Piacenza (Italy), carrying out oral surgery, periodontology and digital techniques.

Andrea Baruffaldi, DDS

Graduated in Dentistry and Dental Prosthodontics from the University of Insubria, with a thesis on "Guided surgery in modern digital dentistry".
Lecturer at national and international courses and conferences.
Trainer in the field of photography and CAD-CAM techniques.
His practice specializes in prosthodontics and smile-design.

Livio Yoshinaga

Smile architect specializing in high tech projects and international private dentistry consultant. Co-founder of DSD-Digital Smile Design with Christian Coachman.
Creator of the SKYN Concept method used in private offices, digital laboratories and training centers in more than twenty countries.
He has developed various applications for CAD-CAM and for digital dentistry, including 3Shape Smile Design

WITH THE COLLABORATION OF

Pasquale Romano

Qualified as a dental technician in 1994. He collaborates with the main companies in the sector (3Shape, Exocad, DentsplySirona, Kuraray Noritake). Since 2017 he has been a certified SKYN-Concept Technician.
Actively involved in the development of the DIGIT technique by Dr. Alfonso Baruffaldi.
Works in the Digital Dental laboratory.

Foreword

Dentistry is undergoing a profound change. The progress of diagnostic technologies and the evolution of implant prosthodontics inevitably require us to take important decisions on how we intend to pursue our profession and manage our practice and the relationship with our patients.

The digital revolution is like the toll booth of a ring road that allows the motorist to leave the rural road and join the motorway. Going digital therefore means choosing how we want to run our practice and live out our mission, today and tomorrow. And if we failed to reflect on the momentous significance of the term "digital" and, consequently, on all the practical and concrete implications it entails, we would not be able to constructively consider one of the current debates, which concerns the nature of our profession.

This wonderful book, which I have the pleasure and honor to preface, is a work produced with great intelligence, cultural erudition and sophisticated pedagogical methodology, providing the reader with a highly valuable educational tool.

The Authors have masterfully illustrated modern digital implantology in this extraordinary book evidenced by a clinical case history unique in its quality and innovations.

The Authors' merit is to have combined at the highest scientific levels an "all-round digital vision" with everything that can currently be clinically achieved. This is distilled in a modern book which allows the reader to acquire sound clinical and scientific knowledge.

The thoroughness which underlies the whole work derives from the Authors' ability to apply the principles of scientific methodology to clinical research and its innovative applications.

This work confirms that a deep knowledge of dental disciplines is the indispensable basis for an ethical and modern "digital implant treatment". The layout of the chapters enables both the experienced clinician and the student to access the world of modern implantology through a consistent educational pathway.

The book combines the aims of a students' textbook with those of a valuable refresher tool for the professional with clinical experience wishing to further explore the frontiers of digitization through rational and innovative workflows.

Finally, I would like to reiterate my appreciation for the Authors, whose efforts have resulted in a work that will contribute to improving our patients' health, the ultimate goal that all clinicians must strive for.

I am certain that this masterly work will withstand for many years the physiological obsolescence of publications, due to the innumerable surgical-prosthetic innovations it puts forward and the rational and consistent digital flows it describes.

I am also confident that this book will have the success it deserves in the professional and academic fields.

Tiziano Testori
Adjunct Clinical Associate Professor
Department of Periodontics and Oral Medicine
The University of Michigan, School of Dentistry (Ann Arbor, Mi)
Head of the Implant Dentistry and Oral Rehabilitation Section
I.R.C.C.S. Istituto Galeazzi, Milan, Italy
Dental University Clinic

Foreword

In the scientific field, clinicians have always sought to reduce the time requirements of protocols and make their execution easier and more reliable. For this reason digital technologies have now become essential, especially in dentistry and implantology. Making procedures less invasive, reducing execution time frames and increasing precision, have always been primary goals of research in the dental care sector. The immediate placement of an implant on an edentulous patient has been a routine procedure since the end of the 90s. This technique, validated by the scientific literature, has been perfected as a result of digital techniques, which have made it possible to optimize implant placement using surgical guides, designed from 3D radiographic renderings.

In the past, the provisional prosthesis was fabricated from a conventional impression following the surgical procedure then placed afterwards. However, success was not always assured. The cause of these failures lay in the fact that the technique for taking the impression and recording the intermaxillary relations was not always true to the patient's reality. The use of intraoral scanners was put forward in order to reduce these disadvantages but unfortunately new problems arose. Firstly, in the precise repositioning of the surgical guide in mucosal contact, following changes to the anatomy brought about in the surgical stage, but also in the use of the digitalized impression, which has shown its limits especially in the fully edentulous patient. The accumulation of these inaccuracies underlay the onset of complications, such as fractures of the components, detachment of the screws and occlusion errors.

The originality of the technique put forward in this book lies in its ability to maintain the same anatomical references for surgical guide placement as well as for provisional prosthesis insertion, thereby reducing prosthetic complications.

Another strength of this book is the consideration of the patient specific factors when customizing the therapeutic plan. This engages the patient even more and turns them into an extremely valuable ally for the dentist.

This new procedural method will undoubtedly be an important step towards the use of digital technologies in implantology.

Pascal Valentini
Chairman Post Graduate Oral Implantology
University of Corsica

Preface

In 1985 I graduated in Medicine with the aim of practicing Oral Surgery and Dentistry, and later specializing in Odontostomatology. At that time, the doctrine of osseointegrated implant surgery was taking hold in Italy. Bone regeneration techniques were introduced a few years later. I immediately took an interest in these techniques and soon became a teacher in these disciplines. Since then, I have never stopped teaching, in universities as well as privately, while practicing the dental profession. Indeed, I believe it is essential to convey what you have learned to your colleagues, while still being open to exchanges of views. It has been a real privilege to have had this opportunity for all these years, as it is a privilege to have the opportunity to see in print one of the results of this continuous search for professional growth and improving techniques.

As mentioned above, at the beginning of my career I dealt almost exclusively with implantology and oral surgery. However, as I was working alongside professionals who then had to finalize the surgeon's work into prosthetic products, with the aim of achieving an aesthetically beautiful – but above all functional – final result, I was forced to change my initial approach. This meant starting from the end of treatment, i.e. from the prosthesis, and moving backwards, in order to insert the implants where they are actually useful functionally as well as aesthetically. In light of this, the advent of digital technology – in prosthetics as well as in radiology – turned my way of working upside down, giving me the opportunity to design the final prosthesis virtually, and then go through the process in reverse, until the most suitable implant positions for each case are identified and the expected results achieved. Digital implantology has made it possible to transfer the design from the computer to the oral cavity in an extremely precise manner, through surgical guides that lead the surgeon to insert the implants exactly in the planned position. The same technology allows us to follow all stages of prosthesis fabrication, from preparation to finalization. However, that has all required a lot of effort, intense study and tireless research. Having embarked on this journey about 14 years ago, when these techniques were still "immature" — although even then one could already guess their significance in terms of the change they would actually bring about today – I needed to delve into the mechanics of how they worked so I could contribute to their improvement.

One of the results I obtained was the development of chair-side systems, jointly with the Skyn Concept method developed by Livio Yoshinaga and, even more so, the DIGIT method, developed to assure more precision, predictability and less invasiveness in the treatment of complex cases, such as rehabilitation with immediate loading of full arches.

This book is the result of the development work carried out over all those years. I was joined on this professional journey by two dentists, my sons Andrea and Martino, but also by my daughter-in-law Maria Giulia, in her role as dental hygienist and, more recently, also by my son Daniele, as a dental technician, who has joined Pasquale Romano and Ardian Sheu in the laboratory. Each one of us has a specific scope of action and seeing so much passion and skill fills me with pride and love at the same time. It has also enhanced the digital transition in our clinical practice.

I must also point out that this publication was made possible thanks to the enthusiastic daily work of our staff, dental assistants and administrative personnel who are always ready to eagerly welcome new innovations with curiosity. Therefore, we would also like to thank Alessandra Bernini, Martina Nicolini, Elena Velluti, Elena Bratescu, Silvia Huian, Chiara Gallinari and Valentina Amadei.

Our heartfelt thanks are also due to Professor Massimo Gagliani who, with his acumen and experience, spurred us on to tackle this remarkable endeavor.

Alfonso Baruffaldi

Table of contents

Introduction

Alfonso Baruffaldi

The DIGIT technique (Dental Implant Guided Immediate Therapy)

Since its invention and subsequent improvements, implantology has become an integral part of the conventional concept of prosthesis. Placement of the implant in the bone to meet biological, biomechanical and esthetic requirements has always been a challenge since the very beginning. In the past, the placement site and angle were dictated by the amount of available bone, based on panoramic X-rays and intraoperative probing. This could lead to esthetic or functional compromises.[1]

The wish to achieve more predictable results in prosthetics has led to the development of prosthetically driven implantology. This concept is based on proper implant placement in the diagnostic stage, using the design of the final prosthesis as the guiding factor (📷 1-2).[2] In the field of prosthetically driven implantology, the use of radiographic and surgical templates, in combination with Cone Beam CT, plays an important role, increasing the predictability of results compared to the conventional technique.[3] Currently, **prosthetically driven implantology** makes it possible to treat the most diverse cases of edentulism, and can also be applied in full arch cases (📷 3-7).

The evolution of technologies in the dental field has led to the development of integrated implantology systems capable of simplifying the key steps of this practice, which by becoming part of the routine in clinical activity, provide undoubted advantages for the patient as well as the dentist.

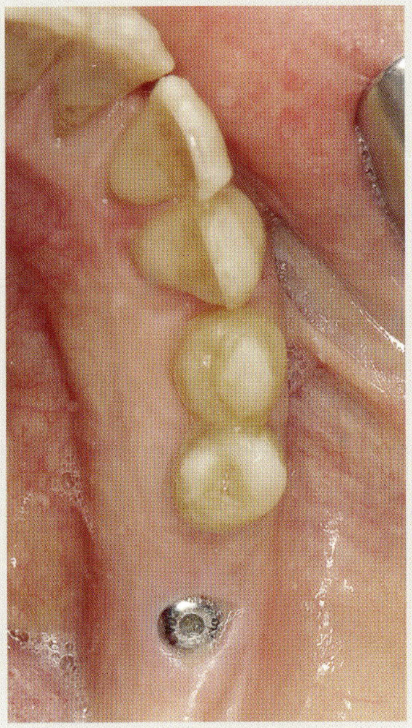

1 Implant inserted in an excessively distal position.

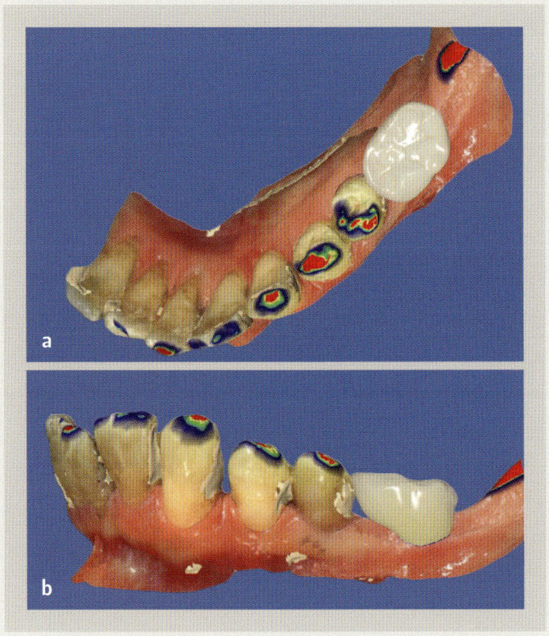

2 a,b) Failure to perform planning and consequent incorrect implant placement in position 36 led to the fabrication of an defective restoration from a functional and esthetic point of view.

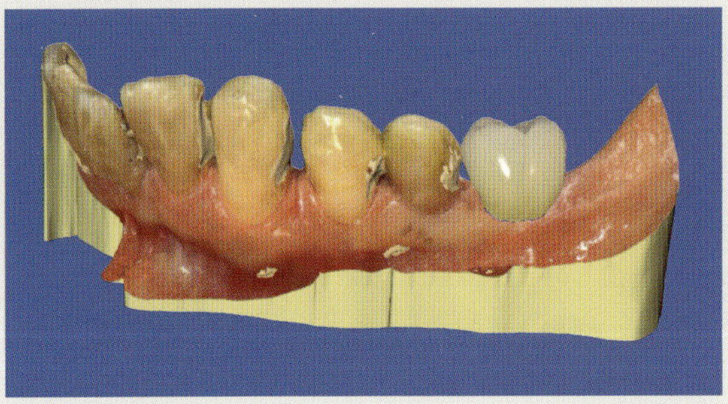

3 In the same case, proper planning would have led to the fabrication of a suitable final element.

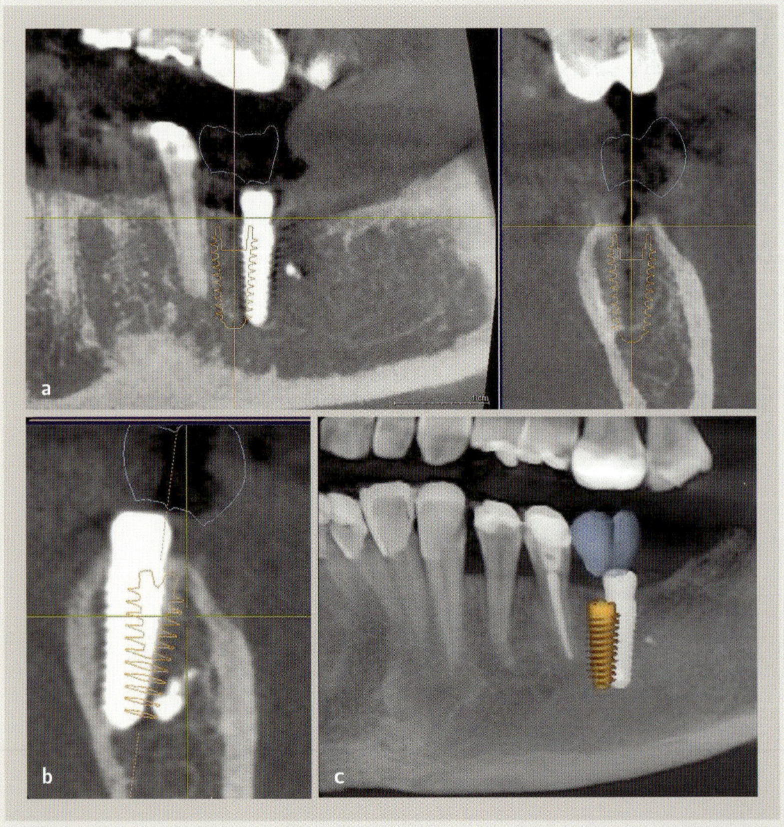

4 a–c) Comparison of proper planning and incorrect implant position after free-hand placement. The difference between the actual implant position and the position dictated by CAD planning can be observed. Esthetic, as well as functional, future errors are evident, deriving from failure to adhere to the possible indications provided by the virtual wax-up.

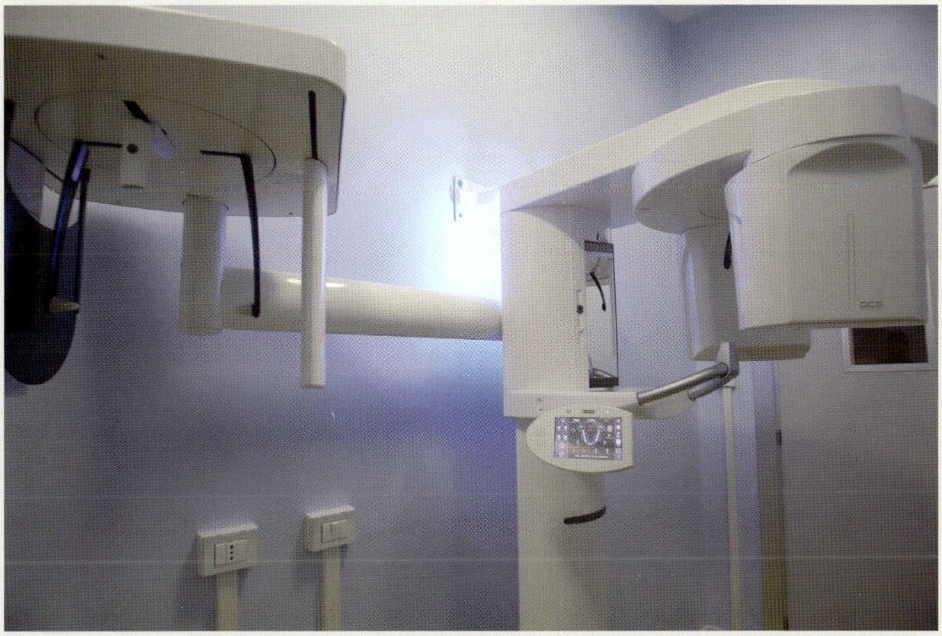

5 Cone Beam CT (CBCT).

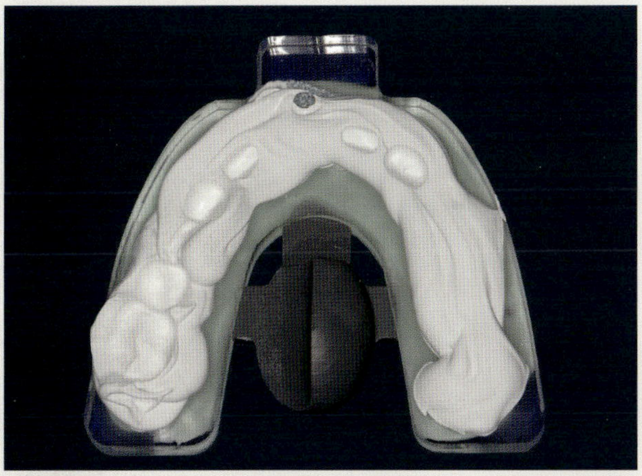

6 Example of indexed custom radiographic template.

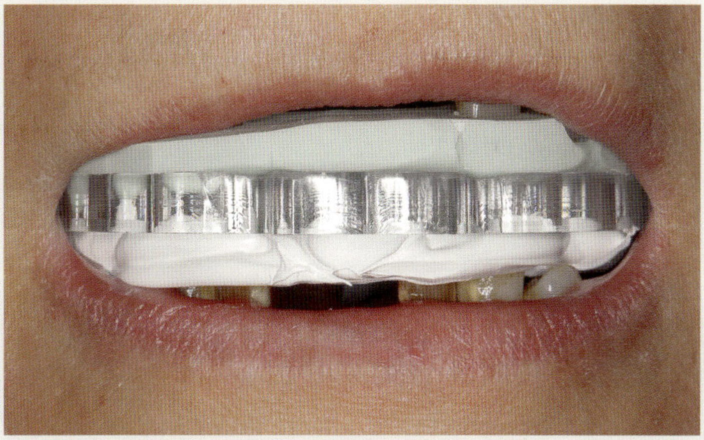

7 The template placed in the patient's mouth, in a definite and reproducible position, during the X-ray investigation with CBCT.

Prosthetically driven implantology, like other dentistry techniques, is about to be revolutionized by digitization processes. While it is not hard to predict the digital conversion of the dental sector, it is less straightforward to estimate when this is going to happen.

The lengthening of the average life expectancy increases the likelihood of treating patients with terminal dentition, characterized by chronic periodontal disease, unstable teeth, poor occlusal relations and unfavorable alveolar anatomy. In these patients, generalized impairment, combined with the lack of stable anatomical references, makes implant-prosthetic procedures more complex.

This is particularly evident in the case of a **"digital" approach**, where guided surgery techniques are used, as the lack of fixed and repeatable reference points makes surgical and prosthetic procedures more complicated (8, 9) for the following reasons:

- it is generally accepted that guided procedures are more accurate in partially edentulous patients than in fully edentulous patients, and that tooth-supported guides are considered more accurate than bone- and mucosa-supported models used in fully edentulous patients;
- digital scanning of an entire edentulous arch still poses a challenge, due to the difficulties in capturing movable soft tissues when scanning smooth surface textures entirely covered by saliva and due to the lack of reference points;
- in some cases, the osteoplasty procedures performed to mold the bone architecture and normalize the vertical dimension before implant insertion may further contribute to the loss of the remaining reference points.

Deviations from the virtual design reflect the sum of all the errors that occur in digital scanning and radiographic capture, to transformation of the design into a surgical stent and its improper placement during the surgical procedure.

The accuracy of surgery guided by digital systems therefore depends on the cumulative effect and interaction of all the errors made throughout the workflow.

As already pointed out, "imprecise" implant placement may have a negative impact on the biomechanical outcome of the provisional prosthesis, fabricated on the basis of the virtual plan before the surgical procedure.

The literature has reported an incidence of 18.8% and 12% respectively for early and delayed prosthetic complications in particular, when stereolithographic guided surgery is followed by an immediate provisionalization with a fixed bridge prepared in the laboratory beforehand.

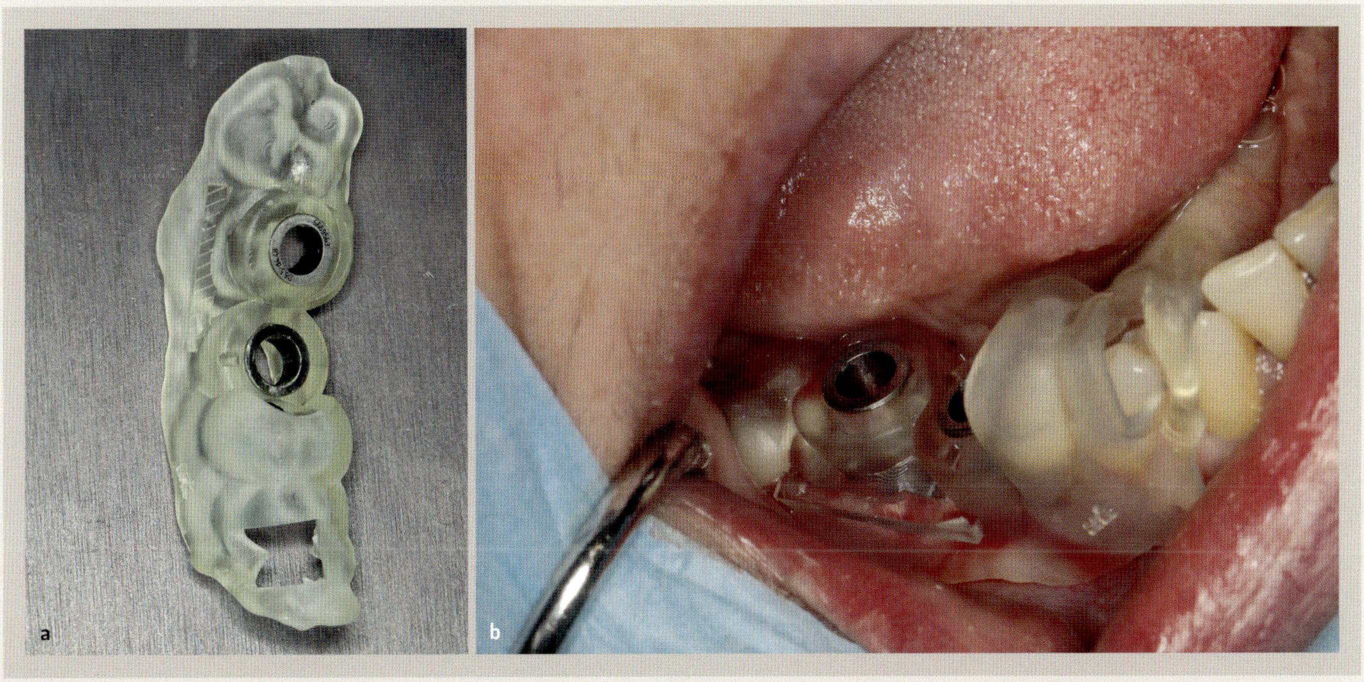

8 **a,b)** Example of tooth-supported template.

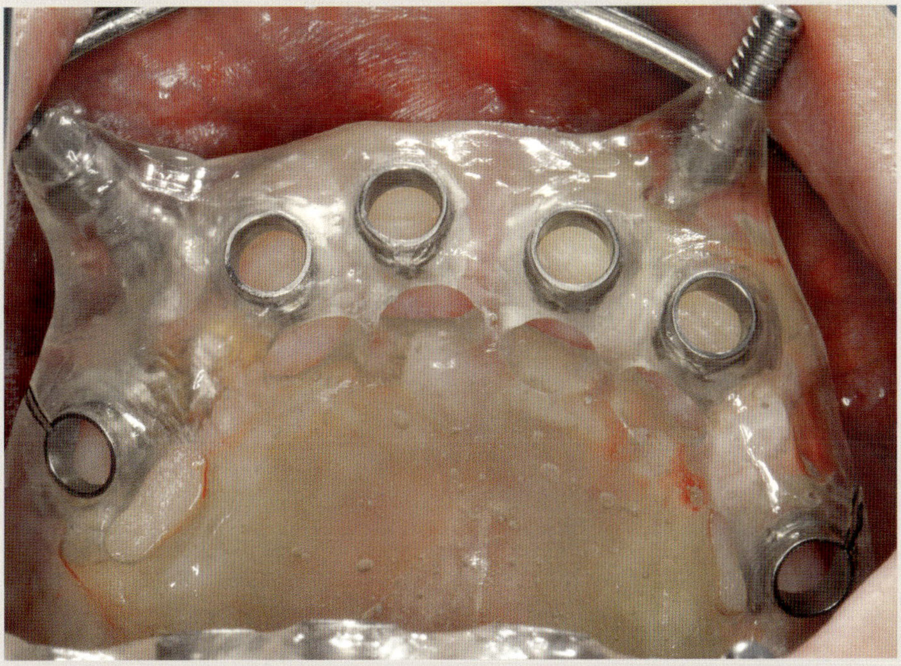

9 Example of mucosa-supported surgical template.

Prosthetic complications reported in the literature include fracture of the prosthesis, screw loosening, screw or implant abutment fracture, mismatch at the time of connecting the superstructure and the need for considerable occlusal adjustments after superstructure placement (10).

The **prefabrication of the prosthetic restoration** and subsequent implant anchoring **cannot therefore be viewed as a perfect procedure**.

In this sense, during realignment procedures in immediate loading protocols, the difficulties in stabilizing the temporary prosthesis in the correct position may play an important role in the occurrence of prosthetic complications. The critical step arises between surgical guide removal and provisional prosthesis fixation, after all the reference points have been completely lost.

In order to achieve the maximum level of precision in repositioning the prosthesis on the implants, we have developed a technique that makes it possible to use the same **"bone pins"** used during surgery, to anchor the guide, in order to stabilize the prosthesis in the proper position during the subsequent prosthetic procedures.

This is achieved by transferring the same three-dimensional position and the same angle of the guide sleeves used to anchor the surgical stent to the temporary prosthesis, by means of protective acrylic resin guides.

Using this technique, the position of the temporary prosthesis should be the same as that of the surgical guide (11,12).

Hypothetically, this method allows the operator to constantly reproduce the transfer of data relating to the temporary fixed prosthesis with the same means

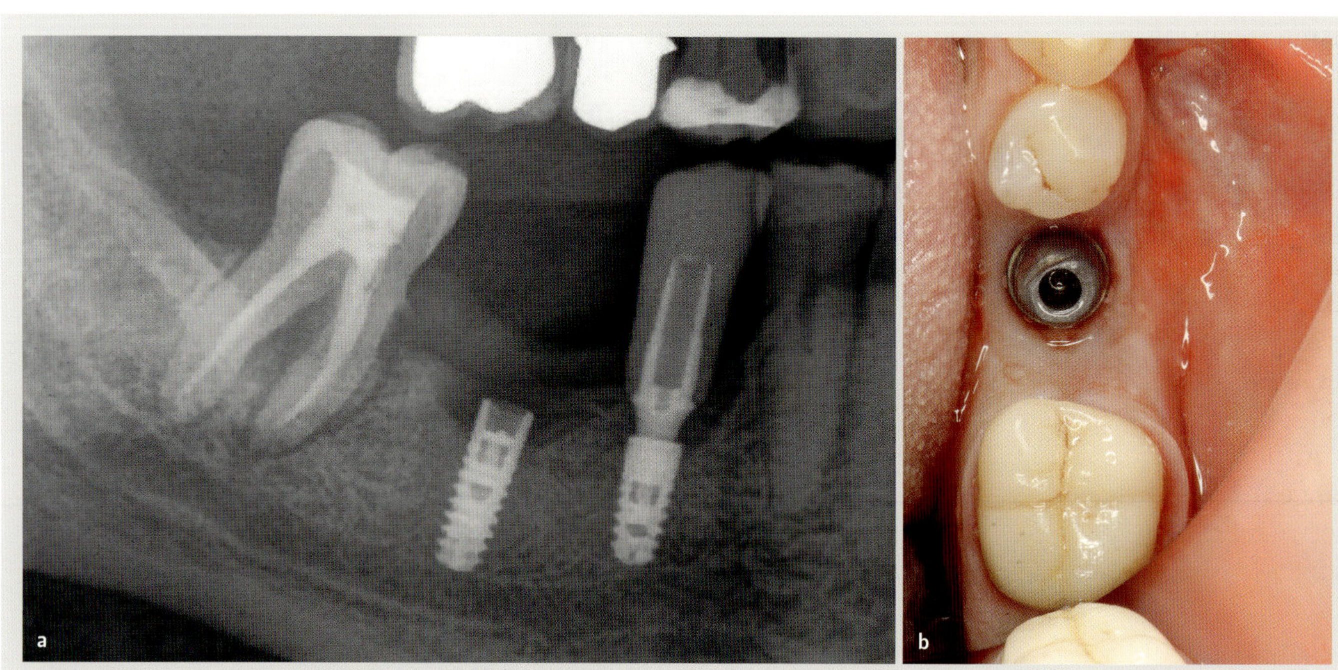

10 a,b) Fractured implant abutment: picture and X-ray of the abutment.

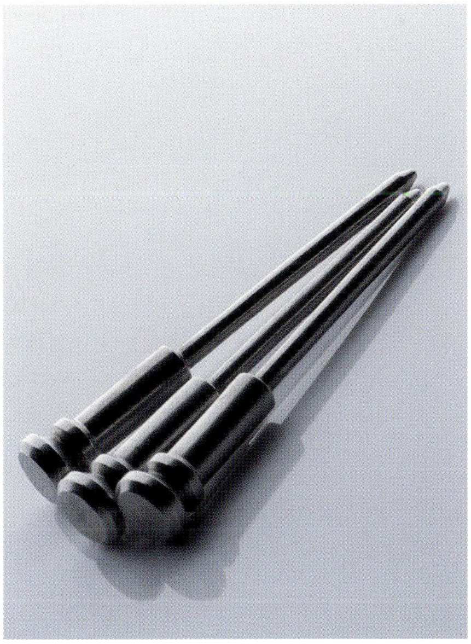

11 Bone pins.

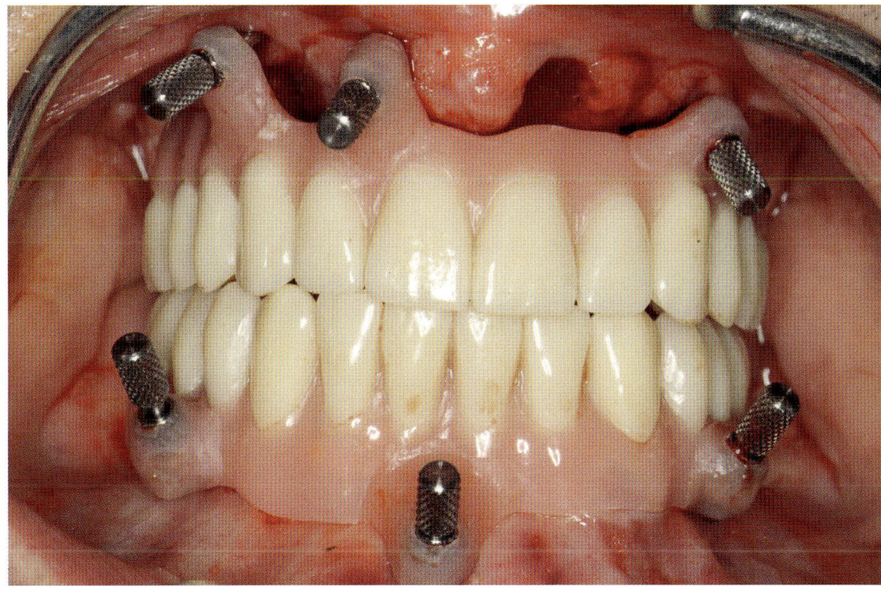

12 Bone pins used to anchor the prosthesis in position during the relining stage.

used for the surgical template, so that the prosthesis is accurately placed with respect to the implants, according to the existing reference points.

However, once the surgical stent is removed, it may be difficult to succeed in repositioning the bone pins in the same holes, because errors are cumulative and interactive and every additional step introduced into the procedure has the potential to increase the imprecision of the workflow.

Other factors that should be taken into account are bone resilience and resistance, shrinkage of the mucosa, poor visibility due to bleeding and encumbrance of the prosthesis, as well as potential interference with implant components.

Assuming that all phases of the protocol must be carefully managed to minimize any imprecision, the aim of this work is to offer **an alternative solution that increases accuracy in the transition from the surgical to the prosthetic stage, so as to reduce the risk of prosthetic complications in immediate loading protocols**.

In recent years, the use of the Toronto type bridges has grown considerably, owing to the fact that the success rate for implant immediate loading has been found to equal that for delayed loading (13, 14).

Although the one-year survival rate of implants placed by guided surgery ranges from 89% to 100%, the corresponding prosthesis showed a survival rate between 62% and 100%.[4] This discrepancy may be due to a variety of factors, which can be classified as postoperative complications, such as, for example, fracture of the prosthesis, loosening of the screws, poor precision in connection to the superstructure, or the need to resort to extensive occlusal retouching.

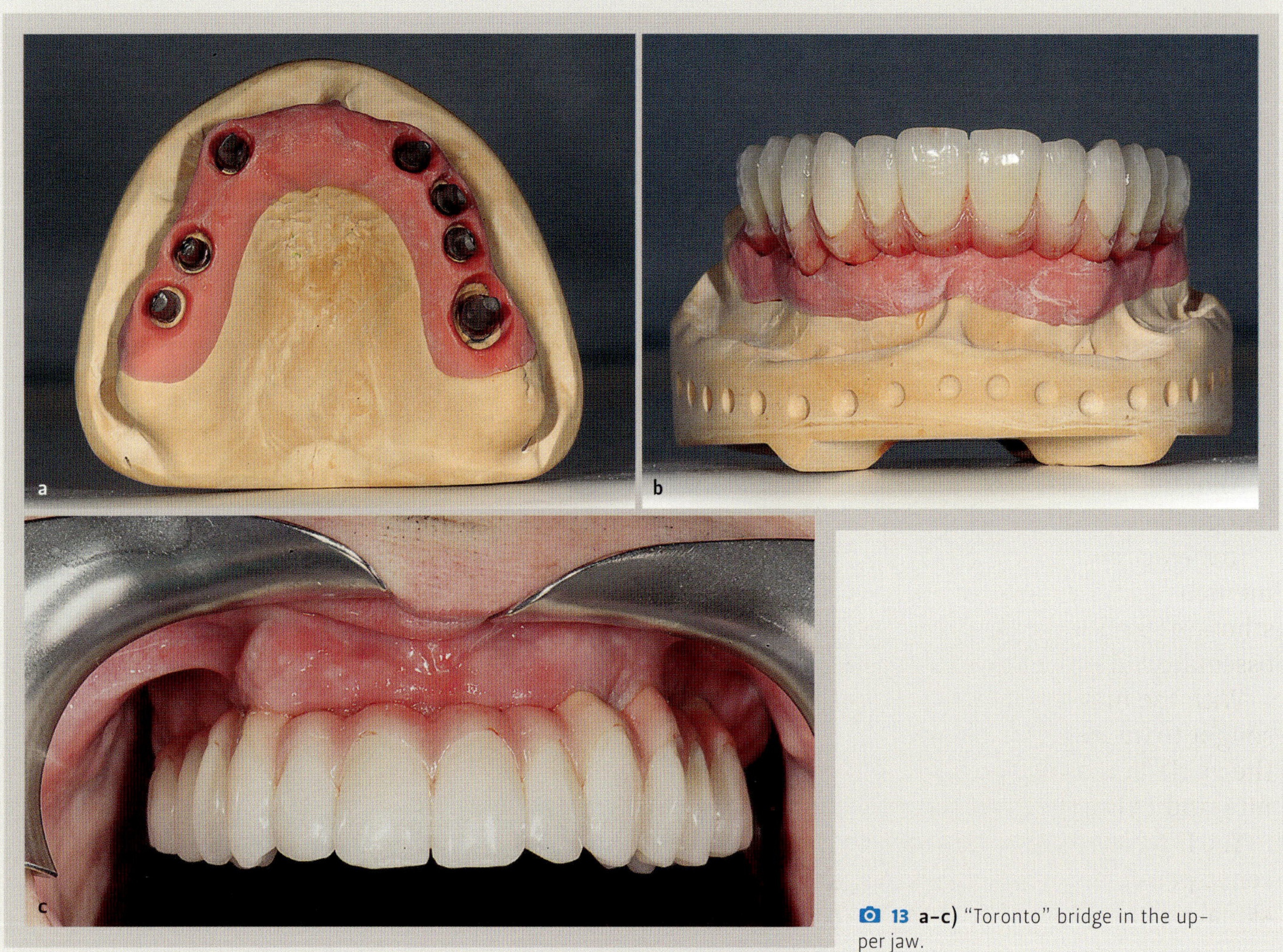

13 **a–c)** “Toronto” bridge in the upper jaw.

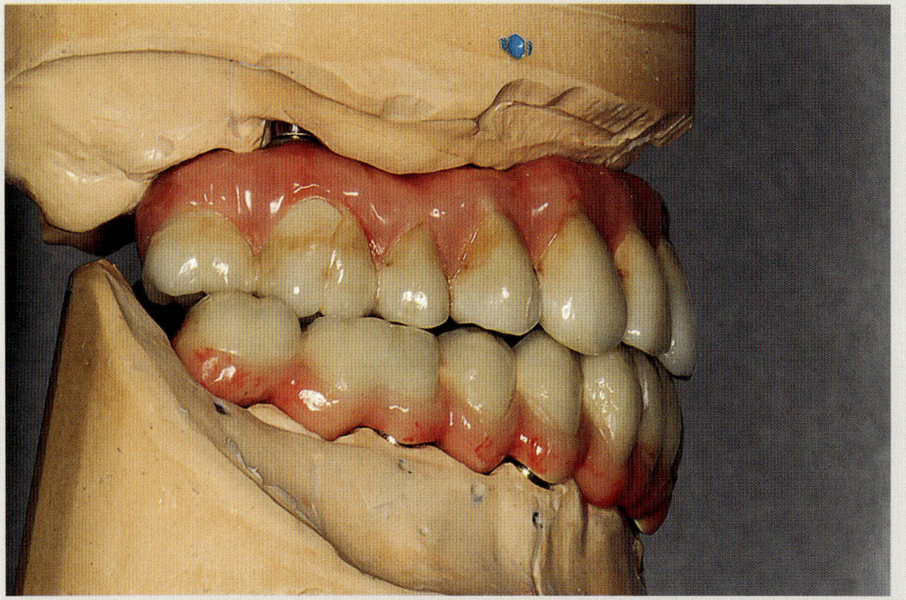

14 “Toronto” bridges in the upper and lower jaws.

Another possible explanation involves the difficulty in correctly placing the prosthesis during relining procedures. Generally speaking, provisional prostheses either wholly made of resin, or including metal reinforcement structures, are delivered to the patient immediately after the procedure. The unavoidable, slight inaccuracy between the implant position defined in pre-surgical planning and the eventual actual position is compensated for by a small space between the abutments and the prosthesis, which will then be filled in the relining stage.[5] However, in the case of going from partial edentulism to total edentulism following the extraction of teeth or implants, all the points of reference taken in the design stage are lost due to the changes that occur in both hard and soft tissues. Specifically, it might be hard to establish the proper vertical dimension and balanced occlusion during the relining procedures of the provisional prosthesis.

Another factor to be taken into account is the likelihood of the patient not being fully cooperative owing to possible sedation and anesthesia.

Incorrect placement of the prosthesis might lead to the buildup of twisting moment and high load stress, which cause multiple complications of a prosthetic as well as biological nature (bone remodeling, micro-fractures, loss of osseointegration) and could account for the high failure rate.

With the first working hypothesis described in a scientific publication,[6] we sought to address this possible problem by using the same pins that stabilize the guide in the surgical stage and the prosthesis during procedures for relining and fixing the conometric retention copings in the structure.

The DIGIT technique has been developed as a solution to maintain the reference points normally lost in the transition from surgical template to provisional restoration placement.[7]

REFERENCES

1. **Orentlicher G, Horowitz A, Kobren L.** Computer-Guided Dental Implant Treatment of Complete Arch Restoration of Edentulous and Terminal Dentition Patients. *Oral Maxillofac Surg Clin North Am* 2019;31(3):399-426.
2. **Al Yafi F, Camenisch B, Al-Sabbagh M.** Is Digital Guided Implant Surgery Accurate and Reliable? *Dent Clin North Am* 2019;63(3):381-397.
3. **Patzelt SB, Vonau S, Stampf S, et al.** Assessing the feasibility and accuracy of digitizing edentulous jaws. *J Am Dent Assoc* 2013;144(8):914-920.
4. **Beretta M, Poli PP, Tansella S, et al.** Virtually guided alveolar ridge reduction combined with computer-aided implant placement for a bimaxillary implant-supported rehabilitation: A clinical report. *J Prosthet Dent* 2018;120(2):160-172.
5. **Beretta M, Poli PP, Maiorana C.** Accuracy of computer-aided template-guided oral implant placement: a prospective clinical study. *J Periodontal Implant Sci* 2014;44(4):184-193.
6. **Baruffaldi A, Poli PP, Baruffaldi A, et al.** Computer-aided flapless implant surgery and immediate loading. A technical note. *Oral Maxillofac Surg* 2016;20(3):313-319.
7. **Baruffaldi A, Baruffaldi M, et al.** A suggested protocol to increase the accuracy of prosthetic phases in case of full-arch model-free fully guided computer-aided implant placement and immediate loading. *Oral Maxillofac Surg.* 2020;24(3):343-351.

Immediate loading implant prosthodontics

Alfonso Baruffaldi

Definition and scientific evidence: surgical and prosthetic indications

Implantology and osseointegration: the biological foundations

Implantology is a branch of dentistry that in recent years has made it possible to achieve extraordinary results, solving esthetic, functional and psychological problems in cases of partial as well as total edentulism.

The development of new technologies and the state of the art of materials have made it possible today to bring forward prosthetic loading, up to the application of a prosthesis in the same appointment at which the implants are inserted, thus increasing patients' confidence in and attitude to implant treatments.

The universally recognized mechanism underlying modern implantology is osseointegration.

Osseointegration refers to a direct bone-implant connection with no soft tissue in between.

Osseointegration is an event characterized by a series of processes driven by a specific pool of proteins and cells and is the end result of a complex system of events, which occur throughout the life of an implant.

The bone and the implant interface are two dynamic entities subject to continuous changes induced by biological as well as mechanical stimuli.

The phenomenon of osseointegration has been the subject of considerable interest and research. A number of studies in the literature have different positions on the mechanism of formation.

Some authors[1] believe that bone growth is a process that may occur from the implant towards the bone at two distinct times, referred to as "distance osteogenesis" and "contact osteogenesis". Others, however,[2] claim that new bone formation proceeds from the bone towards the implant.

After preparing the osteotomy site and inserting the implant, a bone-implant "space" is created, which can be considered to be comparable to a normal surgical wound. Such space is immediately filled with blood, forming a clot, following activation of the coagulation factors.

The phenomenon through which osteogenic cells tend to deposit new bone tissue in the space surrounding the implant, is divided into two distinct processes, which are called:

- distance osteogenesis;
- contact osteogenesis.

In the process of distance osteogenesis, new bone tissue is formed on the surface of the existing bone towards the implant.

In the process of contact osteogenesis, the new bone forms directly on the implant surface. This phenomenon depends only on the migration of osteogenic cells towards the implant surface, associated with the differentiation process from potentially osteogenic cells to mature osteoblasts, capable of producing the extracellular bone matrix.

The second stage of contact osteogenesis then begins, i.e. the phase called "*new bone production*", which in its turn is divided into four different processes. The last one of these processes results in the production of collagen proteins and their subsequent mineralization.

Following this cascade of biological events, the bone layer rich in collagen fibers is separated from the underlying implant surface by a layer of mineralized tissue, the protein matrix of which is not formed by collagen fibers, but by a fibrillar network of proteins, osteopontin and bone sialoprotein. This layer is called "cementum" and is the actual contact surface between bone tissue and implant.

According to Thomas Albrektsson, Biomaterials Department of the University of Göteborg, Sweden, however, the bone mineralization process takes place from the bone margins towards the implant.

Osteoblasts initially produce the bone matrix, rich in collagen fibers, which are deposited in the immediate vicinity of the implant surface. After that, the bone matrix undergoes mineralization during the osteogenesis process. The collagen fibers nearly reach the implant surface, leaving a space of between 20 and 50 nm, which is filled by a layer of proteoglycans produced by the osteoblasts. The mineralized matrix reaches the immediate vicinity of the implant, and is only separated by a 20-50 nm thick, non-mineralized layer of proteoglycans.

The cells involved in the bone remodeling process that occurs after the placement of one or more endosseous implants are: osteoclasts, pre-osteoblasts, osteoblasts and osteocytes.

Bone tissue undergoes continuous remodeling, which changes constantly in response to the mechanical stimuli it is subject to. This process is called skeletal homeostasis, and is a consequence of the activity of osteoblasts, osteocytes and osteoclasts.

Osteoblasts are cells originating from the perivascular connective tissue, after a first differentiation phase. These cells have a high metabolic activity, and are capable of synthesizing the organic matrix and regulate the deposition of the inorganic one. After a period of synthesis of the organic matrix, they are trapped in their own matrix, which undergoes a mineralization process; at this stage they are called osteocytes.

These oblate shaped cells, collected in cavities called bone lacunae, feature branched cytoplasmic extensions, which allow them to network with the other osteocytes and to open to the vascularized surfaces of the bone tissue (haversian canals and medullary cavities). Thanks to the presence of extensions and canaliculi, osteocytes can have metabolic exchanges with one another and with the circulatory system.

While osteoblasts perform a role in osteoneogenesis, osteoclasts carry out bone matrix degradation. They are syncytia (they have up to 100 nuclei) and are the cells of choice in bone resorption areas. Their catabolic activity is carried out by releasing a whole range of hydrolytic enzymes. A number of studies have shown that osteoclasts derive from the fusion of mononuclear macrophages, which reach the bone tissue via the blood. It has been observed that the implant surface, in some points, can be separated from the mineralized matrix by a layer of non-mineralized tissue, that is, the implant may not be completely surrounded by mature bone tissue, but by a non-mineralized matrix consisting of collagen fibers arranged parallel to the implant itself. The origin of this tissue has been attributed to the activity of some osteoblasts, found in proximity to the implant surface. Furthermore, through their extensions, some osteocytes found in the peri-implant bone tissue reach the surface of the implant. However, there are few multinucleated cells similar to osteoclasts in this area. The finding of bone-related cells close to the implant suggests that continuous remodeling takes place here like in other areas of the bone tissue. The mechanical stress derived from the masticatory load would therefore be transformed into a direct stimulus to the cells that carry out bone turnover. In particular, continuous bone remodeling takes place in the first millimeter around the implant, which ensures 80% of bone mineralization is never exceeded and which probably enables the healing of the micro-fractures that would be created at the bone-implant interface caused by the different modulus of elasticity between these two entities.

Peri-implant bone healing can be divided into different stages:

- formation of the clot between implant and bone tissue;
- build-up of algogenic and mesenchymal cells;
- release of mediators from the traumatized bone tissue;
- differentiation of mesenchymal cells into osteoblasts and organization of the clot;
- neoangiogenesis;
- new bone deposition;
- bone remodeling.

The various surgical steps cause trauma to the alveolar bone and to the epithelial-connective tissue, which results in an impressive release of pro-algogenic mediators. An inflammatory process is thus triggered which attracts lymphocytes, platelets, osteoclasts and macrophages into the tissue. Approximately seven days after the procedure, the clot contracts, and is progressively replaced by mesenchymal tissue. Osteoblasts begin depositing osteoid matrix. Bone proliferation thus starts migrating towards the implant surface.
One month after the implant insertion, the formation of lamellar bone tissue can be observed, whereas the subsequent bone remodeling may take up to 12 months.

From classic implantology to immediate loading

The surgical procedures put forward by Brånemark entailed a first surgical procedure with submerged fixture for 3-6 months and a second surgical stage of exposure, implant activation and soft tissue treatment (📷 1.1).

The basic elements of this method were:

- reducing the risk of infection to the minimum;
- preventing apical migration of the mucous epithelium along the titanium surface;
- reducing the risk of early implant loading to the minimum.

Brånemark believed that an implant should not receive any load until 3 months after its insertion, when placed in the mandible, and up to 6 months in the case of implants placed in the maxilla. Brånemark's studies3 represented the transition from pioneering implantology, considered as a sort of "experiment", which only few experts were able to implement, to a more modern vision. The application of this protocol, together with continuous scientific research, has turned implantology into a more than valid therapeutic alternative to conventional prosthetic rehabilitation, allowing to replace extracted or lost teeth with functional, esthetic and highly predictable implant-prosthetic solutions. However, the numerous scientific studies conducted on the topic were able, over the years, to modify the original Brånemark protocol and put forward the search for valid alternatives, to address patients' growing esthetic needs, while respecting the time frames and long-term success of implants.

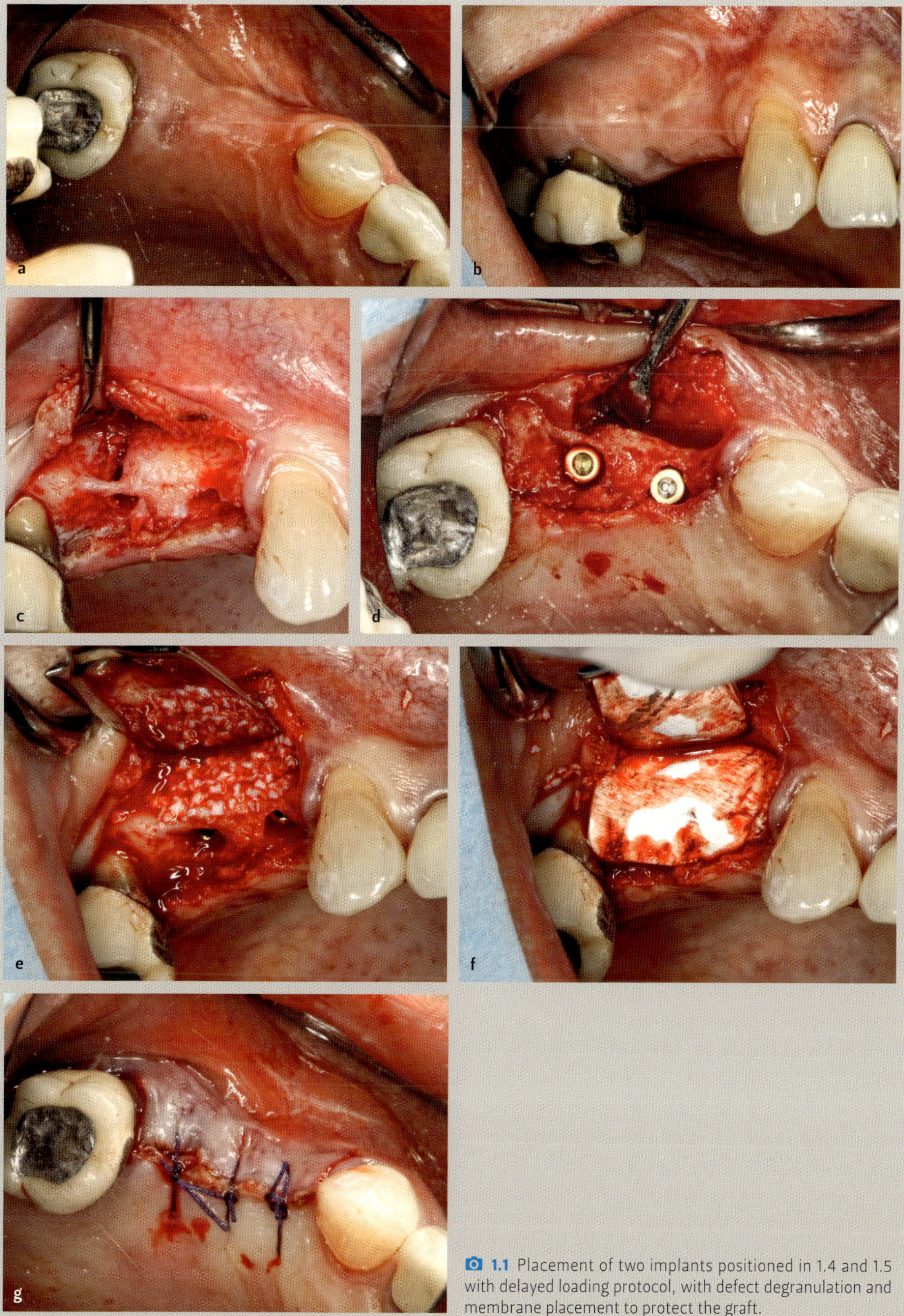

1.1 Placement of two implants positioned in 1.4 and 1.5 with delayed loading protocol, with defect degranulation and membrane placement to protect the graft.

The first researchers who offered new perspectives to modern implantology were Gotfredsen and Buser,[4] who already in the early 1990s compared the behaviour of some implants positioned according to the original Brånemark protocol (standard submerged technique, with two-step surgery), with that of implants inserted with non-submerged technique (protocol with one-step surgery), and did not find any differences between the two groups, thus paving the way for one-step surgery implant placement protocols.

Subsequently, a number of studies were also conducted on humans, showing no statistically significant differences between the success rates that can be obtained with either technique. This early alternative to the original Brånemark protocol immediately showed its advantages (📷 1.2):

- elimination of the second surgery step;
- reduction of the number and extent of post-surgery complications;
- reduced healing time;
- healing of peri-implant soft tissues with better integration of the prosthesis in the morpho-functional architecture of tissues;
- more rapid functional recovery.

The immediate prosthetic rehabilitation of the implants has an extremely positive psychological impact on the patient's emotional sphere, who immediately sees the first results of their therapeutic choice.

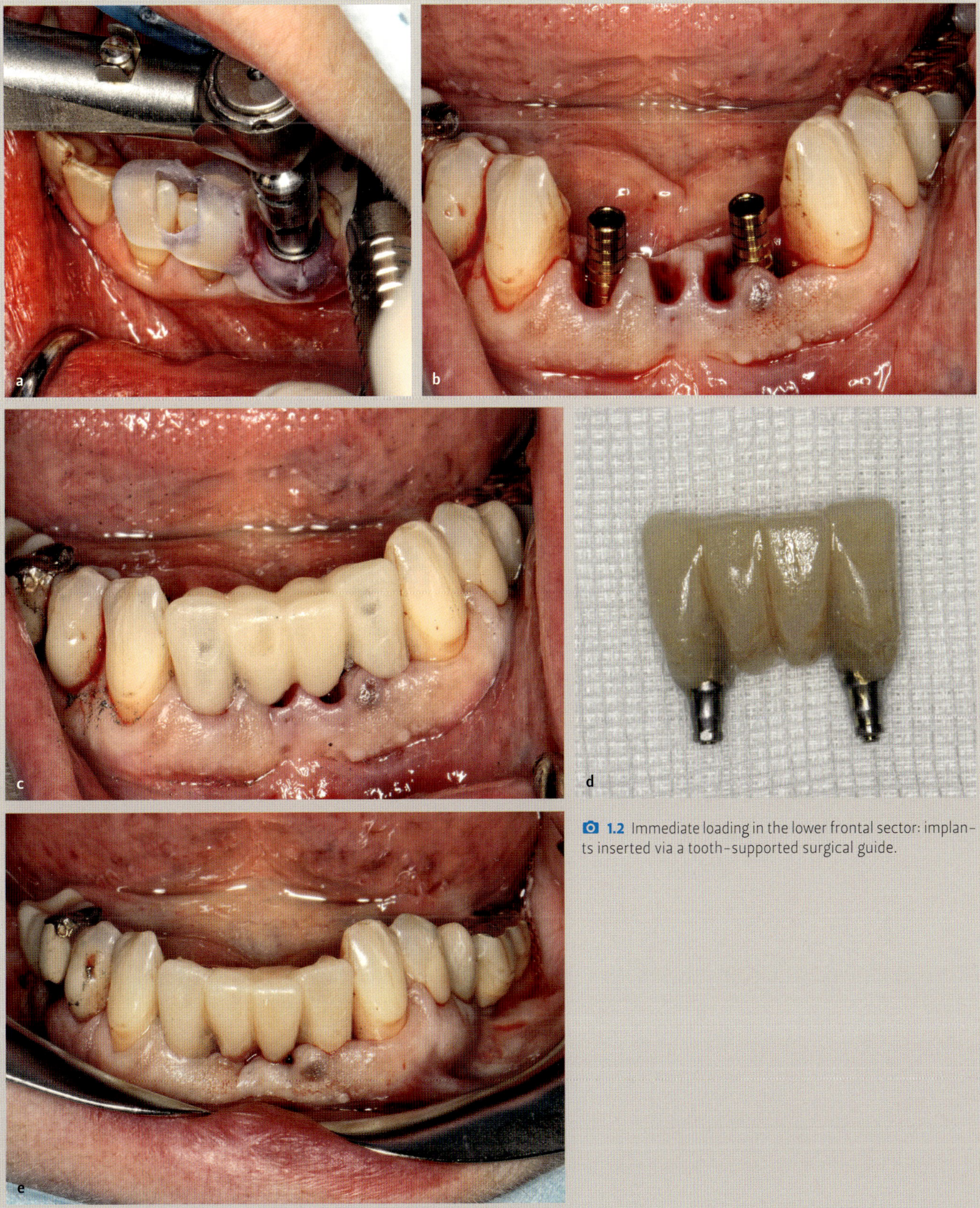

1.2 Immediate loading in the lower frontal sector: implants inserted via a tooth-supported surgical guide.

Biological principles of implant surgery for immediate loading

Following the bone remodeling induced by surgical trauma, the interface between implant and bone tissue is weaker and at greater risk of mechanical overload, particularly in the period between the third and fourth week after implant placement. The risk of failure of immediate loading implants exists especially at this time. In order to minimize surgical trauma, excessive stress on the bone tissue that is in the process of healing must be avoided; when we adopt an immediate loading protocol, implant site preparation must be the least invasive possible.

Surgical trauma is the consequence of a thermal and mechanical trauma caused by implant site preparation.

During preparation of the surgical socket, the temperature of the bone tissue around the drill ranges between 38° C and 41° C and beyond, and requires a time ranging between 34 and 58 seconds to go back to the physiological value of 37° C. Since bone cells die at around 40° C, the preparation and the search for primary mechanical stability – essential for immediate loading – will inevitably result in an area of peri-implant bone remodeling. Implant success or failure will be determined by its extent. During site preparation and implant placement, the bone is prepared through a sequence of drills of increasing diameter, thus producing an area of 1 mm or more of non-vital bone, being replaced, around their flutes. Excessive surgical trauma from a mechanical and/or thermal point of view can lead to overabundant necrosis, with subsequent fibrous sclerosis of the peri-implant bone tissue: the fibrointegration that will take place instead of osseointegration will result in failure of the implant, which will be mobile and painful.

The variables that may affect the extent of the necrosis are (📷 1.3):

- morphology of the implant surface;
- implant length and, consequently, depth of the site to be prepared. The depth of the site is inversely proportional to the amount of irrigation in the apical area, consequently causing more pronounced necrosis;
- type of bone;
- thickness of the cortical bone.

Two histological-functional types of bone tissue can be found at the bone-implant interface:

1. **Woven bone**, highly flexible and mechanically weak, featuring a disorganized and poorly mineralized structure;
2. **Lamellar bone**, very strong and resistant to the mechanical load caused by occlusal contact, featuring a well-organized and highly mineralized structure.

Therefore, the rationale for the clinical application of immediate loading must aim at the least invasive site preparation possible, so as to reduce not only the risk of fibrous sclerosis of the peri-implant bone, but also the formation of woven bone, while promoting lamellar bone, which is better able to withstand mechanical stress and ensure implant stability.

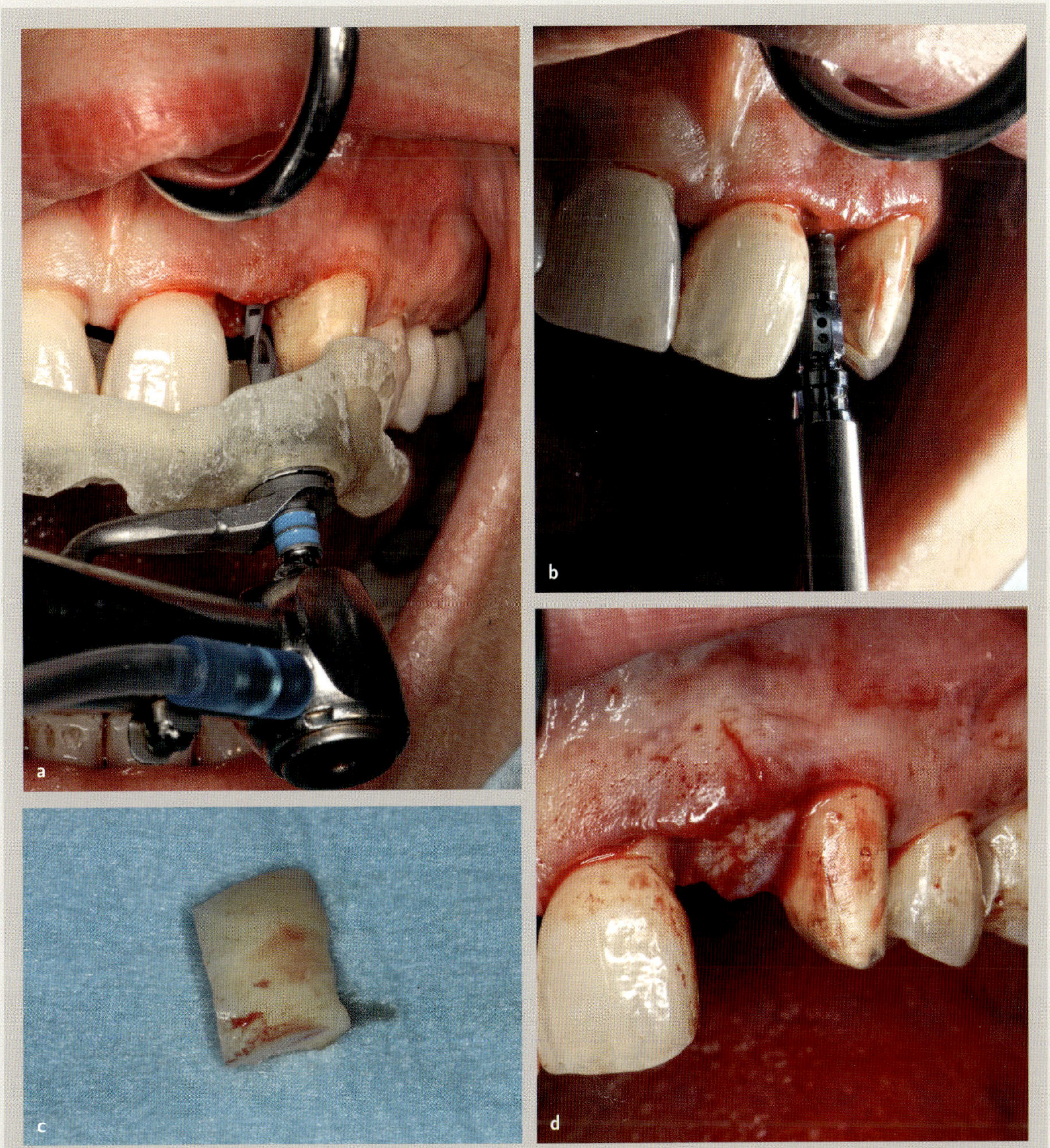

1.3 Preparation of the implant site and insertion of a fixture measuring 3 mm in diameter, to replace a lateral incisor. At the same time, a connective tissue graft – harvested from the palate – is also applied, to increase the thickness and stability of soft tissues.

Continues

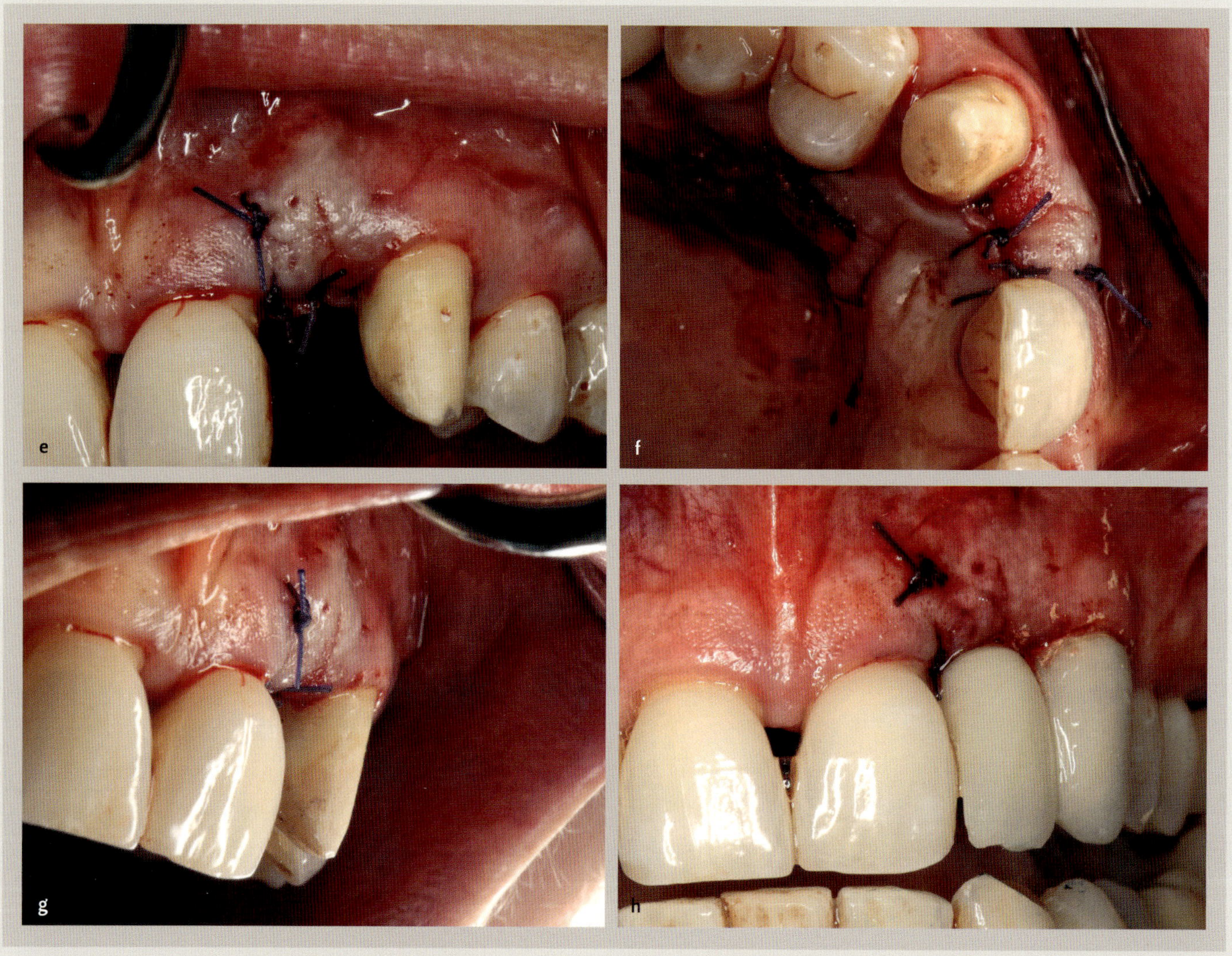

1.3 *Continued*

Definition of immediate loading

When speaking of immediate loading, a distinction must be made between immediate loading and immediate function. In the latter, provisional crowns only perform an esthetic and phonetic function, but have no occlusal contacts. This is the case of provisional crowns used in single edentulism and/or partial edentulism, in esthetic areas. Conversely, immediate loading entails occlusal contacts, hence also the masticatory function. Immediate or early loading of implants poses a challenge to the clinician, which involves biological and biomechanical aspects at the same time. In immediate or early loading protocols, the forces derived from chewing and other oral functions (speech, swallowing) are conveyed though the implant fixture to the surrounding tissue in the process of healing. In order to safely apply immediate/early loading protocols, the bone tissue in the process of healing must be adequately protected from mechanical insults derived from occlusal forces. The only effective protection consists in the reduction of the micro-movements that occur at the bone-implant interface. It has been demonstrated that micro-movements are not harmful and do not impair healing, provided their extent is included within a range of 50 to 150 µm. It has been clinically proven that implant stability plays a significant role in establishing the success of the treatment. Furthermore, the main clinical parameter that determines implant loading protocols is primary implant stability (📷 1.4).

Although implant stability is sometimes described as "absence of clinical mobility",[5] in practice a clinically mobile implant would be so clearly unstable that thinking of loading it would be wholly irrational. Hence, the absence of clinical mobility is not a useful definition for determining the success of the treatment. What is more, an implant that is sufficiently stable to be loaded will still not be 100% immovable. It may be rotationally mobile owing to the fact that when an implant has just been inserted, the bone has not formed yet and is not interacting with the implant surface. Over time, bone formation will lead to greater integration with the implant surface and to a stronger bone-implant interface. An implant will also feature a certain degree of lateral micro-mobility. The extent of lateral micro-mobility in the various stages of treatment is precisely what seems to have a decisive effect on the outcome of the treatment.

Implant stability is a combination of mechanical, or primary stability, and biological, or secondary stability.

Primary stability may be defined as friction between the implant surface and the surrounding bone and is due to mechanical compression of the bone, which holds the implant firmly on site. Primary stability is generally high immediately after insertion of the implant and tends to decrease over time. It is affected by the quantity, but above all by the quality of the bone (understood as the relationship between cortical portion and cancellous portion) in which the implant is inserted.

Secondary stability, on the contrary, is the result of osseointegration and formation of new bone cells in the implant site. Therefore, it does not take place immediately after placement, but it becomes evident over time. It is affected by primary stability itself, by new bone formation and by bone remodeling.

Stability does not remain constant after the implant is inserted. In general, an initial decrease in stability occurs, followed by an increase, when the implant becomes biologically stable. During healing, the cumulative stability of implants may undergo significant decreases, even going below the critical micro-mobility threshold, thus undermining success and resulting in fibrointegration. This makes it clear how it would always be appropriate to pursue the maximum possible primary stability, in order to hyper compensate for the natural decrease in fixation of the implant in the bone undergoing remodeling. The gradual change from primary to secondary stability is critical between the

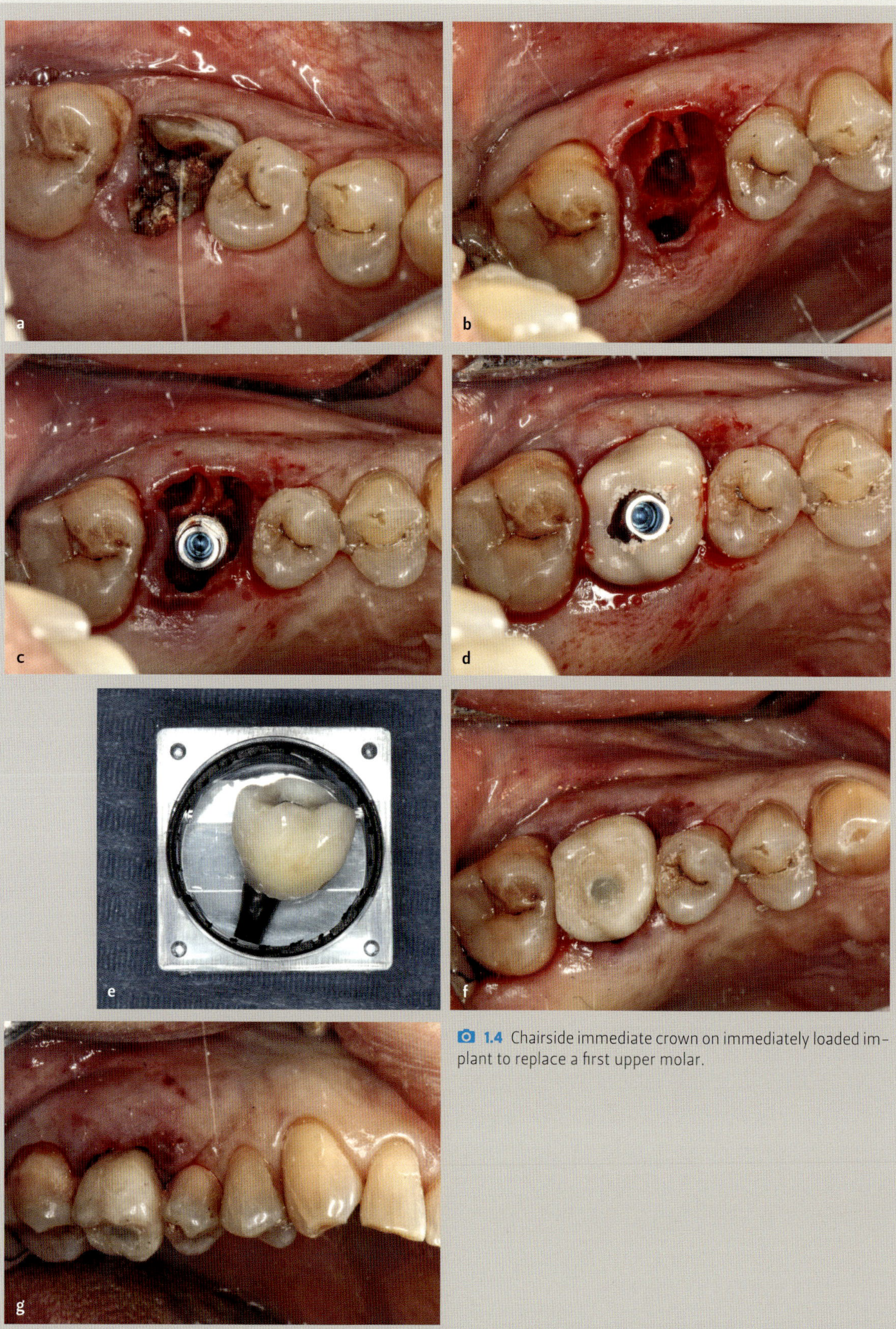

1.4 Chairside immediate crown on immediately loaded implant to replace a first upper molar.

second and third week. It has been demonstrated that this is the time of least stability, in which the viscoelastic distension stress of bone, which develops during remodeling, results in a loss of primary mechanical stability, but still with a low degree of secondary stability or osseointegration (1.5).

The parameters that affect implant stability (either primary or secondary) can be broken down as follows:

- **Patient-related parameters**: an evaluation of patient-related parameters must absolutely include the quantity and quality of the residual bone. The latter factor is linked to the patient's systemic conditions, sex, bone metabolism regulation factors, related medications. All these considerations are becoming more and more common, since an increasing number of patients can undergo implant treatment (1.6).
- **Surgical parameters**: the surgical technique plays an important role in determining implant stability and consequently, in the outcome of the treatment. The most evident affecting factor is the diameter of the drills used in relation to implant diameter, that is to say, the extent of possible undersized osteotomy preparation. Other factors are the depth of preparation and any tapping

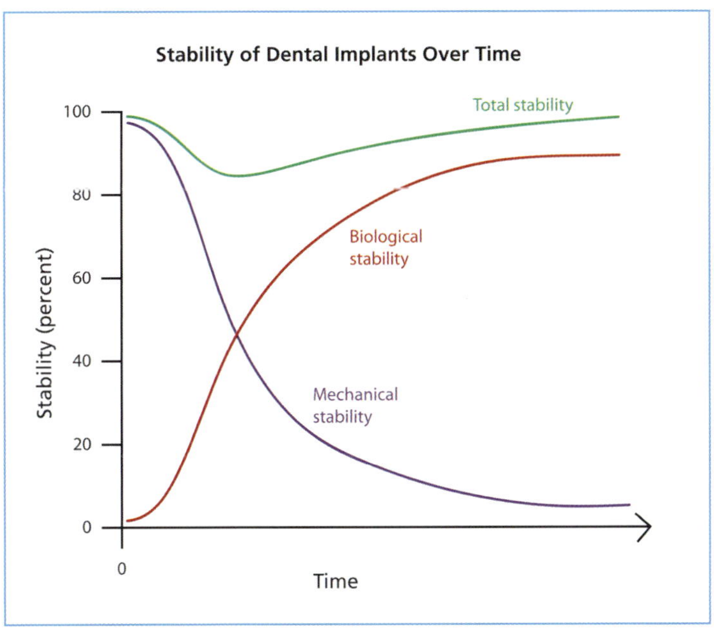

1.5 Graph of implant stability resulting from the combination of primary and secondary stability.

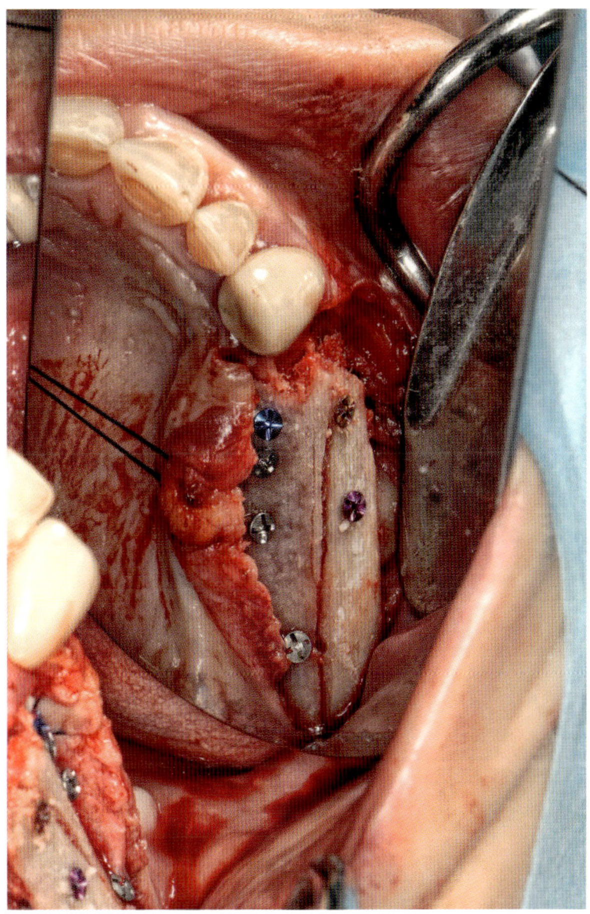

1.6 It is absolutely advisable to resort to delayed loading for the implants placed in regenerated bone, in this case obtained by harvesting from the iliac crest, as its density is usually very low.

of the site. The risk factors concern mainly the cases of traumatic surgical technique, which may cause damage to bone through "compression-related bone necrosis".

- **Implant-related parameters**: in general, an implant body may be divided into a crest module (cervical geometry), a body and an apex.
- Each of these parts has features that are favourable for achieving good implant stability. The implant-related parameters that influence implant stability include crest module, implant design (conical or cylindrical shape and any apical holes), length, diameter, surface type, self-threading ability and flute geometry. The crest module of an implant withstands most of the implant load and seems to play an important role in implant stability. It should be slightly wider than the outer diameter of the threaded implant body, since the seal created by a larger crest module determines greater primary stability of the implant, especially in unprepared, softer bone, because it compresses the crest bone region (1.7).

Implant design does not only govern primary stability, but especially determines the percentage of BIC (Bone Implant Contact), a value that expresses the extent of implant surface in direct contact with bone, and the location of the contact available for the actual transfer of force to the bone after occlusal loading. The objective measurement of implant stability is a valid tool to consistently achieve good results, especially because, as stated above, stability plays a significant role in achieving a successful outcome.

The objective measurement of implant stability is associated to the following advantages:

- it supports decision-making on optimal loading time frames;
- it allows the most suitable protocol for each individual patient to be chosen;
- it indicates situations in which loading should be performed.

Being able to quantify the primary stability of the implant after it has been inserted is therefore of the utmost importance.

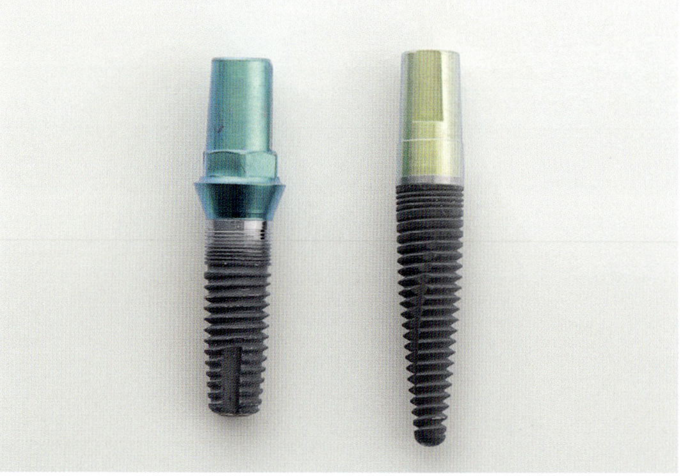

1.7 A comparison between the two most widespread implant types: on the left a cylindrical implant, on the right a conical one.

A one-step protocol offers clear advantages for the patient as well as to the professional: fewer appointments are required and the clinical time frames are shorter. With objective measurement of implant stability, however, the surgeon is able to make informed decisions on the choice of the appropriate protocol for each individual case. In other words, a low implant stability measurement indicates that immediate loading might undermine the result, and one might opt for the two-step protocol.

Over the years, many methods have been used to measure implant stability with varying degrees of success. What follows is an examination of a few of them.

THE CLINICAL PERCEPTION BY THE IMPLANTOLOGIST

One method to assess implant stability is simple perception by the surgeon. This is often based on resistance upon insertion and on torque at the end of insertion, during implant placement. A perceived "good" stability may be strengthened by the feeling of a sudden stop when the implant is inserted. The geometry of an implant with a given neck creates this stopping feeling, hence, the perception of high stability.[5] The perceptiveness of a skilled surgeon is logically priceless and should not be underestimated. On the other hand, it is obviously not possible to quantify a perception so that this method can be taught to others, in a reproducible and effective manner, or be used as a basis for future comparisons. Especially in high-risk cases, relying on perception alone is often not enough to assure a successful outcome of the treatment. What is more, it is difficult to communicate a person's perception to others. Even more importantly, this type of measurement can only be carried out when the implant is inserted and cannot be used subsequently, for instance, before loading the implant.

PERCUSSION TEST

The percussion test is based on the use of an instrument to check the stability of an implant. This method entails percussion with an instrument, such as the handle of a mirror, and listening in order to hear a (good) clinking sound. Electronic devices are also available for this purpose, such as the Periotest or the Dental Mobility Checker. This type of test is highly subjective and has been strongly criticized. As indicated by Sennerby and Meredith, "the percussion test probably provides more information relating to the instrument used for percussion and, at best, it can only provide lower quality information".[5] The cons of the electronic percussion test consist in the non-sensitivity to variations in implant stability and by the fact that the results are operator dependent.

RADIOGRAPHY

A radiographic assessment is a semi-invasive method, that may be performed at every stage of healing. X-rays may provide other information, such as implant position, but do not make it possible to establish the bone quality and quantity or implant stability. Plus, changes in bone mineralization cannot be radiographically detected before several months have elapsed and before de-mineralization has reached 40% (1.8).

INSERTION TORQUE

Measuring the insertion torque when an implant is inserted is an attempt to quantify the surgeon's tactile perception. The method provides some information concerning the energy used when inserting an implant. One disadvantage of this method consists in the fact that the insertion torque varies according to the cutting properties of the implant and the presence of fluids in the preparation. As for the surgeon's perception, measurements of the insertion torque can only be used when the implant is inserted and are not possible at a later stage. Although ISQ (Implant Stability Quotient) and ITV (Insertion Torque Value) provide quantifiable measurements of implant stability, they evaluate different aspects of stability. ISQ measures the implant axial stability, ITV measures its rotational stability. Both measurements jointly provide the clinician with important elements for a better understanding of implant stability.

RESONANCE FREQUENCY ANALYSIS (RFA)

The RFA technique is essentially a bending test of the bone-implant system in which an extremely small bending force is applied by stimulating a transducer. In terms of direction and type, it is equivalent to the application of a fixed lateral force on the implant, measuring its displacement. In this way, clinical loading conditions are effectively reproduced, albeit on a smaller scale. The RFA method may potentially provide important clinical information on the state of the bone-implant interface at every stage of treatment.

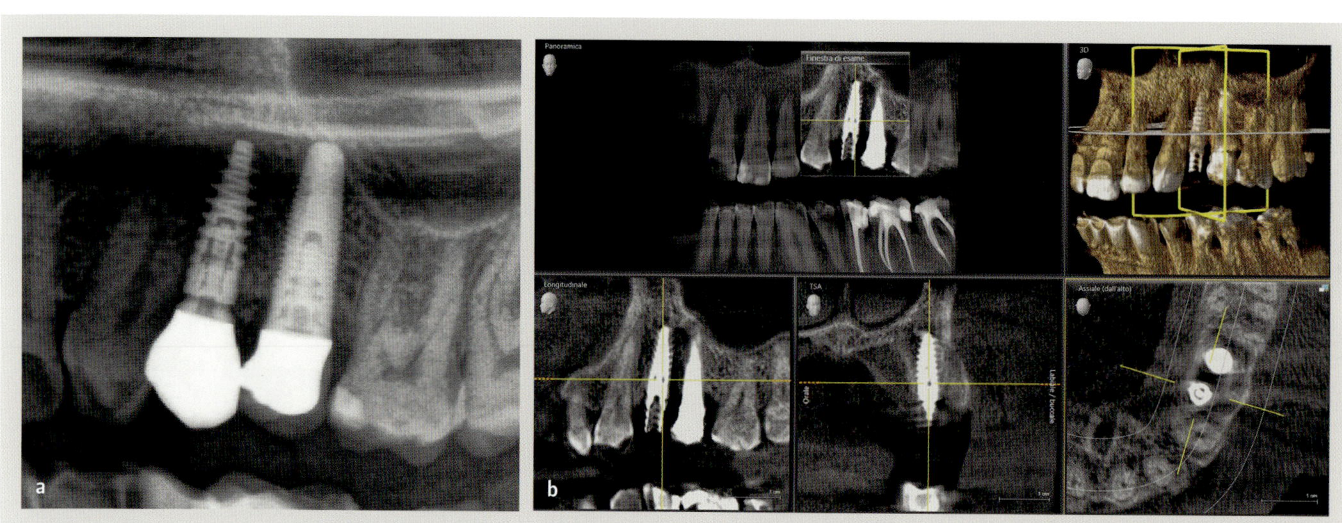

1.8 View under panoramic radiography and CBCT of an implant in the second quadrant.

IMPLANT STABILITY QUOTIENT (ISQ)

The resonance frequency analysis is a method that provides objective and reliable measurements of lateral micro-mobility, at the various stages of implant treatment. The method evaluates the first resonance frequency of a small transducer attached to the implant or post. The unit of measurement is the ISQ (Implant Stability Quotient). Although it is potentially objective, accurate and useful, this method has traditionally been subject to a few drawbacks. The first transducer models had the disadvantage of being sensitive to implant stability based on the direction it was fitted. Since the transducer could be fitted in any direction, if there was enough space, and since stability differed in different directions, the result might vary if the transducer was fitted in a different direction. The original transducer has now been replaced by a multi-directional version. Other recent developments have mitigated the other disadvantages. The Implant Stability Quotient is an almost linear mapping of the resonance frequency, measured in kHz at the most clinically useful scale of 1-100 ISQ. The higher the ISQ reading, the more stable the implant. Currently, different implants require different transducers (Smartpeg), but all Smartpegs show comparable ISQ values for the same degree of stability, even when implants from different systems are measured. This is obtained by developing the design of each new Smartpeg type, by comparing its ISQ with existing Smartpegs. The development of the ISQ makes it possible to determine a standard clinical range within which the stability values should be, to obtain a successful end result. Many studies provide good indications on the fact that the acceptable stability range is between 55 and 85 ISQ, with a medium level of 70 ISQ. The ISQ supports decisions on the optimal loading time frames, allows the most suitable protocol to be chosen for each individual patient, indicates situations in which it is best to discontinue loading, provides better documentation of the case. The high initial stability (ISQ values greater than or equal to 70) tends not to increase over time, despite the fact that high initial mechanical stability decreases and is replaced by increased biological stability. The lower initial stability normally increases over time, because the lower mechanical stability is increased by the bone remodeling process.

Values equal to or lower than 55 ISQ should be considered an alarm signal and in that case, actions should be taken to improve stability (larger implant diameter, longer healing time, etc.). The general average value in all implants is approximately 70 ISQ. If the initial ISQ value is high, normally there is a small drop in stability over time. A marked drop in stability or a continuous decrease should be considered an alarm signal. The lower values should get higher after the healing period. Otherwise, this might indicate a failed implant and the clinician should weigh what actions to undertake (📷 1.9).

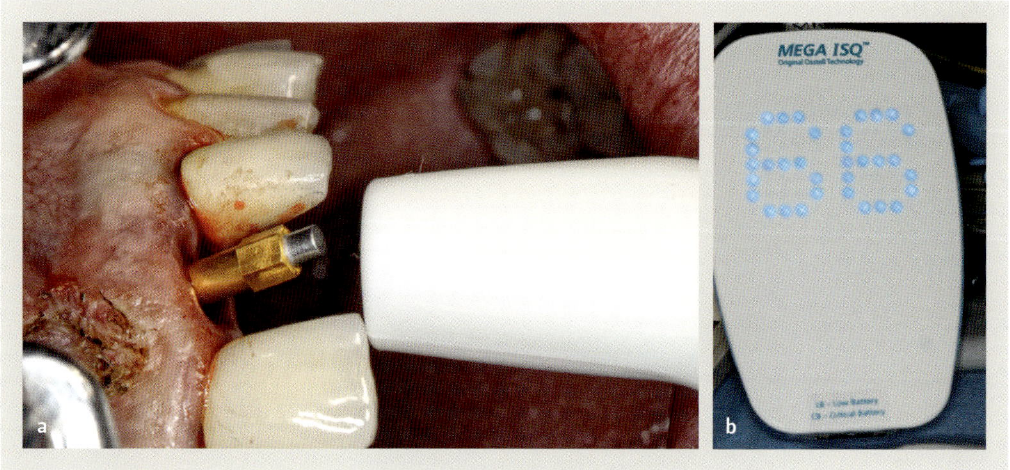

1.9 Measurement of the ISQ of an implant positioned in 2.1.

Factors determining immediate loading success

The implant surface and the quality of micro movement along the bone-implant interface are the main elements affecting the success or failure of an immediately loaded fixture.

Both elements are also conditioned by a variety of factors such as:

- bone quality;
- implant surface treatment;
- implant shape;
- prosthesis-related factors.

However, all factors that guide the surgical approach in general must be considered first, hence:

- factors linked to the patient's general conditions;
- factors linked to the patient's dental conditions;
- factors linked to the implant site (bone quality and quantity);
- implant-related factors;
- prosthesis-related factors;
- factors linked to the clinical management of the patient.

FACTORS LINKED TO THE PATIENT'S GENERAL CONDITIONS

- General condition, nutritional status, age, lifestyle (smoking, alcohol);
- pharmacological treatments in progress;
- metabolic disorders;
- hemopathies;
- heart and circulation disorders;
- bone turnover disorders.

FACTORS LINKED TO THE PATIENT'S DENTAL CONDITIONS

- Availability of an amount of bone allowing no interference with anatomical structures (inferior alveolar nerve, maxillary sinus, nasal cavities, mental foramen, periodontal spaces, contiguous roots);
- inadequate functional occlusal conditions;
- parafunctions;
- pathological findings of the maxillary bones;
- previous Roentgen therapy on the jaws;
- disorders of the oral mucosa;
- xerostomia;
- macroglossia;
- less than ideal conditions of the residual dentition;
- poor oral hygiene.

FACTORS LINKED TO THE IMPLANT SITE (BONE QUALITY AND QUANTITY)

Bone quality

For the implant-supported prosthetic therapy to be successful and even more so, in the event that the implants are loaded immediately, bone quality must be adequate. Bone quality is expressed by density, which depends directly on the level of stress the bone is subjected to: the higher the stimulation, the greater the density. It is a well-known fact that when a tooth is lost, therefore physical stress is no longer transmitted to the supporting bone, the alveolar process begins to undergo remodeling which leads to bone resorption. To confirm the importance of bone quality, it is appropriate to underline a study carried out by Jaffin and coll.,[6] who subjected a group of partially or totally edentulous patients to implant surgery with immediate loading. The classical criteria that guide implant surgery were used. Furthermore, the patients needed to meet certain specific bone conditions, that is: adequate bone density and adequate bone volume. The bone crest needed to be able to hold at least four 10 mm long implants in the mandible and at least 6 implants in the maxilla. This implied a crestal bone height between 12 and 14 mm. Bone density needed to be higher than 350 Hounsfield units, hence, according to the Misch classification, bone with D2 density. The implants were loaded 72 hours later, with metal reinforced provisional crowns. The patients completed the treatment with the placement of the final structures. The operators reached the conclusion that, with adequate bone support, implants placed in the oral cavity can be functionalized early.

Also Balshi and coll.,[7] after placing 130 implants, in a study conducted on ten patients aged between 45 and 70 years old, reached the conclusion that, in addition to implant length and the type of implant surface treatment, the quality and quantity of the bone holding the implant structure play an essential role. D1 bone, the hardest type, is like drilling oak or maple wood; type D2 bone is like drilling pine or fir wood; type D3 bone is like drilling balsa wood; type D4 bone is like drilling a piece of polystyrene. These four differences may also be arranged in degrees ranging from the densest to the least dense, considering the histological structure.

- **D1 bone** - Corresponds to compact bone. This type of bone is not commonly found in the jaws, as it can only be found in the anterior area of a highly resorbed mandible or at the level of the symphysis menti. The cause of the presence of such compact bone must be due to the high concentration of torsional forces, which are concentrated there during chewing, stimulating the formation of more resistant bone, as well as to the stresses of the muscles that are inserted there. The advantage of this type of bone is to be able to provide excellent primary stability and a percentage of bone contact close to 90%. An implant placed in this position will have a success rate that exceeds 94%. However, this type of bone may also have a few drawbacks. Often, the amount of bone available in a highly resorbed mandible does not allow long implants to be used, with the danger of obtaining a crown-root ratio greater than 1.25. Furthermore, a very dense bone risks being more easily overheated during the osteotomy procedure. In that case, both external and internal irrigation is recommended, in order to reduce the heat generated by drilling and allow the drill to be lubricated. Finally, D1 bone is less vascularized and its supply of nutrients depends almost exclusively on the periosteum.
- **D2 bone** - The density of this type of bone is a combination of dense compact bone and trabecular bone, the trabeculae of which (📷 1.10) appear to be very thick. D2 type bone is found more frequently in the anterior portion of the mandible, rarely in the posterior one; occasionally, it may be found in the anterior portion of the maxilla, although it is more easily found in the palatine process. This type of bone is able to provide excellent primary stability to the implant. The percentage of bone-implant contact exceeds 70% and it also has an adequate blood supply.
- **D3 bone** - It corresponds to the density provided by porous-type compact bone and trabecular bone, with thin trabeculae. This type of bone is found especially in the posterior portion of the mandible and in the anterior and posterior portion of the maxilla. The lack of bone consistency can easily lead to perforation of the compact bone, especially in the anterior portion of the upper jaw. The primary stability provided is limited. In this connection, it is indeed recommended not to use the last drill for more than one pass; in addition, self-tapping implants should be preferred over those that require tapping. One way to increase primary stability is to use a significant number of implants that will be splinted by the prosthetic bridge. The percentage of bone-implant contact is also reduced to less than 50%.
- **D4 bone** - This type of bone is by far the least dense and corresponds to trabecular bone, the trabeculae of which are extremely thinned. It is found especially in the posterior portion of the upper jaw which has been edentulous for a long time. Primary stability is extremely low and can only be increased with special surgi-

cal measures. The percentage of bone-implant contact is less than 25% (1.11).

Classification according to Lekholm and Zarb

In 1985, Lekholm and Zarb developed a classification of maxillary bone based on quality and shape, to be used in order to analyze implant anchoring.

They described four groups of bone quality:

- **Class I**: almost all the maxillary bone consists of homogenous compact bone;
- **Class II**: a thick cortical layer surrounding dense trabecular bone;
- **Class III**: a thin cortical layer surrounding a dense trabecular bone core;
- **Class IV**: a thin cortical layer surrounding a low-density trabecular bone core.

The authors also described five groups of shapes of the mandibular and maxillary cross section:

- most of the alveolar crest is present;
- moderate resorption of the residual crest;
- advanced resorption of the residual crest (only the basal bone remains);
- initial resorption of the basal bone;
- extreme resorption of the basal bone.

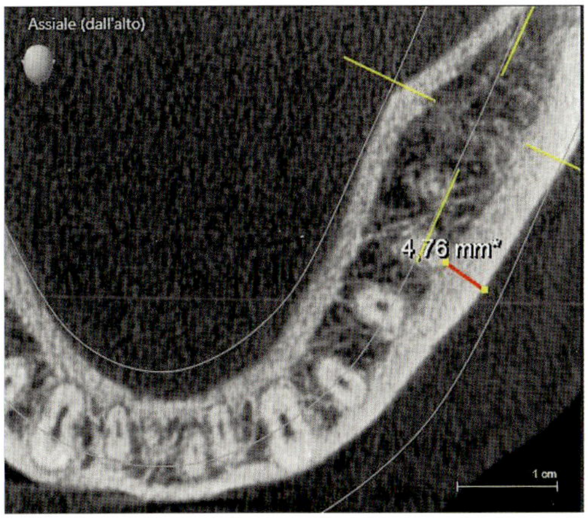

1.10 Axial section of a mandibular CBCT where the high thickness of the vestibular cortical bone can be observed.

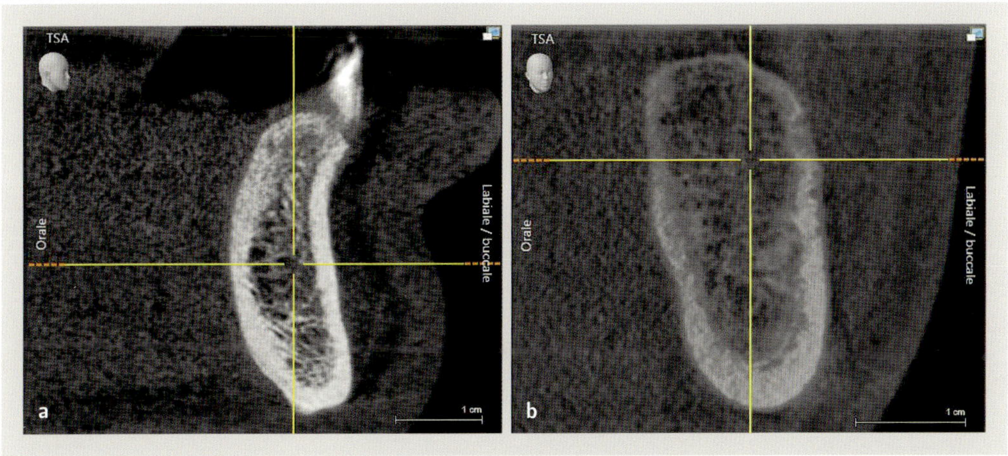

1.11 Cross sections of a type D1 and type D4 bone showing the different density of the cancellous bone.

Quantity of available bone

The quantity of available bone is measured by thickness, height, width. The height of the bone is measured from the edentulous crest to the opposite limit, be it the maxillary sinus or the mandibular canal, in the posterior region. Anteriorly, the limits consist of the floor of the nasal cavity and the lower mandibular margin. Many authors agree on the fact that the minimum length required for an implant is 10 mm, since a higher failure rate has been documented in the literature for implants shorter than 10 mm, regardless of shape, surface features or insertion method.

The thickness of the available bone consists in the distance between vestibular cortical bone and lingual or palatine cortical bone of the crest. It is advisable to have a bone peri-implant thickness of at least 0.5 mm on each side of the implant at crestal level, because the bone widens as one moves apically and these minimum dimensions increase rapidly. Adequate bone thickness ensures implant stability and integration.

The bone width in the mesial/distal direction between implants or between implant and natural tooth should also adhere to precise distances, in the order of 3 mm, again to avoid unpleasant failures due to reduced blood supply in the peri-implant area and also in order to ensure a certain degree of esthetics and greater functionality to the prosthetic work.

Implant-related factors

A number of studies have shown that the shape and the surface treatment of an implant influence the success of the implant surgical treatment, hence significantly promote and boost its osseointegration.

Much research work has been carried out in order to ascertain which implant morphology is most suited to replace the tooth roots unfortunately lost. Thanks to the results of these works, companies specializing in the sector were steered towards the development of a whole range of implant systems, capable of addressing most clinical requirements.

Implant surface

In recent years, researchers' efforts have focused on understanding which implant surface was best in terms of osseointegration speed and amount of bone-implant bond. What is more, these factors are the main elements that, jointly with implant immobility, promote the osseointegration of an implant with immediate loading. The market offers several titanium implants, which undergo treatments capable of modifying their surface features, in order to achieve greater osteoconduction. Surfaces may be: sandblasted, etched, smooth machined (subtractive technique), covered by hydroxyapatite, by titanium plasma spray, by bioactive glass (additive technique). A smooth implant surface will cause the detachment of the fibrin molecules, even if it undergoes a micro-movement of just over 50 µm (minimum threshold); an uneven surface will not allow it to detach even if it undergoes a micro-movement just under 150 µm (maximum threshold), precisely owing to its adhesive capacity. The absence of migration of osteogenic cells has the end effect of a slower and qualitatively worse bone production. Clearly, the osseointegration of an implant subjected to immediate loading is linked to the balance of two factors: the surface and the micro-movement it is subjected to. In the case of a smaller micro-movement an implant with smooth surface may be used; in the case of a larger micro-movement an implant with uneven surface must compulsorily be used (1.12).

PROSTHESIS-RELATED FACTORS

Prosthesis-related factors include:

- possibility of rigid connection of implants;
- wide distribution of prosthetic loads;
- absence of tension bearing on the structure;
- bio-integration and maintainability of the item;
- materials.

Despite the high success rates achieved by implant therapy, the risk of failure is always real. The two most important etiological factors in implant failure are considered to be:

- infection of peri-implant tissues;
- excessive loading.

Failure from overloading occurs more frequently during the healing period or in the first year of function. The loss of peri-implant marginal bone is closely related to the biomechanical ability of the bone to adapt and react to the micro-movements that occur at the bone-implant interface. That is why the extent of bone resorption has been correlated with: poor initial bone quality, excessively aggressive surgical phase, excessive early loading, incorrect design and/or fabrication of the prosthesis. The forces generated at the occlusal level are discharged on the implant structure, from there to the bone-implant interface, hence to the peri-implant bone tissue. Depending on the intensity, direction and frequency of the forces that develop on the occlusal table, peri-implant bone tissue may repair the micro-fractures that occur at the interface, with formation of new bone, or, undergo fibrous sclerosis, with loss of peri-implant

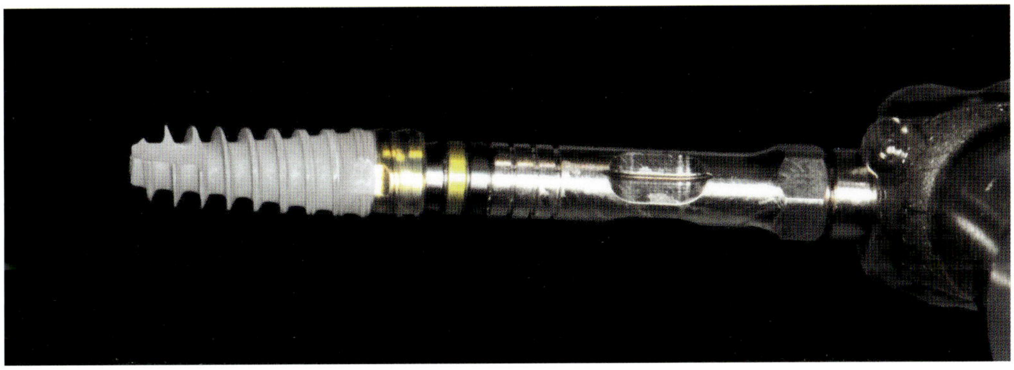

1.12 Implant surface alternating the machined neck to the rough body to combine less aggression by the biofilm in the coronal section with more stable osseointegration in the most apical part.

bone and subsequent apical migration of the junctional epithelium. Mastication induces vertical and transversal forces on the prosthesis. They result in axial loads and bending moments, which cause continuous stress on the implant and therefore on the surrounding bone tissue. A bending moment is induced by a force applied at a given distance from the longitudinal axis of the implant. The development of transversal forces (lateral) is mainly due to the inclination of the cusps, following mandibular movements. These loading situations are amplified by the reduced number of exteroceptors found around the implants: there will be a reduced neurophysiological feedback compared to a tooth and this situation may lead to the development of excessive masticatory loads by the patient, who may not notice it. Indeed, over time, a significant increase is observed in the average closing forces in treated patients: up to 40% more in 3 years (📷 1.13).

Excessive masticatory forces on implant-supported prostheses may not only cause the mechanical components of the implant-prosthetic complex to break, but also damage the bone and prevent osseointegration.

Below a certain threshold, bone deformation due to mechanical load might be repaired by bone remodeling. However, when the deformation exceeds that limit, the reparative mechanism might not be activated, consequently leading to irreversible bone damage. In view of the fact that the presence of bending micro-movements will be inevitable during normal masticatory loads, at this point it is important to emphasize the need to implement all precautions aimed at reducing tensions to the minimum during the prosthetic surgical stage (📷 1.14).

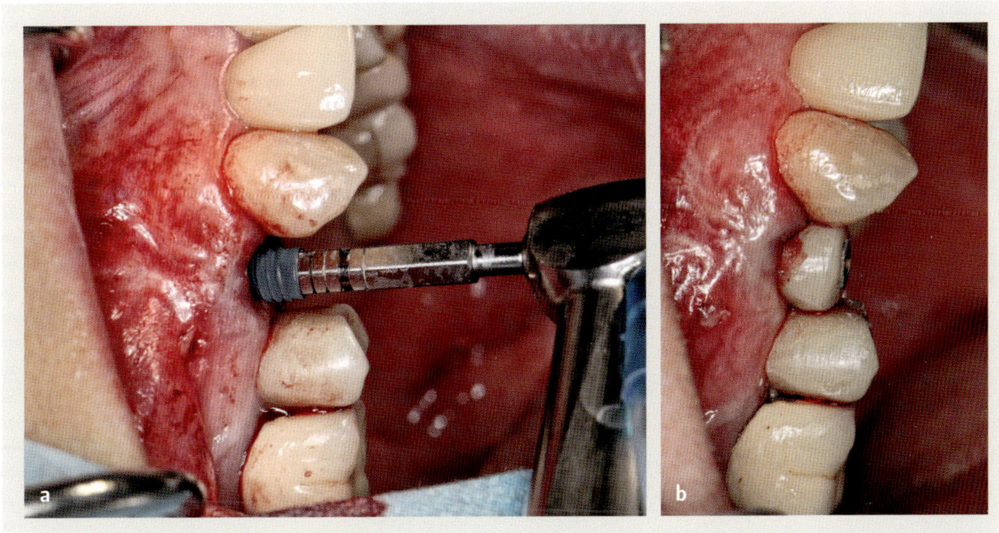

1.13 Another option for conditioning tissues around an implant that is still not ready to withstand the masticatory load is to fabricate a custom healing abutment.

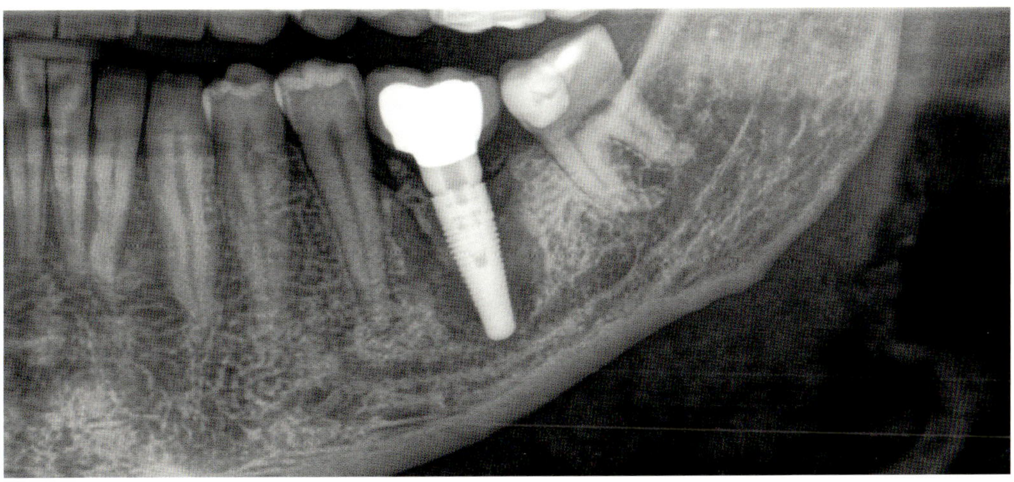

1.14 X-ray showing the presence of advanced peri-implantitis around the implant positioned in 3.6.

Prosthetic solutions for immediate loading

The choice of the type of prosthetic rehabilitation depends on multiple factors, which must be accurately assessed in the diagnostic stage. They depend on the type of edentulism, on the conditions of the anatomical site, in terms of tissue quality and quantity, on the interarch ratios, on integration with the prosthetic context, on functional factors and, above all, on the patient's esthetic and personal needs.

A number of works in the literature have compared the medium and long-term results of screw-retained vs. cemented implant-prosthetic rehabilitations, in terms of biological and mechanical results, as well as with regards to the onset of possible complications. However, few works have analyzed the comparative results between these types of prostheses and conometric prostheses, the use of which has become widespread among clinicians in recent years - due to their easy removal, absence of cements and possibility of re-intervention. The clinical decision on which retention system best suits the individual patient depends on a variety of factors. A detailed overview of the elements that might potentially affect the choice between screw- or cement retention should be taken into account. These factors include individual indication, pros and cons of the different retention mechanisms, the retention provided, the possibility of re-intervention, the provisional crown, esthetics and clinical performance, including failures and complications. The choice of the type of retention might not influence the overall survival of the prosthesis, but it may cause the onset of certain complications. The decision may depend on technical feasibility and the assessment of the pros and cons in each individual clinical case. A work published in 2008,[8] for instance, observed as many as 1939 dental implants, placed in a group of 527 patients requiring implant-prosthetic rehabilitation. The following factors were analyzed:

- esthetics;
- possibility of removing the prosthesis;
- passive behaviour of the structure;
- occlusion;
- ease of execution;
- cost;
- retentive ability.

In this study, 762 cemented prostheses were applied on 1551 dental implants. The success rate of the implant-prosthetic structure of this type of prosthesis was 98.4%, with an average follow-up of 34.7 months. Eighty-four screw-retained prostheses were placed on 330 dental implants and the success rate of this type of rehabilitation was 100%, with an average follow-up of 44.3 months.

In conclusion, the two types of prosthetic rehabilitation examined both featured advantages and disadvantages. The clinician should be able to assess the limitations and drawbacks of each type of prosthesis and appropriately make the best choice for every clinical situation.

In a recent systematic review of the literature on this topic, the Prosthodontics group of the University of Geneva headed by Irena Sailer analyzed 59 clinical studies.[9] For cemented single crowns, the estimated survival of the rehabilitation after 5 years was 96.5%, for screw-retained single crowns it was 89.3%. The 5-year survival for cement-retained fixed partial dentures (FPD) was 96.9%, similar to that of screw-retained FPDs, at 98%. For cemented full arch prostheses, the 5-year survival was 100%, slightly higher than screw-retained full arch prostheses, at 95.8%. The estimated cumulative incidence after 5 years of technical complications was 11.9% for cemented single crowns, and 24.4% for screw-retained crowns. On the contrary, in FPD and full arch prostheses, the trend appeared to be towards a lower complication rate in the screw-retained ones compared to the cemented ones (cemented FPds: 24.5%, screw-retained: 22.1%; full arch cemented prostheses: 62.9%, screw-retained: 54.1%). Biological complications (marginal bone loss >2 mm) occurred more frequently on cemented crowns (incidence after 5 years: 2.8%) compared to screw-retained ones (incidence after 5 years: 0%). This systematic literature review shows that the two types of rehabilitation affected the clinical results differently, but neither method is significantly more advantageous than the other. Cemented rehabilitations showed more severe biological complications (implant loss, bone loss >2 mm); screw-retained rehabilitations showed over time the onset of more technical problems. Screw-retained prostheses can be removed more easily and re-intervention is easier than with cemented rehabilitations; what is more, the technical complications and any biological ones can be treated more easily. For this reason and due to their apparent higher biological compatibility, these rehabilitations seem to be preferable (1.15 and 1.16).

A recent study by Bressan and Lops [10] however, evaluated the reliability of conometric systems for fixed retention of full arch prostheses with 4 implants supporting a conometric prosthesis, after 5 years of service and follow up. Twenty-five patients with total mandibular edentulism were treated. At the 5-year follow-up, no significant changes were found in the Modified Bleeding Index, nor with regard to the average probing depth.

In immediate loading procedures, a distinction must be made between the

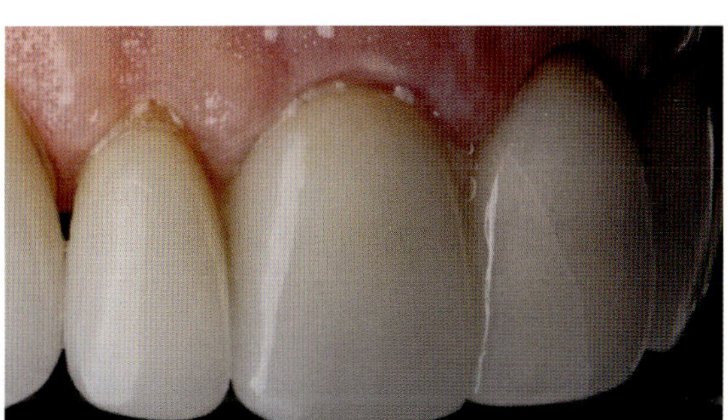

1.15 Fractured cement-retained ceramic crown on an implant in position 21.

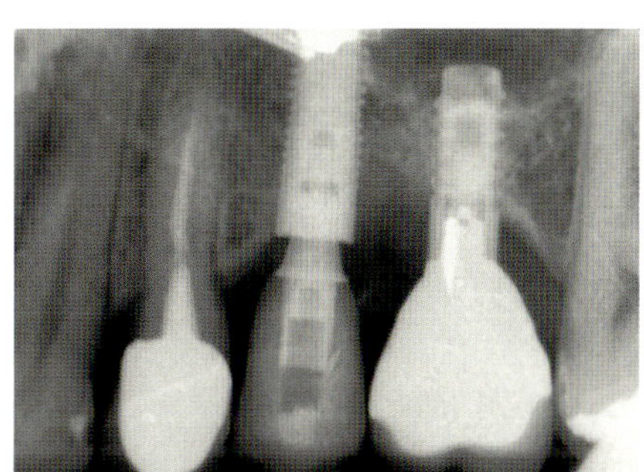

1.16 Fractured prosthetic connection screw on 26.

rules that must be respected in the sites having high esthetic value and in the posterior sites, however, the treatment plan should also be contextualized according to the type of edentulism. Immediate restoration on an immediate post-extraction implant in the esthetic area follows wholly different principles from FPDs on short implants in the mandibular arch or a full arch on zygomatic or pterygoid implants. The key to success lies in the customization of the treatment plan, based on the parameters collected in the assessment of the levels of complexity, already mentioned in the previous paragraph. New technologies and digital workflows, moreover, allow to design and resolve conditions even at the limit, in patients with significant dental-bone atrophy – making it possible nowadays to find solutions for rehabilitation with ultra-performing and extremely predictable materials.

One of the principles on which the DIGIT technique described here is based, is case pre-visualization and planning, through a digital technique, allowing the clinician to assess prior to surgery every specific complex condition, any procedural or anatomical risk – and above all, to decide the prosthetic steps upstream, in terms of indications as well as of materials. In accordance with the latest literature reviews and his clinical experience, the Author recommends following the scheme below in immediate loading procedures.

Upper or lower esthetic area

The proper choice for immediate loading, in the largest majority of cases, means using a screw-retained prosthesis. Proper implant placement, pre-established by digital technology and implant planning systems, makes it possible to position the fixtures three-dimensionally and to predefine the mucosal tunnel and emergence profile of the provisional crown. The great challenge of esthetics and soft tissue management is played out on this aspect. A number of works in the literature have reported the rules for emergence profiles management in the esthetic area in case of immediate loading implants, in immediately post-extraction sites as well as on mature bone. The rule to be followed is that of establishing, through proper shaping of the provisional crown, the dominance of shapes, which in its turn shapes and outlines the critical and sub-critical areas, useful for perfect esthetic integration. This makes it possible to outline the level of the zeniths, the course of the gingival contours, the three-dimensional profile and the progressive shape of the papillae and the margin of tissue space – in order to obtain a stable structural conformation of tissues. The choice of the screw-retained technique is therefore indispensable and recommended in this procedure, due to its ease of execution, as well as for the absence of cements that might, unless properly removed, cause complications, and for proper management of the immediate work steps. Using a cemented technique would often require use of an abutment in the immediate stage, the customization of which might be complex and inconvenient. On the contrary, the use of modern anchoring devices for screw-retained prosthesis, with dynamic abutments and angulated screws, opens up more clinical possibilities and ease of execution (📷 1.17).

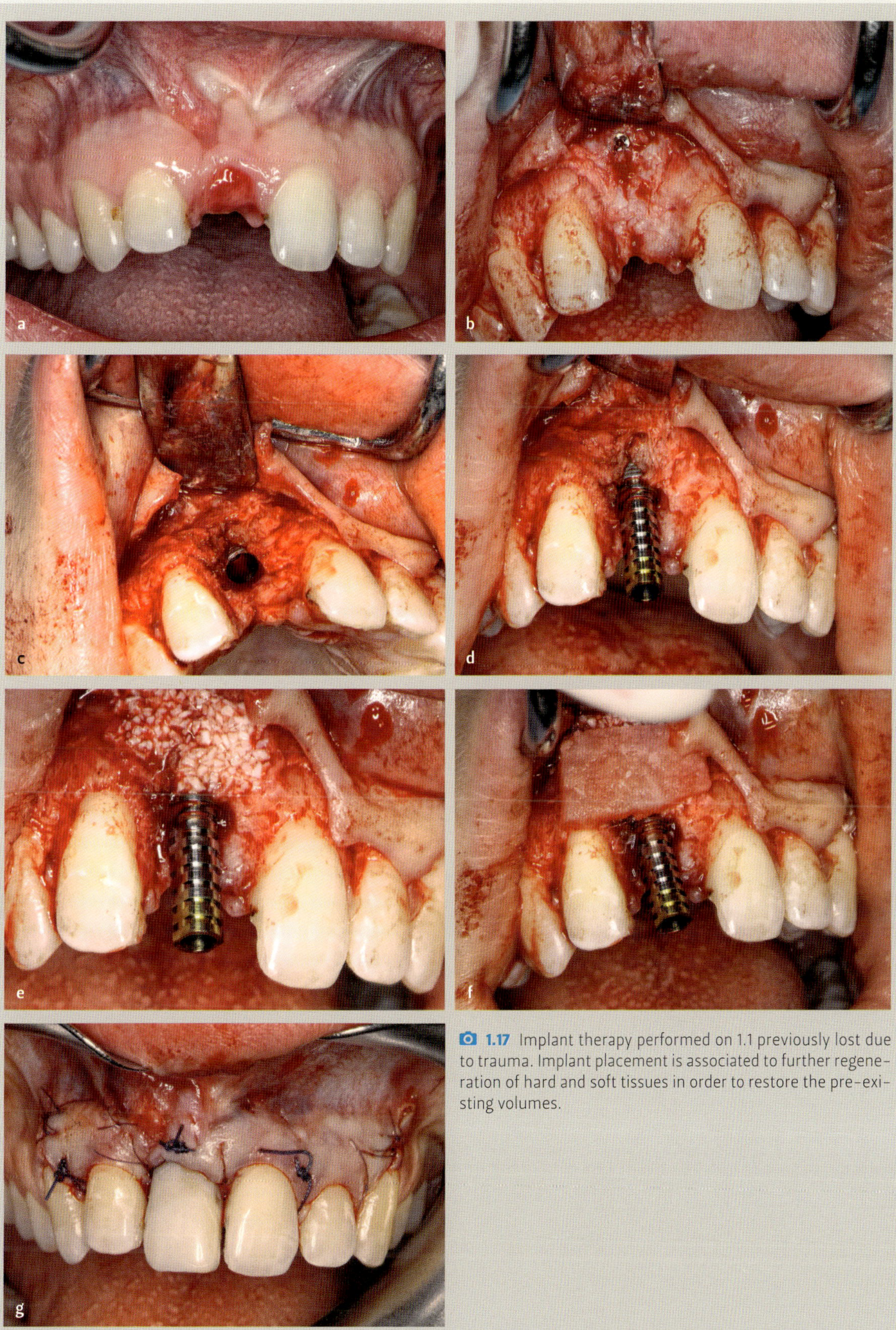

1.17 Implant therapy performed on 1.1 previously lost due to trauma. Implant placement is associated to further regeneration of hard and soft tissues in order to restore the pre-existing volumes.

Posterior area

The immediate loading of the teeth in the anterior-posterior premolar sector, entails the same application rules that are valid in the esthetic area. In this case, it is essential to define a prosthetically guided implant position. In the large majority of cases, the position of the insertion hole in single implants is not significant, as one often chooses not to have any functional contact and to resort to a non-functional prosthesis. The purpose of the provisional crown will mostly be esthetic, while also making it possible to pre-shape the emergence profiles and tissue healing.

In the case of implant-supported FPDs, the screw-retained solution with immediate loading is a solution that can be pursued with greater safety than the cemented one, although in recent years, the clinical use of the conometric solution is becoming widespread. The need, in the case of several teeth, to provide the immediate prosthesis with a prosthetic contact, albeit very free and with progressive dynamics, is often made complicated by the presence of access holes. It is, however, always advisable for occlusal contacts to match the axial centre of the implant position. This is especially valid for short implants, all the more so if loaded with single crowns, in which the relationship between crown and fixture length is crucial (1.18).

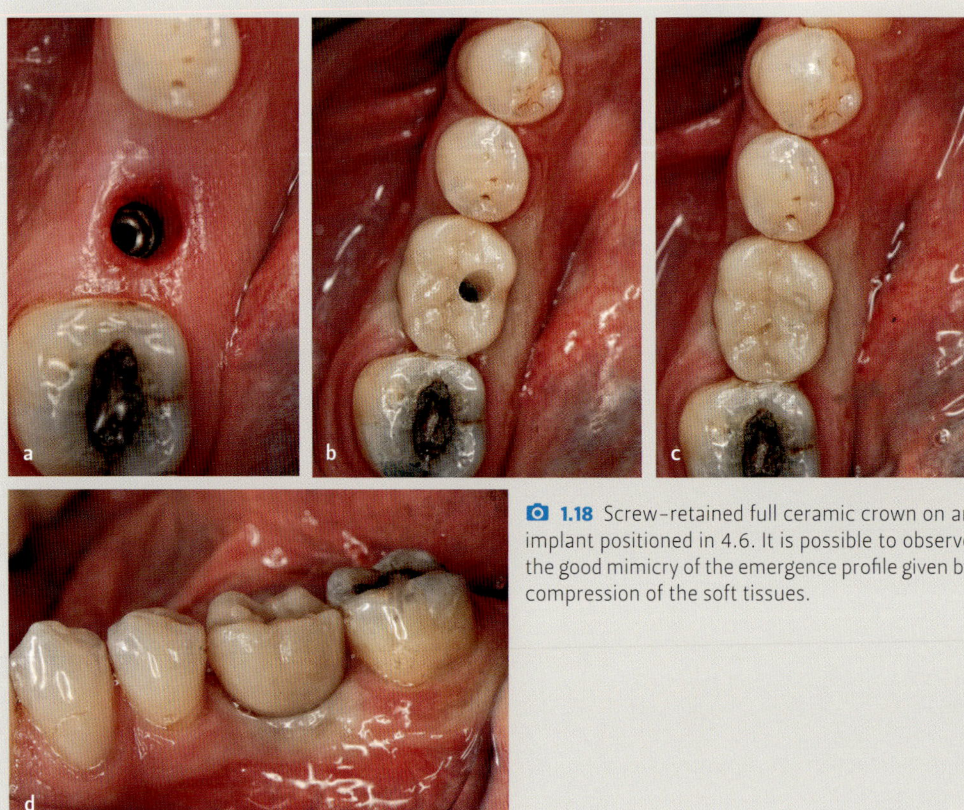

1.18 Screw-retained full ceramic crown on an implant positioned in 4.6. It is possible to observe the good mimicry of the emergence profile given by compression of the soft tissues.

Full arch

From a prosthetic point of view, immediate loading has several advantages: the improvement of the chewing function, the stability of the temporary prosthesis, the reduction to the minimum of the uncontrolled transmucosal load (caused by a transitional complete denture), the preservation of the bone and the stimulation of bone remodeling, the improvement of gingival profiles, better esthetics, as well as an extraordinary improvement in the psychological impact. The mechanical stability of the arch is the essential requirement in a full arch provisional prosthesis and it must be achieved by using rigid, "bilaterally splinted" frameworks. Splinting the implants helps to counteract the bending effect of lateral forces, thus reducing unfavourable stresses and distributing the chewing forces evenly over a larger area. Restoration of the transversal arch requires adequate passive adaptation, which protects from excessive micro-movement and provides the stability required for osseointegration (📷 1.19).

Micro-movements underneath a removable prosthesis during the healing stage is one of the main causes of fixture failure, leading to fibrointegration of implants, rather than osseointegration. When implants are splinted with a provisional prosthesis fitted with a rigid framework, the issue of micro-movement is reduced to the minimum, to less than 100 µm. The presence of a rigid structure seems to be important in conditioning the response of the peri-implant tissue, because the mechanical stress acting on implants is reduced, stability is increased and micro-movement at the interface can be kept below the critical threshold. Therefore, screw-retained provisional prostheses are recommended. It is important to avoid any cement residue that interferes with tissue healing, as it may cause inflammation and impair the healing process of bones and soft tissues. Furthermore, in the event of divergent implants, it is easier to restore with a screw-retained prosthesis. Angular corrections with screw-retained prostheses range between 40° and 90°, whereas with cemented prostheses they range between 10° and 30°. With regard to occlusion, there is disagreement on when and how to provide occlusal contacts, but all authors agree on only maintaining centric contacts.

Provisional prostheses should have a slightly smaller occlusal surface on posterior teeth compared to natural dentition. In conclusion:

- it is advisable to place occlusal contacts within the diameter of the implant;
- the provisional crown should have flat cusps in order to reduce lateral forces to the minimum and spread them over a large area;
- good symmetrical distribution of masticatory forces is important, especially in the early stages of healing;
- exposure to para-functional forces may interrupt the osseointegration process;
- there must not be any excessive cantilevers in order to prevent the presence of non-axial forces;
- patients should modify their diet, and avoid hard foods during the early healing period (approximately 4 weeks);

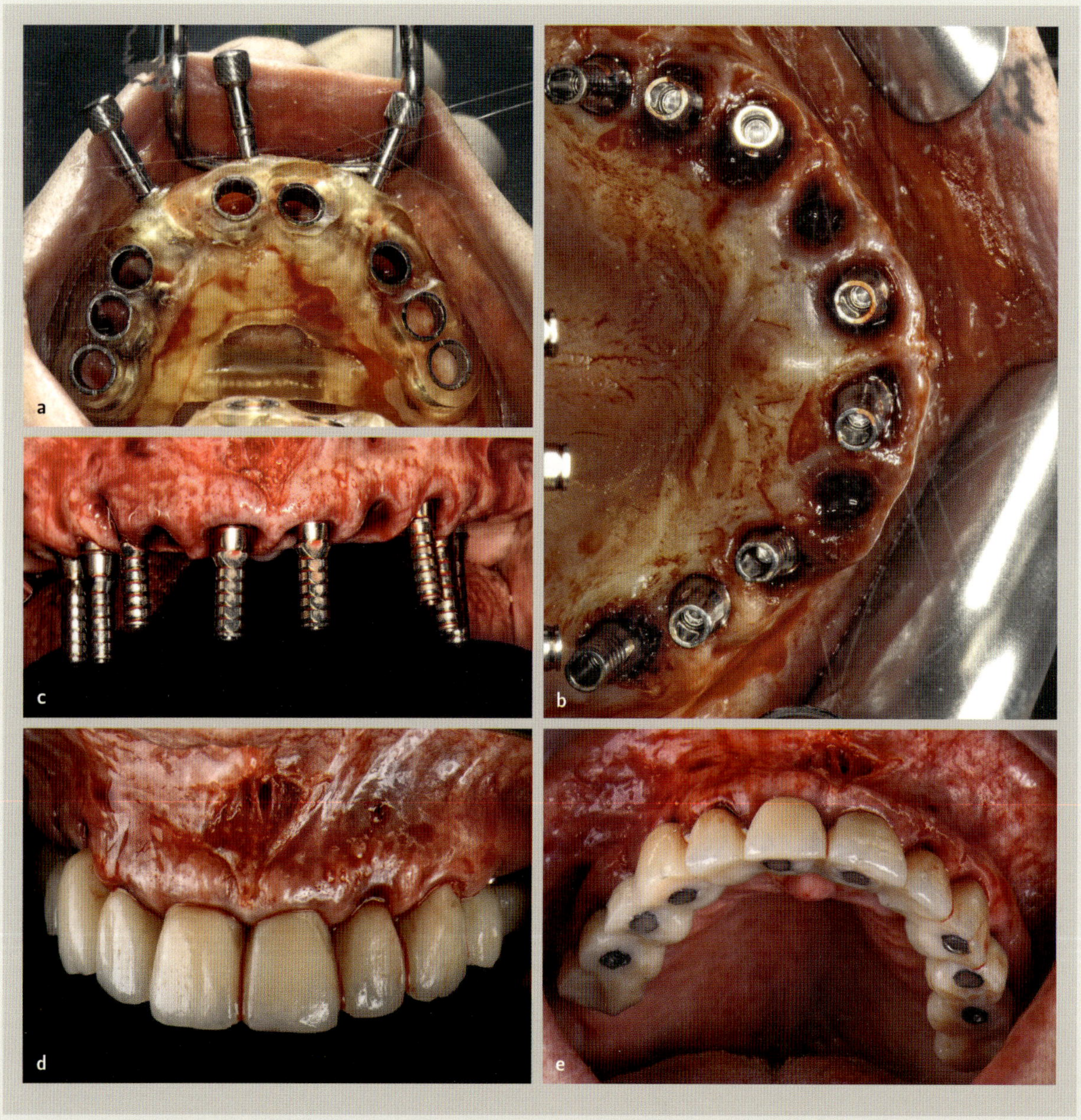

1.19 Immediate load Toronto bridge prosthesis on 8 implants placed on the upper arch. The small size and not too prominent anatomy of the occlusal table of the teeth in association with proper implant placement thanks to the surgical guide ensure an ideal distribution of masticatory forces.

- control of the functional forces is one of the important factors to achieve success in immediate loading. Therefore, it is recommended to start by regulating occlusion with progressive function, especially in the early healing stages. This is very important to avoid complications such as fracture and peri-implant bone loss.

Screw-retained prosthesis

This technique has a number of advantages in immediate prosthetic procedures as well as in definitive rehabilitations. Most certainly, the greatest benefit, which also supports its greatest indication at the moment, is the possibility of easily removing the restoration in case of need. This enables the clinician to monitor very carefully all work phases and to perform the procedures for finalization or impression for the final restoration. Regardless of the chosen type of implant connection, fixed prostheses can be screwed directly at the level of the fixture platform, through an occlusal access hole, or indirectly, through mesostructures. In the latter case, the prosthesis will consist of two components: a mesostructure the provides support to a superstructure, which is the visible part of the restoration.

The choice of using a screw-retained prosthesis is normally taken in the design stage based on:

- available interocclusal space (if it is exceedingly small, there is less retention, which is required for cementation);
- degree of disparallelism in the case of multiple implants;
- ratio between implant length and prosthetic clinical crown;
- possibility of inserting implants in the prosthetically correct position, with the emergence of the screw hole near the centre of the occlusal table of posterior teeth or on the lingual/palatal side of anterior teeth.

Performing a screw-retained prosthesis requires adequate implant placement, in order to avoid the presence of excessively palatal or vestibular access holes, which might undermine the esthetics and function of the restoration. Should the position of the implants require significant prosthetic compensation, it is generally preferable to use prostheses that include intermediate components, such as mesostructures, or prostheses cemented on abutments. In recent years, the development of angulation control systems and dynamic abutment systems, combined with the progress of CAD-CAM technologies, has made it possible to solve a number of issues linked to disparallelism and the placement of the access hole, enabling to opt for screw-retained solutions in many cases. The indications for the procedure must in any case be customized on the basis of the clinical case, also assessing the patient's local and global biomechanical features, from static and dynamic forces to the existing muscle pattern.
Another parameter to be taken into account in the analysis of the screw-retained prosthesis is represented by the materials. Recent systematic literature reviews have shown that there are no statistically significant differences

in the comparison between various types of fixed screw-retained prostheses, directly or by means of mesostructures (single crowns, bridges, full arches), performed in various types of materials (porcelain fused to metal, porcelain fused to zirconia), neither comparing cemented prostheses with screw-retained ones. The comparison between screw-retained and cemented prostheses has not highlighted any biological complications, in terms of bone loss over time, although the incidence of cement-related peri-implantitis plays a decisive role in opting for the screw-retained prosthesis.

In many studies, technical complications such as chipping or alterations of the superstructure have been highlighted, more frequent in screw-retained prostheses than in cemented prostheses, while the total number of complications, in screw-retained prostheses, remains lower (1.20).

From the clinical point of view, it is appropriate to analyze the behaviour of prosthetic types based on the degree of edentulism and type of material.

In the case of single implants, the issues reported in the literature relating to the incidence of screw loosening are presumably caused by inadequate screwing torque of the abutment on the implant and by the use of imprecise anti-rotational components. By applying an adequate torque (25-35 Ncm) and prosthetic components with a higher degree of precision, the problem of screw loosening in single restorations is markedly reduced, regardless of the type of connection. In the event of screw loosening, there is no clear scientific evidence of how micro-movements have an influence on the stability of bone and of soft tissues. Screw-retained prostheses seem to offer excellent functional performance, easy removability and the possibility of inspection. It should be underlined that the production of implant and prosthetic components entails surface treatments that improve the performance in implants with internal connection as well as those with external connection. Indeed, screws that undergo these surface treatments make it possible to achieve, with torque being equal, higher preload values. Compared to restorations on individual teeth, fixed partial prostheses or extensive, implant-supported rehabilitations are more susceptible to chipping phenomena and framework fractures, but less subject to loss of retention linked to the fastening screws coming loose. A relatively frequent complication in the prosthesis directly screwed onto multiple implants is the loss of the obturation material of the occlusal access hole. Although this is a minor and easily solved complication, its recurrence over time may cause discomfort to the patient.

When several implants need to be joined, structure passivation is essential. The presence of even small imprecisions, in fact, involves that part of the preload of the fixation screw is dissipated, to completely house the prosthetic structure. In-vitro tests have showed that single, screw-retained directly on implants, PFM (porcelain fused to metal) crowns have less mechanical resistance than cemented crowns in the same material. The most frequent technical complications reported in clinical studies concern the loss of retention, due to the loss of preload in single tooth restorations, chipping of the porcelain veneering and, more rarely, fracture of the supporting framework. Screw-re-

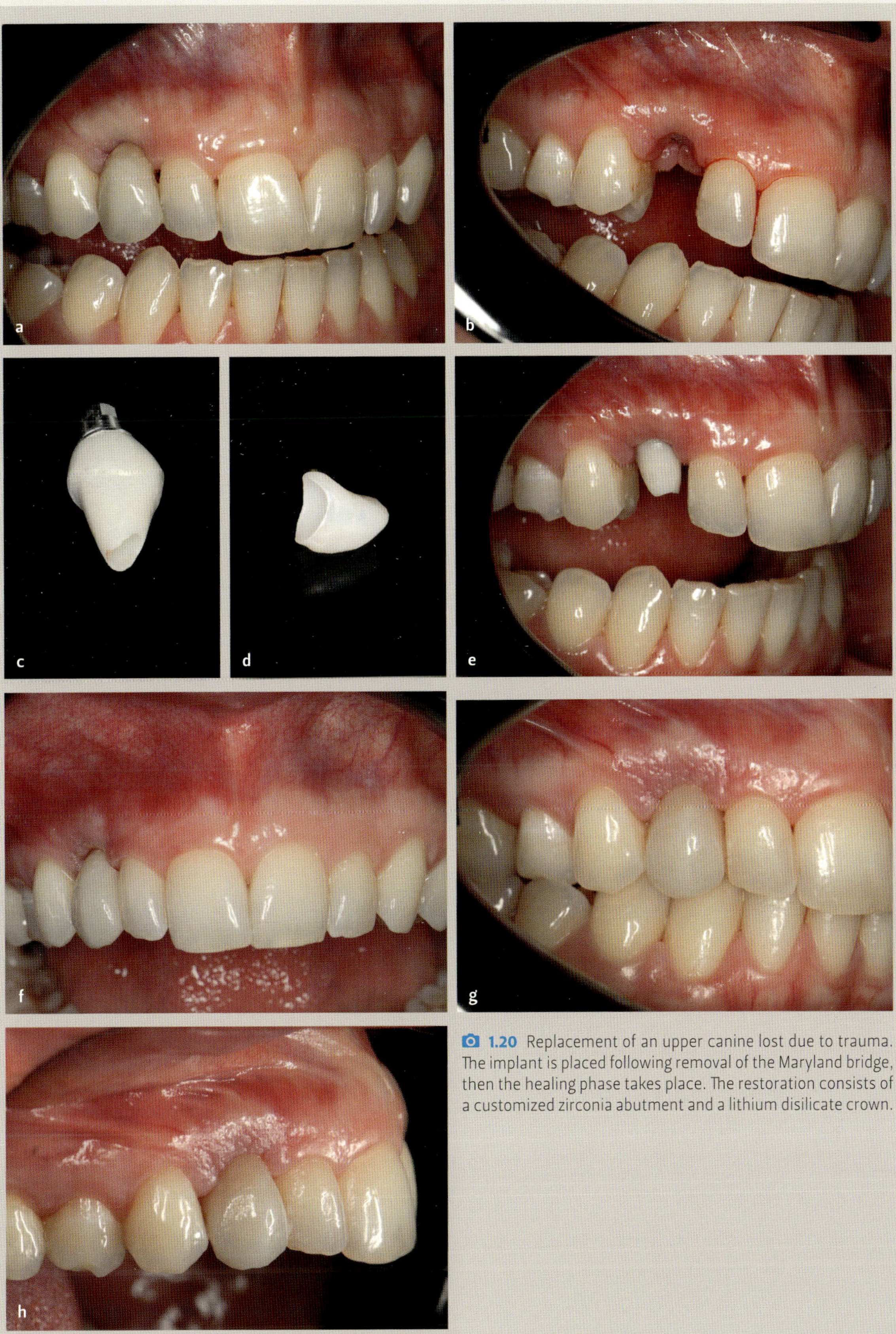

1.20 Replacement of an upper canine lost due to trauma. The implant is placed following removal of the Maryland bridge, then the healing phase takes place. The restoration consists of a customized zirconia abutment and a lithium disilicate crown.

tained directly on implants, layered PFZ (porcelain fused to zirconia) crowns also appear to be less fracture resistant than cemented crowns. In total edentulism or in cases with severe atrophies and high orthopedic component, it is advisable to use mesostructure - or MUA - supported prostheses.

From a biomechanical point of view, it is important to also evaluate the connection.

The internal connection features less intrinsic resistance of the prosthetic component, because the terminal part is smaller than the implant diameter. Furthermore, a wear mechanism of the anti-rotational engagement of the fixtures by the zirconia structures has been hypothesized. This phenomenon might potentially lead to the loss of effectiveness of the anti-rotational device and consequently, an increased risk of loosening of the retaining screws and the opening of undesirable micro-gaps.

The modifications introduced to the design of zirconia structures, aimed at improving the support of the veneering material and fabrication protocols - specifically, about the thermal cycles of items - have reduced the incidence of chipping and of other mechanical complications. Monolithic zirconia products have recently been introduced on the market, which can be directly screwed to fixture or cemented in the laboratory, on specific temporary titanium cylinders. Owing to the absence of veneering material, the chipping problem is thus overcome and the first results seem promising; however, the considerations concerning the mechanical behaviour of zirconia structures remain valid. Furthermore, a form of translucent zirconia has been developed for this type of application, with a better esthetic result (to the detriment of the material mechanical strength, however), which can be treated in order to further improve esthetic integration. Despite the numerous works in the literature, other clinical findings are certainly required over the coming years, in order to establish whether this type of solution is the most appropriate in terms of materials for the fixed prosthesis of the complete arch.

Use of CAD-CAM techniques has introduced new materials that may certainly be high-performing from the esthetic as well as functional point of view (📷 1.21).

From a clinical point of view, temporary solutions for immediate loading must be distinguished from definitive solutions. A second distinction must be made in the choice of restoration material based on all the existing complexity factors and on the level of inter-arch ratio generated by the existing atrophy.

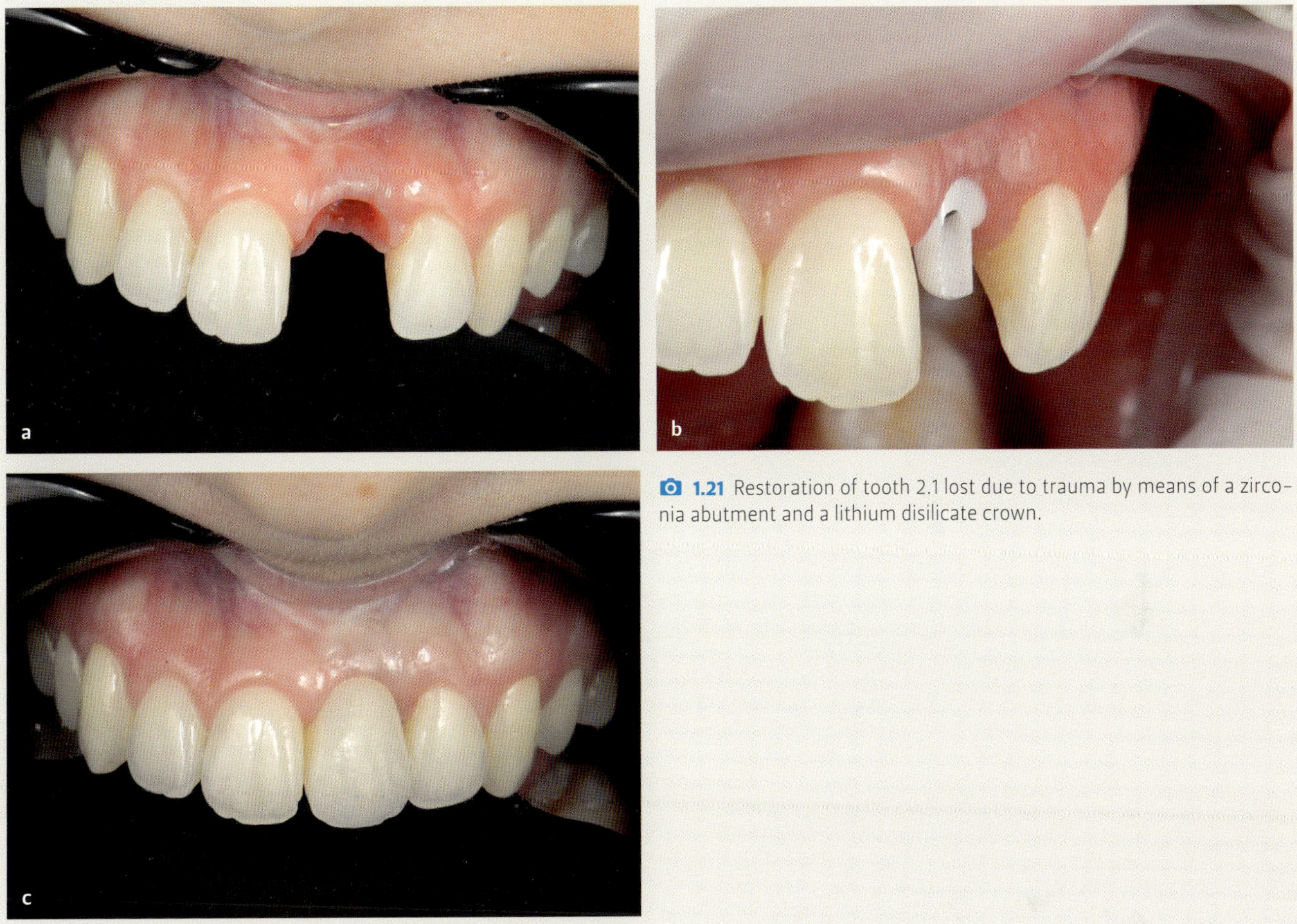

1.21 Restoration of tooth 2.1 lost due to trauma by means of a zirconia abutment and a lithium disilicate crown.

Many works in the literature have in fact highlighted the differences in mechanical and biological terms among prosthetic materials in full-arch rehabilitations, in the case of standard dental prostheses or with high orthopedic component.

In order to simplify the decision making process, we can use the following scheme on the materials to choose in screw-retained prostheses:

- metal-resin: recommended in provisional stages or in immediate loading procedures. Its use over time has unfortunately highlighted a number of mechanical complications, from lesion of the dental components to structure alterations, excessive degradation and pigmentation of the material, infiltration of transition points. There are also many biological complications.

- titanium-composite: better performing than metal-resin solutions; it combines the precision and predictability of CAD-CAM procedures for the framework fabrication with the esthetic-functional performance of composite. Its use over time provides better predictability and esthetic results. Particularly suitable for those patients in whom the presence of parafunctions and TMJ disorders might contraindicate the use of rigid materials. A noteworthy variant of the use of this solution is matching CAD-CAM structures in cobalt-chromium or titanium with superstructures in the monolithic latest generation composite. This solution makes it possible to avoid the phenomenon of the detachment of composite elements, in the case of primary anchoring, but also to reduce infiltration in the case of a layered solution. In the Author's opinion, monolithic solutions ensure excellent biomechanical performance and equally stable esthetic result over (1.22).
- CAD-CAM solutions in PEEK and PEEK PMMA: this CAD-CAM prosthetic solution makes it possible to manage immediate loading procedures in a smooth and effective manner, ensuring good function as well as good esthetic integration. Nowadays, it is one of the most promising solutions for immediate loading procedures with screw-retained technique. PEEK is a high-performance polymer, partially crystalline, thermoplastic and stable at high temperatures, based on polyether-ether-ketone, which is added with inorganic ceramic microparticles, smaller than 0.5 µm in diameter.

Physiological elasticity is thus granted and thanks to the addition of ceramic particles, perfect rigidity has been combined with exceptional polishing properties.

The main features of the material are:

- resilience;
- shock absorption;
- non-abrasiveness on the residual natural teeth;
- elasticity equal to bone tissue;

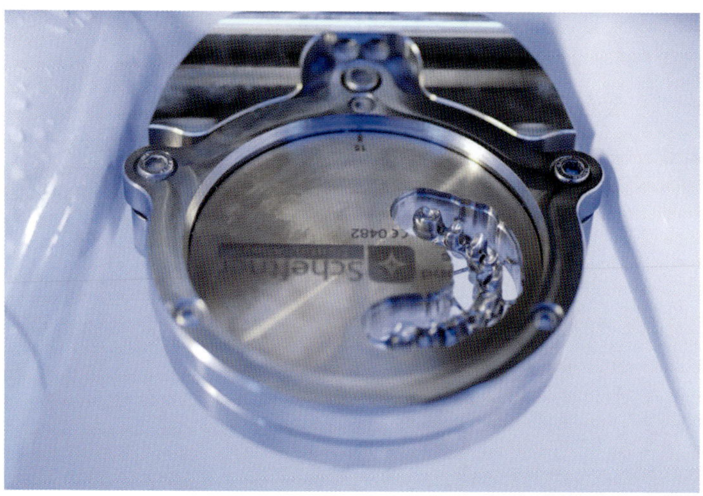

1.22 Milling process for the prosthesis framework, starting from a titanium disc.

- fracture resistance and torsional stability;
- maximum tolerability;
- maintenance of friction values;
- metal free;
- hypo-allergenicity;
- non solubility in water;
- plaque resistance;
- no electrolytic conductivity;
- compared to ceramic, it retains intrinsic resistance;
- no degeneration linked to ageing;
- resistance to gamma rays and X-rays;
- stability from the chemical point of view.

This material, which has already been covered by a number of studies in the literature for years, features an excellent combination of elasticity and rigidity, absorbs shocks, is semi-rigid like healthy bone tissue, and enables the natural, physiological torsion of the maxillary arch. It is resistant to breakage, easy to handle, metal free, hypoallergenic, with no ion exchange, no metal taste, good integration with soft tissues. The biomechanical properties reported in the literature include:

- stability, thanks to its high mechanical resistance values;
- resistance to abrasion;
- optimal and long-lasting esthetic veneering capability.

Its lightness, smooth surfaces and physiological integration in the human body make it possible to maintain good esthetics as well as excellent health conditions of soft tissues.

Cement-retained restorations

The choice of using a cemented implant-supported prosthesis is normally taken in the design stage based on variables such as:

- the available interocclusal space;
- the degree of disparallelism, in case of multiple implants;
- the ratio between implant length and prosthetic clinical crown, and inadequate implant inclination.

Clinical criteria, such as the ability to easily remove the restoration if needed, esthetics, occlusion management, ease, precision and production costs may affect the decision-making process, as a less-than-ideal implant placement may affect the final esthetic result, actually making the screw access hole visible in the case of a screw-retained prosthesis. Furthermore, in case of multiple implants, should the position of the implants require significant prosthetic compensation, it is preferable to use cemented prostheses or prostheses that include intermediate components, such as screw-retained mesostructures, with a cement- or screw-retained superstructure (1.23).

The final esthetic result is one of the main advantages of cement-retained prostheses, ruling out any patient concerns regarding the screw access hole. Better occlusion management of the definitive crowns is another advantage, since the screw access hole, required for the screw-retained solution, often falls within a functional part of the restoration. Although the delivery of a cemented restoration may be easier in situations of limited mouth opening, the greatest drawback of this prosthetic solution is the removal of excess cement. Indeed, a few studies11 showed the permanence of cement residues, notwithstanding the subgingival position of the prosthetic margin, and the fact that these residues are the main cause of peri-implantitis, regardless of the type of cement used. Therefore, careful planning of the abutment design and margin are required in order to make removal of excess cement easier. This may be aided by placement of a retractor cord below the undercut of the prosthetic abutment

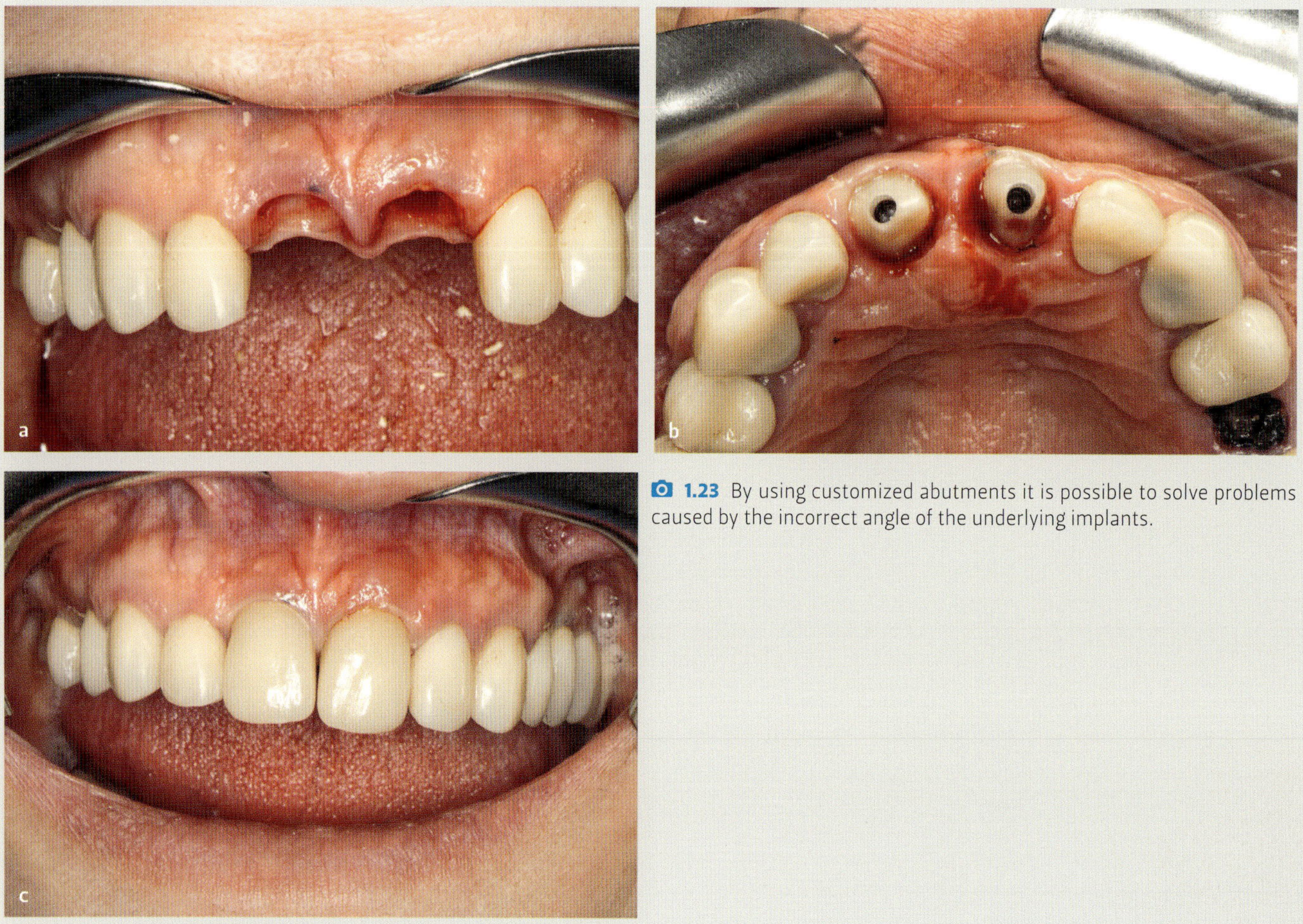

1.23 By using customized abutments it is possible to solve problems caused by the incorrect angle of the underlying implants.

and/or extraoral cementation on a replica of the abutment (1.24).

Further possible complications of cemented restorations are due to inadequate placement of the crown on the abutment during the cementation stage, consequently leading to loss of the proper restoration position, as well as loss of the retention of the crown over time, which mainly depends on the prosthetic abutment. In-vitro studies have shown how the convergence and height of the abutments are essential to maintain the stability of the prosthetic restoration over time. In the literature, it has been put forward to use provisional cement to aid re-intervention at a later time in the event of complications. However, due to the fact that the abutment is tightly attached to the crown, removing the crown without damaging it or avoiding to damage the retention screw was found to be very difficult. The loss of crown retention is a more of a drawback in single crowns than in full or partial arches, as they can rely on more implants. However, any decementation of one of these units may not be perceived, the consequence being incorrect distribution of occlusal forces on the various implants.

One of the advantages of a cemented prosthesis is the greater ease in achieving passivation of the prosthetic components compared to a screw-retained one, thanks to the presence of cement, which seems to act as shock-absorber.

Systematic literature reviews have shown no statistically significant differences when comparing various types of fixed screw-retained prostheses, directly or by means of mesostructures (single crowns, bridges, full arches), performed in various types of materials (PFM, PFZ), nor comparing cemented with screw-retained prostheses.

There is no evidence of a larger extent of bone loss when comparing the two forms of prosthesis,[12] but a higher rate of chipping has been observed in screw-retained prostheses compared to cemented ones.

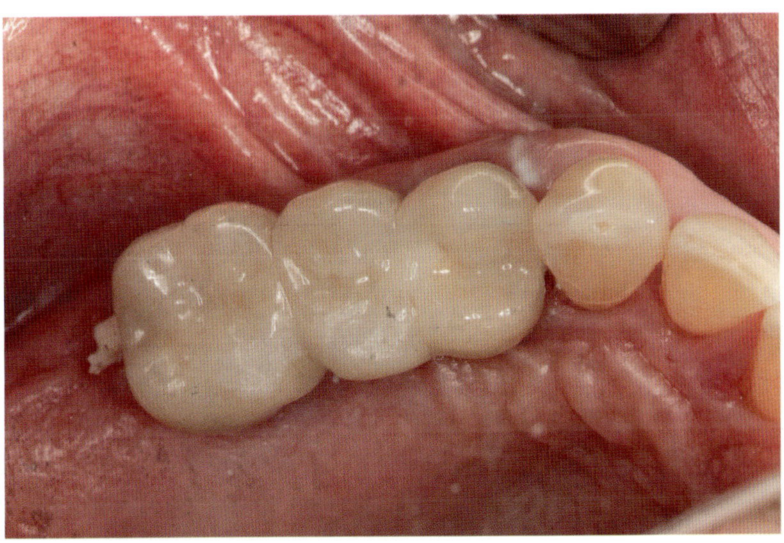

1.24 The removal of excess cement such as shown in the picture is essential to preserve the health of peri-implant tissues.

An essential role is played by the abutment, which may be fabricated, thanks to the new CAD-CAM technologies, in grade 4 or 5 titanium, entirely in zirconia, zirconia on titanium base, lithium disilicate on titanium base, cobalt-chromium on titanium base and composite resin on titanium base. Additionally, grade 4 and 5 titanium abutments are also available on the market, fabricated by milling by implant manufacturers. Esthetic abutments (zirconia, disilicate and composite resin) ensure better colour management of the peri-implant soft tissues. The full zirconia abutment features excellent rigidity and prevents the formation of galvanic currents between different metals, i.e. between implant and abutment; however, cases of fracture of the anti-rotational component of the abutment have been reported. To counteract the incidence of fracture of zirconia abutments, it is possible to fabricate them with a grade 4 or 5 titanium base, on which a zirconia abutment is cemented with resin cements in the laboratory. Monolithic or layered crowns can be cemented on the prosthetic abutment (1.25 and 1.26).

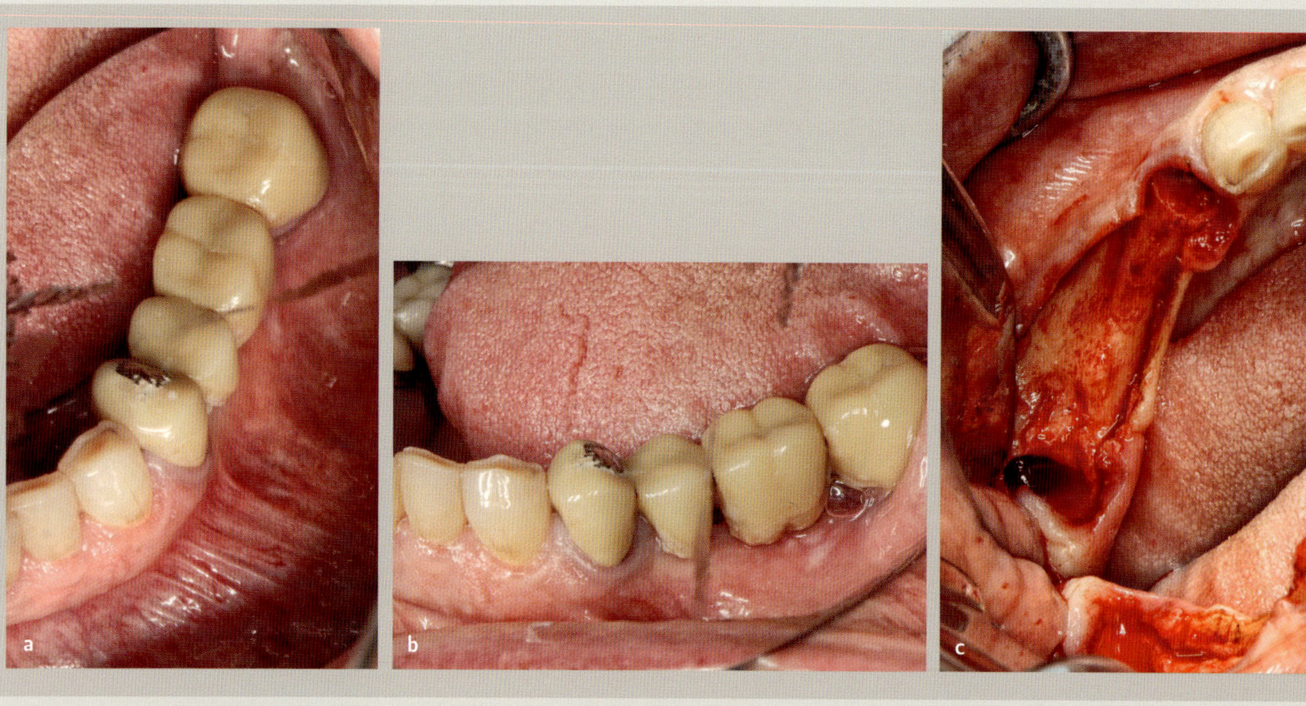

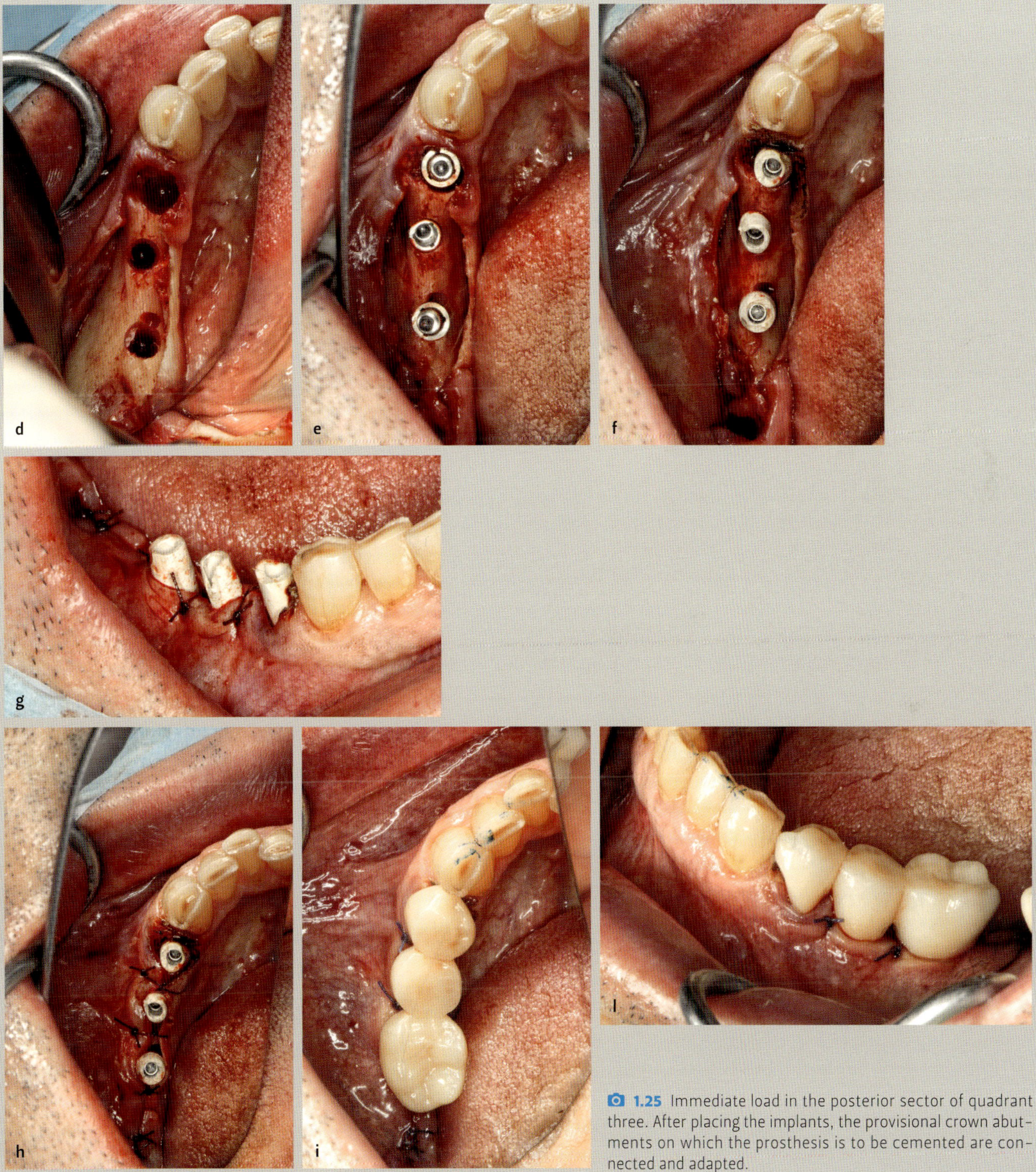

1.25 Immediate load in the posterior sector of quadrant three. After placing the implants, the provisional crown abutments on which the prosthesis is to be cemented are connected and adapted.

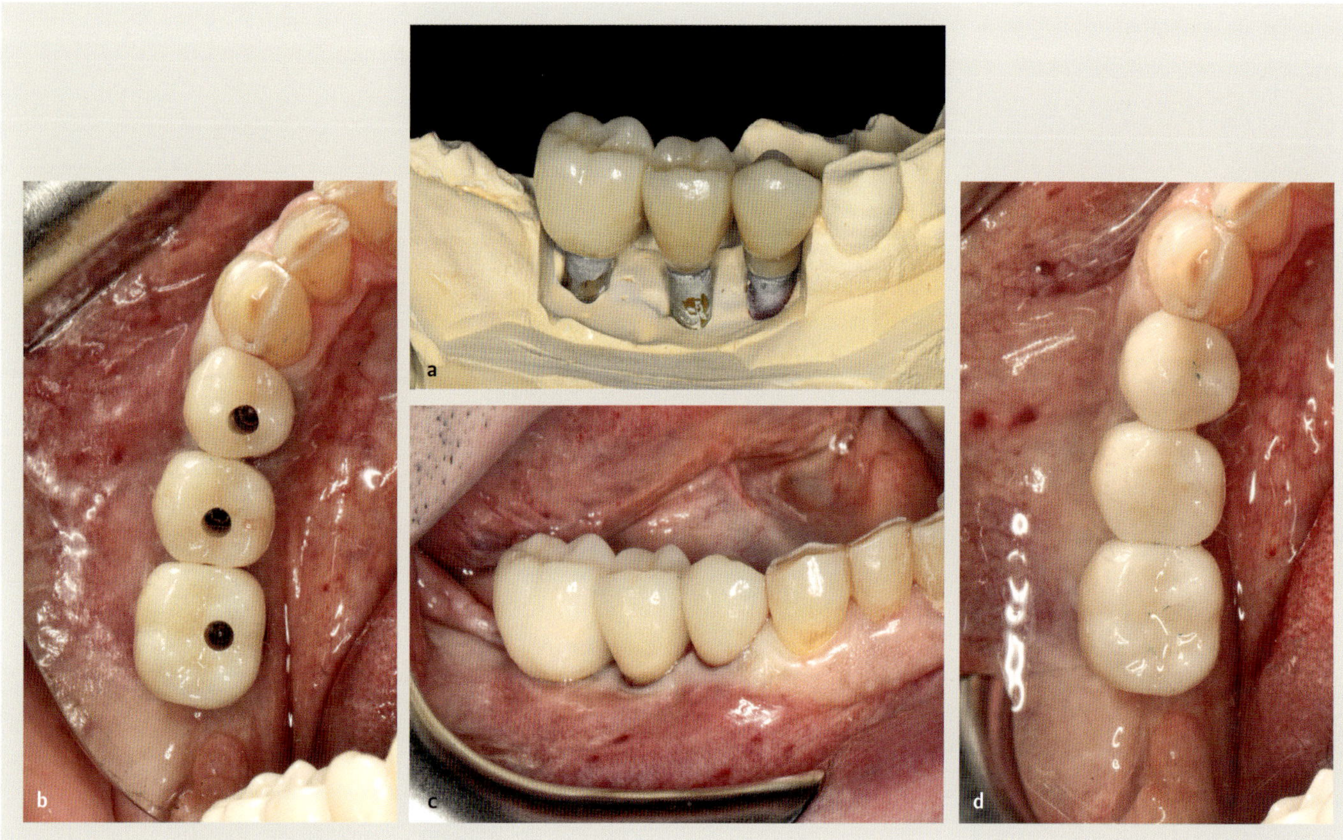

1.26 A screw-retained connection has been chosen for the final restoration.

Conometric prosthesis

A number of studies in the literature and clinical experiences have revived this prosthetic solution in recent years. The main advantages consist in the ease of removal and the possibility of re-intervention, combined with the stability of the fixed prosthesis and the total esthetics of the item, due to the absence of fixation screw holes. What is more, certain works in the literature have reported the excellent stability of soft tissues, combined with the possibility of performing simple and effective professional hygiene procedures.
The introduction of CAD-CAM procedures makes surgical and prosthetic implementation easier, reducing operative difficulties and lack of structural precision. The drawbacks to be listed certainly include the loss of stability and retention over time and the occurrence in various circumstances of mechanical complications relating to the secondary prosthetic components, due to failure or alteration of the materials (1.27 and 1.28).

In a recent study, Albiero and coll.[13] assessed the clinical outcome at the 2-year follow-up of full arch restorations, with immediate loading and conometric support, planned by digital methods. The research included 12 patients who presented with compromised teeth in the maxilla. The chosen treatment plan was implants placement through computer-guided surgery. A total of 72 implants

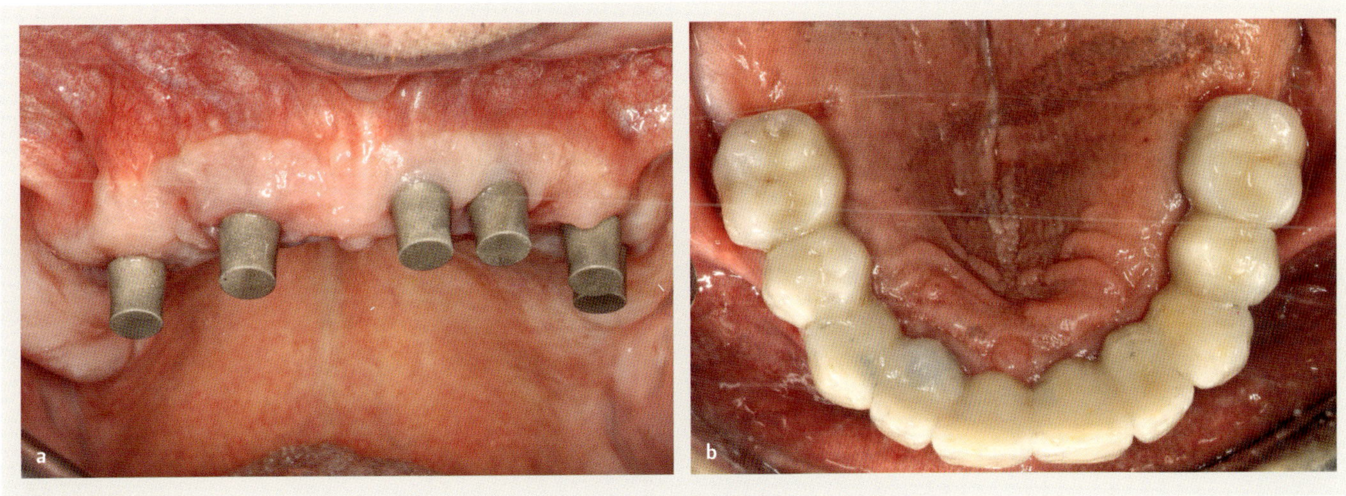

1.27 Condition of the soft tissues underneath an immediate load provisional prosthesis that had been delivered one month before. As it does not require cement, hence removal of excess cement, the conometric retention usually results in much faster healing.

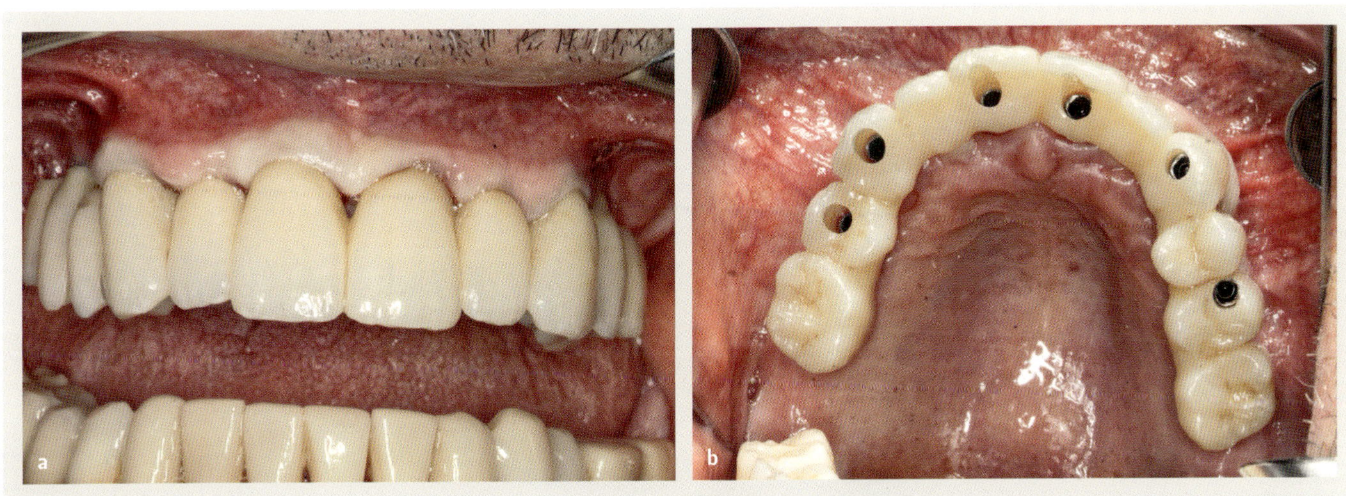

1.28 Example of screw-retained, implant-supported definitive prosthesis, An optimal implant placement, only made possible by guided surgery – especially in cases of complete edentulism – can be observed.

were inserted and immediately loaded with a full arch restoration. The digital scanning technology was used to plan virtually combined conometric- and screw-retention of the structures. The clinical parameters were evaluated after 1 week and at the 1, 3, 6, 12 and 24-month follow-up.

The survival rate after 2 years was 98.6%, because one implant failed during the osseointegration period. No significant prosthetic complications were observed, such as issues of mobility, loosened abutments, disconnected conometric copings and prosthetic fractures. Only one patient reported a biomechanical problem with the prosthesis. It is important to underline the validity of the biological response of this prosthetic solution. In a recent study, Bressan and coll.[14] analyzed in vitro the sealing capacity at the prosthetic connection interface of two conometric systems, with the same design, but different materials, for a total of 24 samples. Each sample was assembled with a conical abutment and respective coping. In group A, the copings were made of gold, whereas in group B they were in PEEK. Three µL of mixed bacterial suspension (species *Aggregatibacter actinomycetemcomitans, Porphyromonas gingivalis and Fusobacterium nucleatum*) were inoculated into the screw hole of the abutment and the coping was inserted onto the abutment. The samples were immersed in culture tubes and incubated for 24, 48 and 72 hours, under anaerobic conditions. The qualitative-quantitative evaluation was performed after 72 hours, using real-time polymerase chain reaction.

The analysis brought to light a microbial dispersal in both groups and no statistically significant difference was observed between the two groups. The microbial concentration determined a presence of less than 1 × 10 copies/µL in all positive assemblies.

REFERENCES

1. **Davies JE.** Understanding peri-implant endosseous healing. J Dent Educ 2003;67(8):932-49.
2. **Albrektsson T,C Johansson.** Osteoinduction, osteoconduction and osseointegration. Eur Spine J 2001;10 (Suppl 2):S96-101.
3. **Brånemark PI.** Osseointegration and its experimental background. J Prosthet Dent 1983 Sep;50(3):399-410.
4. **Gotfredsen K, Nimb L, Buser D et al.** Evaluation of guided bone generation around implants placed into fresh extraction sockets: an experimental study in dogs. J Oral Maxillofac Surg 1993 Aug;51(8):879-84; discussion 885-6.
5. **Sennerby L, Meredith N.** Implant stability measurements using resonance frequency analysis: biological and biomechanical aspects and clinical implications. Periodontol 2000 2008;47:51-66.
6. **Morton D, Jaffin R, Weber HP.** Immediate restoration and loading of dental implants: clinical considerations and protocols. Int J Oral Maxillofac Implants 2004;19 Suppl:103-8.
7. **Balshi TJ, Wolfinger GJ.** Immediate loading of Brånemark implants in edentulous mandibles: a preliminary report. Implant Dent Summer 1997;6(2):83-8.
8. **Cicciù M, Beretta M, Risitano G et al.** Cemented-retained vs screw-retained implant restorations: an investigation on 1939 dental implants. Minerva Stomatol. 2008;57(4):167-79.
9. **Sailer I, Mühlemann S, Zwahlen M et al.** Cemented and screw-retained implant reconstructions: a systematic review of the survival and complication rates. Clin Oral Implants Res 2012;23 Suppl 6:163-201.
10. **Bressan E, Sbricoli L, Guazzo R et al.** Five-year prospective study on conometric retention for complete fixed prostheses. Int J Oral Implantol (Berl) 2019;12(1):105-113.
11. **Staubli N, Walter C, Schmidt JC et al.** Excess cement and the risk of peri-implant disease - a systematic review. Clin Oral Implants Res. 2017;28(10):1278-1290.
12. **de Brandão ML, Vettore MV, Vidigal Júnior GM.** Peri-implant bone loss in cement- and screw-retained prostheses: systematic review and meta-analysis. J Clin Periodontol 2013;40(3):287-95.
13. **Albiero AM, Benato R, Momic S et al.** Guided-welded approach planning using a computer-aided designed prosthetic shell for immediately loaded complete-arch rehabilitations supported by conometric abutments. J Prosthet Dent 2019;122(6):510-515.
14. **Bressan E, Stocchero M, Jimbo R et al.** Microbial Leakage at Morse Taper Conometric Prosthetic Connection: An In Vitro Investigation. Implant Dent 2017;26(5):756-761.

Radiography for dental implantology

Andrea Baruffaldi

Introduction

The Cone Beam Computed Tomography method has revolutionized radiographic diagnostics, making three-dimensional (3D) rendering of anatomical structures possible.

It is used to acquire data and images of a specific volume and, thanks to processing software, it provides diagnostic images in the three planes of space and Volume Rendering (VR) (3D rendered images), plus the advantage of exposing the patient to low radiation doses.

Cone Beam CT (CBCT) offers a number of advantages compared to conventional CT: low cost, precision and convenience of execution.

The basic mechanism is as follows:

- the X-ray source rotates around the patient's facial skeleton; a detector captures the images, and sends them to the workstation for processing.

The exam produces a set of images, which are stored in the computer and are called "basis images" that is, information that is processed and presented graphically in the form of anatomical images (2.1):

- sections of the mandible or maxilla rendered in the three spatial planes: in sagittal, coronal and axial projection;
- sum views, able to make the bone transparent in varying degrees, to highlight the structures within it.

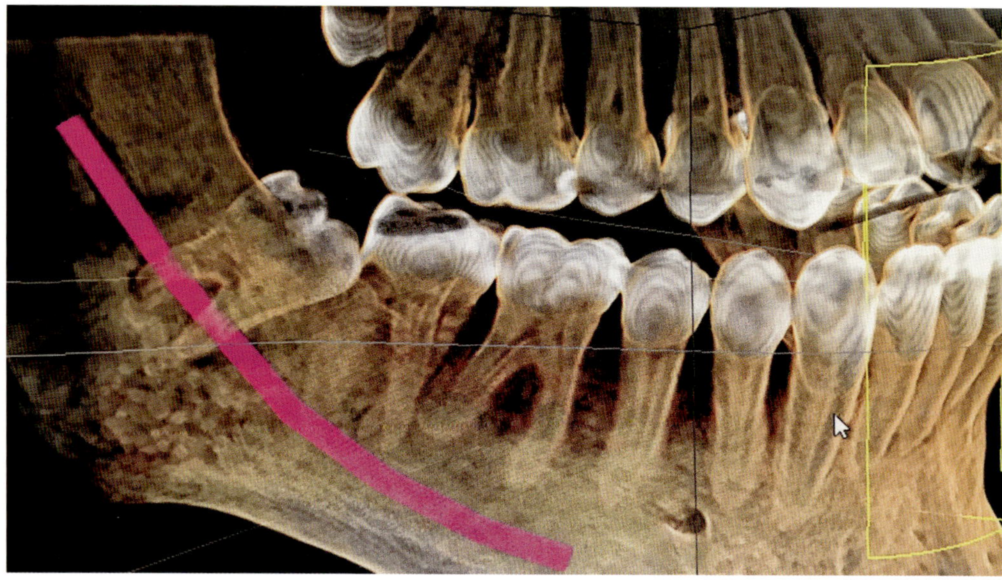

2.1 CBCT allows the analysis of anatomical images.

Cone Beam CT differs from classic spiral CT as it uses a conical radiant beam and a large area detector, thus being able to acquire a large volume of images in a single rotation. In Cone Beam CT, the Field of View (FOV), that is the width of the area exposed to the X-rays, is rather small and is limited to the area of clinical interest only.

CBCT is superior to spiral CT due to the higher definition of its images, lower exposure to radiation doses, and execution times, which are generally shorter.

In implantology, CBTC is used to assess quality and quantity of available bone and to estimate possible causes of failure, thanks to the anatomical assessment of the structures to be avoided when inserting the implants.

Furthermore, the method is indicated in the design of surgical procedures using a "dual scan" protocol, which allows the dentist to undertake an in-depth diagnostic pathway and schedule the placement of implants with the support of specific data processing software.

The main advantage is the option of inserting implant devices with flapless surgery, that is, with the aid of a surgical guide template, fabricated on the basis of the digital design.

This results in greater comfort, with less post-surgery pain, less edema, absence of sutures, better management of surgical processes.

The protocol entails a dual scan: the first of the patient's skull, who is asked to wear a diagnostic template, built on the basis of the desired final prosthetic design; the second is the scan of the diagnostic template alone, outside of the patient's mouth.

This procedure makes it possible to improve the rendering of the radiological image, by more precisely acquiring dental detail, and allows the operator to plan the position of the implants most suited to the prosthetic design on the computer.

Overlapping of the two images is made possible thanks to the presence of asymmetric radiopaque gutta-percha landmarks within the diagnostic template.

A specific software of the Cone-Beam CT equipment recognizes the radiopaque landmarks and overlaps the images.

The CT Scan

Cone Beam CT is a radiological imaging technology that uses a conical or pyramidal X-ray source (hence the name "cone beam"), which makes a single, complete 360° revolution around the object to be examined.

The X-rays passing though the object are then acquired by a detector (usually made with solid state technology) located behind it.

During scanning, the source may emit continuous or pulsed radiation, as in most cases, in order to limit the radiation dose administered to the patient.

The particular feature of having a conical beam, instead of a "fan" one as in the case of spiral CT, allows each exposure to cover the entire field of view (FOV) and therefore, in a single revolution, to acquire a set of complete two-dimensional images of the anatomical part under examination, in the various projections.

The number of images is variable and depends on the operator's choices and on the features of the system: the more images acquired, the better the quality of the end result, but against greater patient exposure to ionizing radiation.

The set of acquired projections is processed by software, which produces a three-dimensional set, which serves as a basis for subsequent re-processing and makes it possible to obtain the renderings in the three orthogonal planes (axial, sagittal, coronal).

The end result is a three-dimensional image, consisting of a set of voxels, the size of which matches the spatial resolution and is intrinsically correlated to the size of the pixels of the detector.

Resolution is usually in the order of 0.09-0.4 mm; this value determines the size of the voxel, which generally has the characteristic of being isotropic. This allows to reconstruct the image on further planes and to obtain three-dimensional graphical models.

As stated above, the typical cone beam of CBCT is able to cover the entire anatomical part of interest (📷 2.2).

In the flat panel detectors, sensors consist of a thin layer of amorphous silicon (a-Si). This detector consists of a scintillator (usually cesium iodide) and a photosensor. The photosensor consists of photodiodes and switching systems.

The scintillator converts the X-rays into an optical signal, which in its turn is translated into an electrical signal by the photodiode (by exploiting the photoelectric effect, whereby a metal hit by electromagnetic radiation releases electrons). Finally, the electrical signal is read by a switching system. The flat panel detector does not generate distortions.

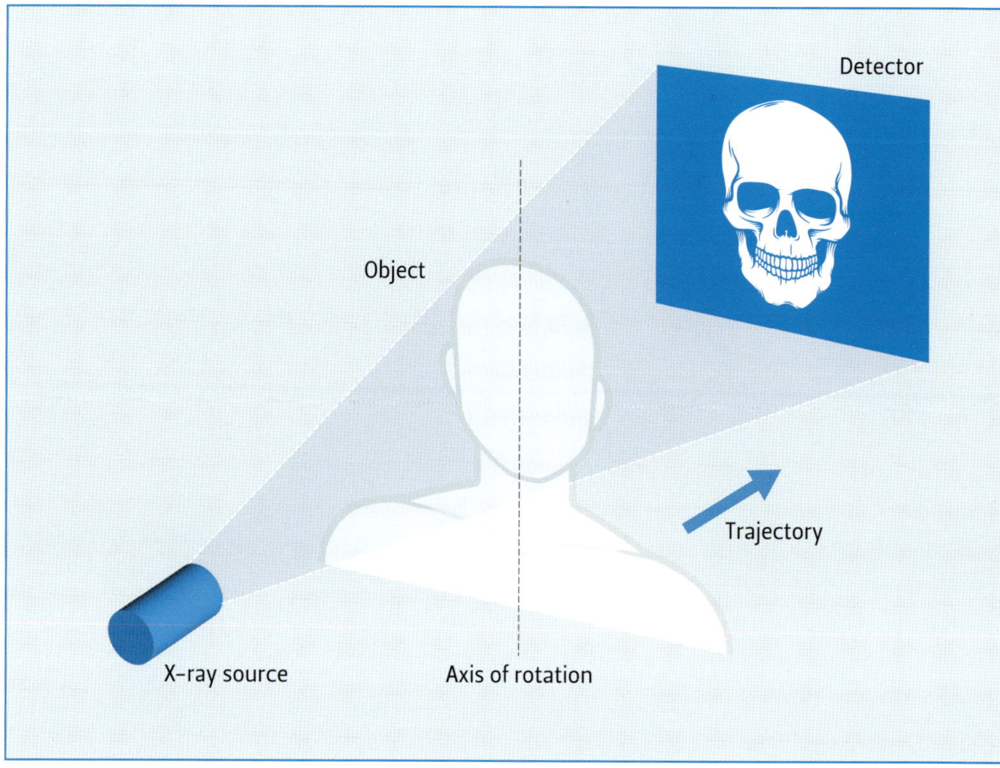

2.2 Diagram illustrating the operation of CBCT.

On the other hand, image-intensifiers work as follows:

- X-rays hit a phosphor screen, which are luminescent. When the phosphors are hit by ionizing radiation, they emit an optical signal (photons) which is then converted into electrons by a photocathode.
- The electrical signal thus generated is weak, therefore, electrons are accelerated and multiplied by an electric field (generated by the so-called diodes) and aimed at a new phosphor screen, placed further inside, which transforms them back into an optical signal, but this time more intense.
- The intensity of the optical signal, thus multiplied, is corrected by an iris diaphragm. At the end, the optical signal is captured by a Charged Couple Device (CCD) sensor.

The complex pathway travelled by the optical signal, however, entails a certain distortion of the image and an increase in glare, which tends to veil the image. In conclusion, flat panel sensors generate less noise than an image intensifier sensor.

Data processing

The photons (quanta of light) that are generated when X-rays strike the scintillating material are captured by the digital sensor, similar to those in digital cameras (CCD, CMOS, amorphous silicon, etc.).

When it is excited by light, the sensor converts the optical signal (photons) into an electrical signal. Therefore, sensors are signal transducers.

The electrical signal is conveyed to a computer, which translates it into numbers and, through the application of mathematical algorithms and by assigning a grey value to each number, allows the object analyzed to be viewed on the monitor in three dimensions.

The numbers assigned may have different grey scales. One of the scales, the one used by some computers and monitors, has shades of grey that range from 0 to 256.

Black colour corresponds to zero value and is assigned to the points where the X-rays hit the sensor without having been attenuated - for example, after passing through air.

The value of 256, which corresponds to white, instead, is obtained when no X-rays reach a point of the sensor, as they have been completely attenuated (blocked) by a dense substance, such as bone.

Thanks to its percentage of calcium, which is a metal and therefore capable of blocking X-rays, bone will appear white, since in that area, the assigned numerical value is 256.

Therefore, the numbers from 0 to 256 indicate the measurement of the attenuation undergone by X-rays in their path through the part of the body being examined. Hence, they provide an indication of the density of the matter that radiation passes through.

Conventional two-dimensional radiographs are represented on the computer monitor as a puzzle of pixels, i.e., many small squares, each with a grey value. Three-dimensional radiography (tomography), however, allows the part of the body under examination to be visualized on the monitor as if it were made up of many cubes, called voxels, i.e. a cube with a specific grey value.

The smaller the voxel, the more precise and detailed the image. The larger the voxel, the more the image appears divided into squares and is imprecise. Once the CT scan has been acquired, some basic processing and measurements on the data may be carried out with the software provided by the manufacturers.

In Cone Beam tomographs, the voxels - the cubes that make up the three-dimensional radiological image - have a much smaller size than in conventional spiral CTs. This means that the Cone Beam CT voxel has a smaller volume, hence the image itself is made up of more voxels. Therefore, the image is more defined and has more details than the image obtained by a spiral CT.

Each voxel has a grey value based on the amount of absorbed radiation, through an algorithm. Visualization is based on the threshold value which defines each voxel as transparent or visible, based on the shade of grey value.

The critical value dividing voxels into visible and invisible is defined.

The result is an image rendered on the screen consisting of all visible voxels. The operator may visualize the set data by looking at the slices or 3D rendered images (📷 2.3).

Computers can reformat the 3D image, allowing the operator to scroll through two-dimensional images in any direction. The most common ones are sagittal, coronal and axial.

Any viewing software makes it possible to scroll through the stack of images. A cursor consisting of 2 crossing lines indicates the precise location in virtual space. Views can also be rotated, panned or zoomed to visualize the region of interest.

A 3D rendered image can be created at each angle, scale or position (2.4).

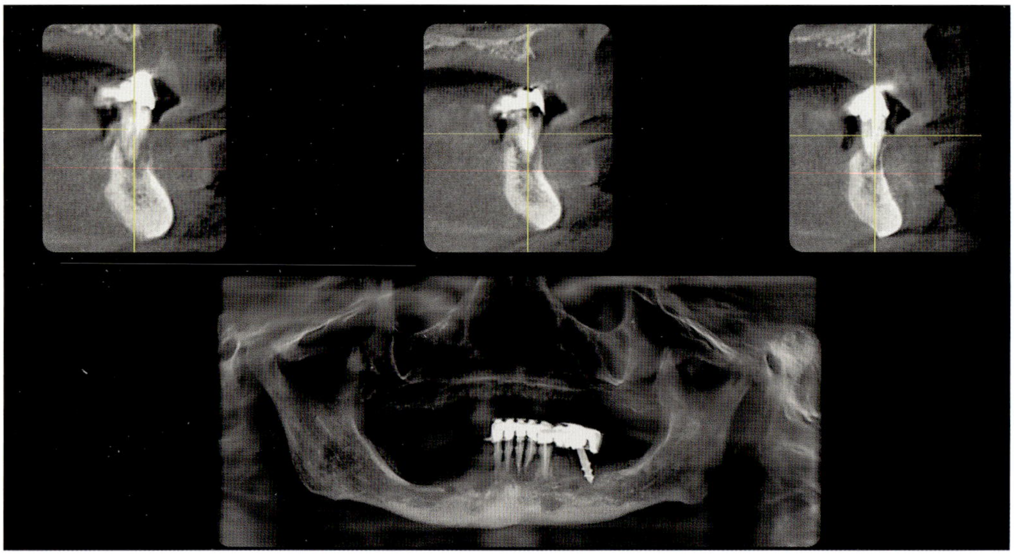

2.3 Image processing enables navigation on several planes.

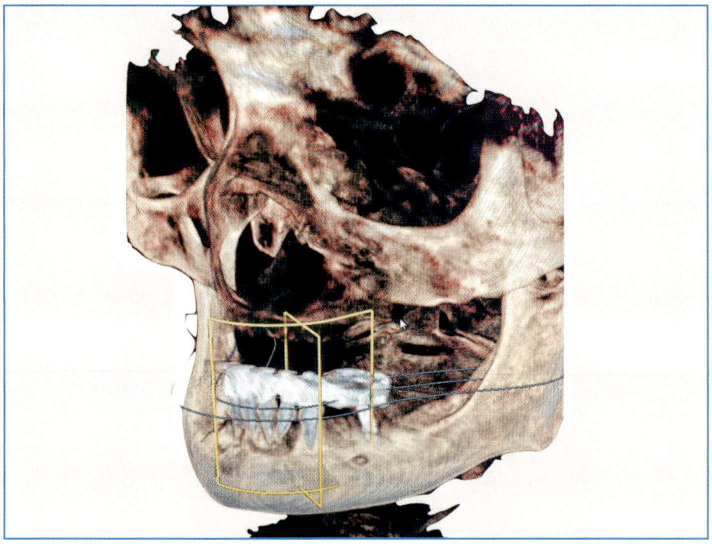

2.4 3D image processing is possible.

Transparency

Transparency is an image fading method, used for a variety of purposes:

- for any text layered over it to be more visible;
- to layer images one over the other;
- to delete or hide a part of the image, i.e. to highlight.

Transparency may also be applied to allow hard tissues to be viewed through soft tissues.

It is also essential to understand that the 3D image in Volume Rendering is the result of a threshold value entered by the user. The operator's visual perception defines what is bone and what is soft tissue, and this may be affected by many factors: image contrast, image noise, individual visual perception and knowledge of anatomy, among others.

Today, three-dimensional images pose many challenges that must still be dealt with, even for a quantitative analysis.

CBCT in implantology

CBCT has been used for pre-and post-operative assessment of dental implants. In the pre-operative stage, it can establish with precision the quantity and quality of the bone available for implant placement.

The three-dimensional images obtained through CBCT accurately depict the anatomy of the jaws, allowing to plan the implant position more accurately, respecting the nerve and vascular structures.

The advantages in the use of CBCT in the pre-operative stage are:

- assessment of the quantity and quality of the available bone;
- location of the vascular-nerve structures (mandibular nerve, mental nerve, lingual artery etc.);
- precise measurements in scale 1:1, with average error of just 0.2 mm;
- planning of computer-assisted implant surgery.

How to perform a Cone Beam CT scan

The structures under study must be in the centre of the exposure field:

- study of the two dental arches: visualization of the two arches, including most of the maxillary sinuses and lower border of the mandible;
- study of the upper dental arch: visualization of the arch, the maxillary sinuses and the incisal margin of the upper teeth;
- study of the mandible: the visualization of the arch must include the incisal margin of the lower teeth and the lower border of the mandible.

As in all procedures, the acquisition of an X-ray also has its operational sequence, which is detailed below.

- **Patient preparation.** Identify the patient, inform them on the radiation risk and have them sign the informed consent; in the case of women of child-bearing age, rule out the possibility of an ongoing pregnancy.
- **Choice of protocol.** Cone Beam CT scans generally feature wide variability in terms of study protocols, exposure parameters (kV, mA), overall duration of pulsed exposure, field of view (FOV) volume and, consequently, radiation dose range as well. In order to determine the extent of the study on the frontal plane as well as on the sagittal plane, laser or placement joysticks must be used.
- **Post processing and visualization output.** One ought to consider that image quality is affected by a whole range of parameters: acquisition and reconstruction parameters, representation and visualization methods, etc. Image definition will depend on the sum of spatial resolution, contrast resolution, temporal resolution, artefacts, noise and the degree of definition.

  For each image it is important to consider the signal-to-noise ratio. Signal is the positive component, the one that actually forms an image of optimal quality corresponding to the acquired volumes. Noise is the component that deteriorates image quality. Its presence is a consequence of the various steps in the chain of events leading to the image production, which involve the various electromechanical components of the equipment. Each component affects the representation of the data of the Cone Beam CT equipment with a certain degree of approximation. As everyone knows, even the best computer processors on the market, however exceptional, always have a margin of error. This means that noise is partly due to the computer calculation errors.
- **Interactive cross visualization.** Image processing software produces a visualization where the display is divided into several quadrants, generally four. The first quadrant displays axial images. By scrolling the mouse wheel, a reference axial image must be selected in which bone and tooth roots are most visible.
- **MPR (Multiplanar Reconstruction).** It is possible to save a multiplanar navigation and 3D processed image, particularly useful in the study of the relationships of the mandibular canal. The reference axial image is shown in the examination display window, starting from which a sagittal image of the area of interest (e.g. right or left side of the arch), a section of interest represented on the coronal plane and a Volume Rendering (VR) of the entire arch are then obtained. At the end of processing, images can be exported in DICOM format (Digital Imaging and Communications in Medicine) (Box 2.1).

BOX 2.1 **FOCUS**

DICOM standard

The DICOM format (Digital Imaging and Communications in Medicine) is a standard, i.e., a set of rules, for transmission between different devices (capture machines, computers, printers, digital archives, etc.) of digital data, such as biomedical images, and medical-health information, by defining a communication protocol and making use of standard networking technologies and protocols.
DICOM files can be exchanged between two entities that possess the ability to receive the information (patient images and data) in the DICOM format. The DICOM format is public, i.e. the definition of the standard is publicly accessible. In essence, a DICOM file can be seen as a container. This standard does not introduce any new image format (such as jpeg, gif). Essentially, a DICOM file consists of a header, made up of a set of attributes containing various types of information, and a body of data suitable to contain one or more images. DICOM elements are classified as:

- mandatory (M): data that must be present;
- conditional (C): data that must be present under certain conditions;
- user-defined (U): they may be present or not.

The commands are all codified with group 0000.
The DICOM standard considers an image as an object formed by a set of attributes: width, height, colour, each with its own code and value.
The images are arranged as tree structures, in which an object contains other objects, and they are archived according to a clearly defined hierarchy. Each patient may have several studies and each set may have several images. Each level of this hierarchy is defined by an UID (Unique IDentifier).
Image information is contained in group 0028. The tag 0028.0101 defines the number of bits allocated for each pixel, hence the available grey tones. The pixel data are found in tag 7FE0,0010, which makes up approximately 95% of the DICOM file size.
If one considers a typical image of 512 * 512 pixel, with 12 bit per pixel, each image occupies 512 * 512 * 2 = 524288 byte. Each study includes several images, hence the usage space may commit volumes of up to 200 MB for each patient.
In order to make image management easier, the DICOM standard supports the main image compression algorithms, which take data from tag 07FE,0010 and compact them in shorter forms. The compression algorithms are divided into two categories:

- lossless or reversible;
- lossy or irreversible.

The use of compression algorithms may generate artefacts or blurs. The choice of the compression algorithm depends on:

- purpose of the images;
- storage;
- available bandwidth.

In the use of lossy algorithms, the following factors are used:

$$\mathbf{Rcomp = Original\ Data\ Size/Compressed\ Data\ Size < 10}$$

Grey levels

The number of grey levels depends on the available number of bits in the DICOM file (e.g. 10 bit correspond to 210 different grey tones), which therefore determine the depth of the image. Formats such as jpg and bmp only support 256 tones of grey.

Data processing

After acquiring the CT scan, some basic processing and measurements on the data may be carried out with the software provided by the manufacturer.

Manufacturers of Cone Beam CT devices offer the option, through their software, to convert their proprietary formats into an exportable DICOM file and this is already a first step in the management of 3D information.

When the services of an imaging and radiology center are used for the Cone Beam CT scan, a CD-ROM containing the DICOM file is provided to the patient or physician. Indeed, the Cone Beam CT software allows to export images in DICOM format.

Usually, the manufacturer's software also includes the tools for visualization, landmarking (establishment of reference points), measurement, recording, superposition, and reformatting of raw data into 3D rendered images (Volume Rendering).

A 3D image consists of a stack of 2D images or slices. Just as a 2D image consists of pixels, a 3D image consists of voxels.

Many threshold filters can be applied to the same image to distinguish between different types of tissue, for instance between hard and soft tissues.

Furthermore, cutting tools are also available: they allow specific regions of interest to be isolated and visualized. The 3D image in Volume Rendering is the result of a threshold value entered by the user.

Measurements

In conventional, two-dimensional X-rays, measurements are made between points of reference, which may consist of:

- an inflection point in a curved line;
- the geometric centre of a structure;
- the superposition of the projections of different structures;
- the tip of a structure;
- the crossing point of two planes.

In rendered 3D images, the same measurements are quite difficult for a number of reasons, such as the difficulty in locating reference points on a curved surface in a 3D image. Secondly, one must always bear in mind that the rendered 3D image depends on many factors, including image contrast, movement during acquisition, the presence of metal that creates noise, the signal/noise ratio and the threshold filters applied by the operator. Owing to all these factors, it makes sense that the points of reference are in the stack of 2D slices rather than in the 3D image.

Segmentation

The Cone Beam CT image segmentation process is an essential step in 3D model generation, in diagnosis and in the definition of the patient treatment plan. The process requires the separation of bone and/or soft structures, as well as the separation of maxilla and mandible.

Segmentation allows the operator to export and import 3D models from/into the software interface. For example, it makes it possible to combine digital models obtained via laser or optical scanners, with the CT data and rendering of soft tissues, obtained through 3D cameras.

These multimodal images are the foundation of digital dentistry, rapid prototyping, computer-assisted design and computer-assisted manufacturing applications.

Once the DICOM package originating from the CT scan has been imported into the software interface, one needs to identify and outline the anatomical structures of interest. The various software programs provide manual, partially automated and fully automated segmentation methods. Fully automated segmentation is preferable for routine clinical use, because it only requires limited interaction with the user and is carried out very rapidly.

A simple way to segment bone structures is by thresholding, which classifies a voxel (volume element in 3D images) according to its intensity in the grey scale.

An intensity interval is described by an upper and lower threshold value. Each voxel belongs to the selected class (bone, for instance) if and only if the intensity level is within the specified range. The appropriate value range must be selected for each patient, because bone density varies between patients and bone strength values may vary in different devices.

Thresholding, hence segmentation, is affected by density artefacts (values very close to the threshold cause "holes" in the condyles and areas with thin cortical bone, for example at the level of the internal branch of the mandible and most of the upper jaw) and metal artefacts (orthodontic appliances, fillings, implants, prostheses with values falling within the threshold range of voxels, causing "star-like" images).

The presence of artefacts entails long and trying manual post-processing work in order to be removed, leading to long processing times.

Visualization

Once segmentation has been carried out, there are two visualization methods in cranio-maxillofacial (CMF) planning software:

- surface-based methods;
- volume-based methods.

The former have the advantage of great sharpness in shading of the facial surfaces and the option to import 3D elements (for example, implants) into the anatomical view, if they originate from triangular mesh processing. Surface-based visualization methods, in fact, mandatorily require the generation of an intermediate surface image with a characteristic triangular mesh.

Volume-based visualization methods are less used in common planning software, because they are limited by the difficulty in establishing boundaries between tissues and assigning the appropriate colour/transparency values in order to achieve the desired visualization.

The advantage of the latter visualization methods lies in the efficient detail and direct visualization of volumetric operations, in 3D as well as directly, on cross sectional reconstructions.

Ultra definition in Cone Beam radiography

CBCT images contain much more information than we can usually see through visualization software. The result we see mainly depends on the range of grey-scale information that video cards and monitors are capable of displaying. If we expand the range by programming our CBCT machines, and have the appropriate software, we will be able to filter the image, reduce noise and focus the results on meeting our diagnostic and planning objectives (📷 2.5-2.11).

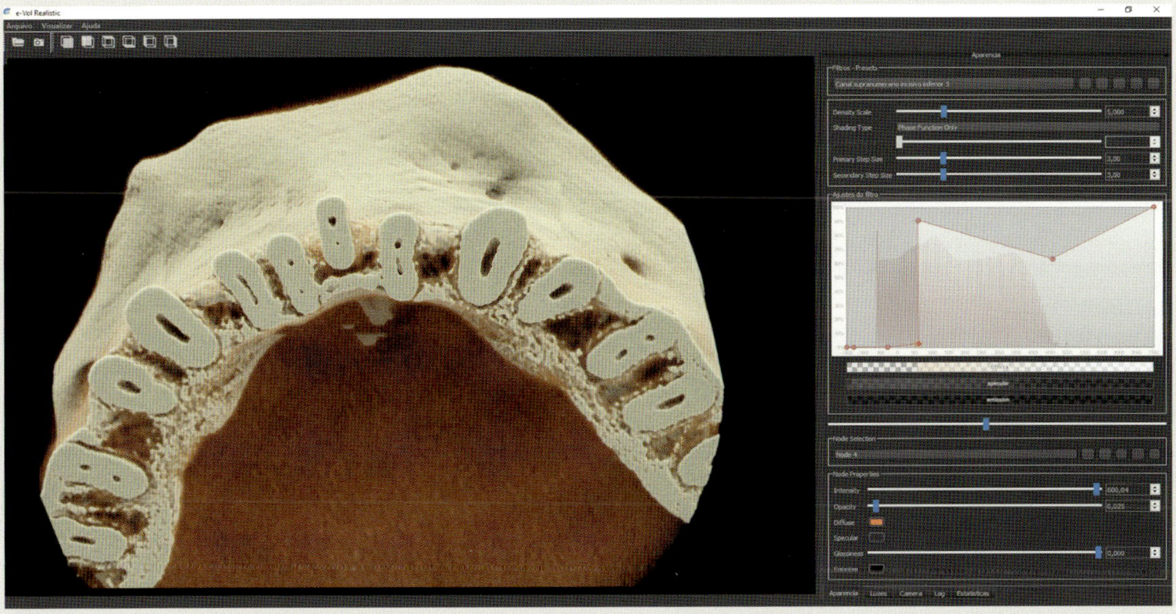

2.5 An UHD (Ultra High Definition) image allows to "magnify" the image without losing quality. Filters enable to focus on what is important, which they make visible in a wholly customized manner, using the optimized rendering technology. (Credits: courtesy of Dr. Mike Bueno, Evol-DX software by CDT.)

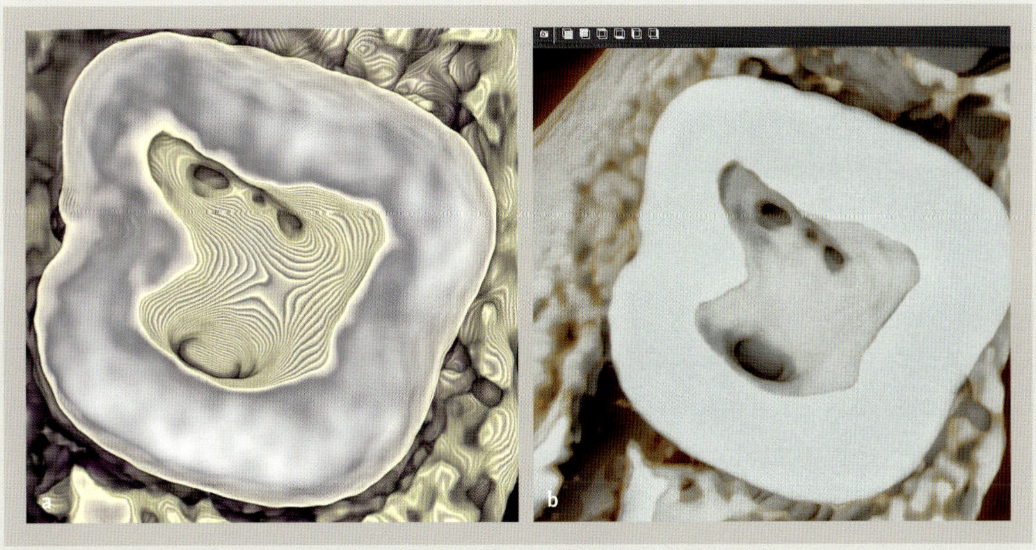

2.6 **a,b)** It is possible to select the colours of a complete 3D image and process it from different angles. In this image, bone and root structure can be observed for a precise analysis. (Credits: courtesy of Dr. Mike Bueno, Evol-DX software by CDT.)

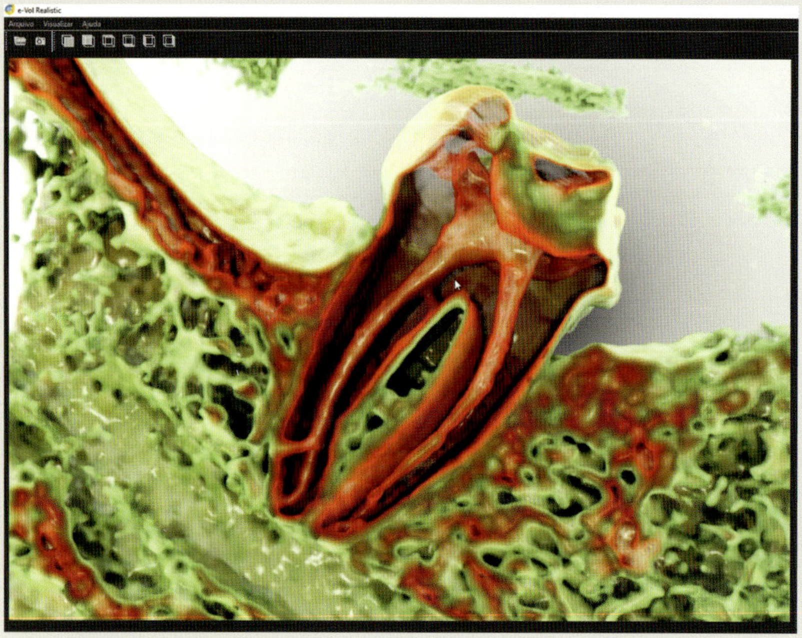

2.7 By applying colour filters, vascular structures may be highlighted. In this image, for example, the colour rendering of a slice with focus on endodontics can be observed. (Credits: courtesy of Dr. Mike Bueno, Evol-DX software by CDT.)

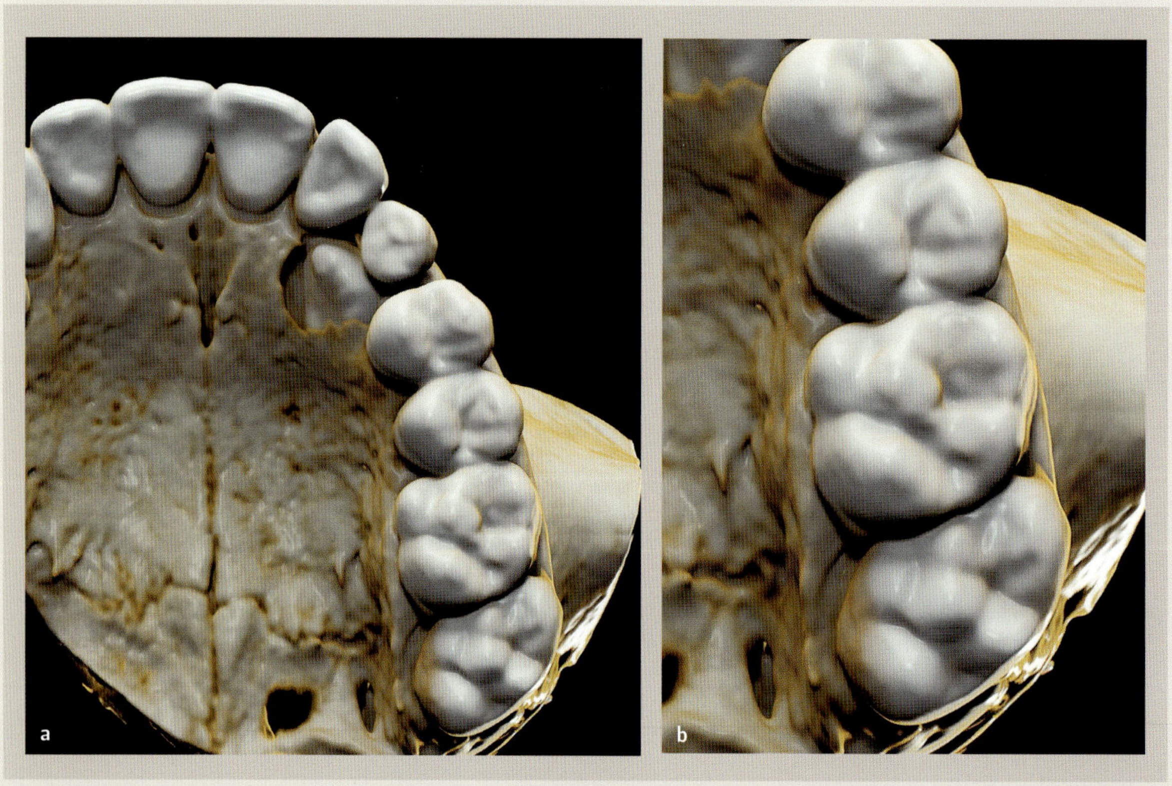

2.8 **a,b)** The photorealistic filter can turn the CBCT image into a realistic model, in which the bone and teeth can be seen in the most accurate possible colour. This application may also provide a detailed 3D picture of edentulous patients, in whom it is difficult to achieve a perfect intraoral scan due to the lack of references (teeth or occlusion surfaces) and in whom it is not easy to obtain an accurate image size, because intraoral scanners cause distortions if not taken with a high-performance brand/model and post-processed with the proper technology. (Credits: courtesy of Dr. Mike Bueno, Evol-DX software by CDT.)

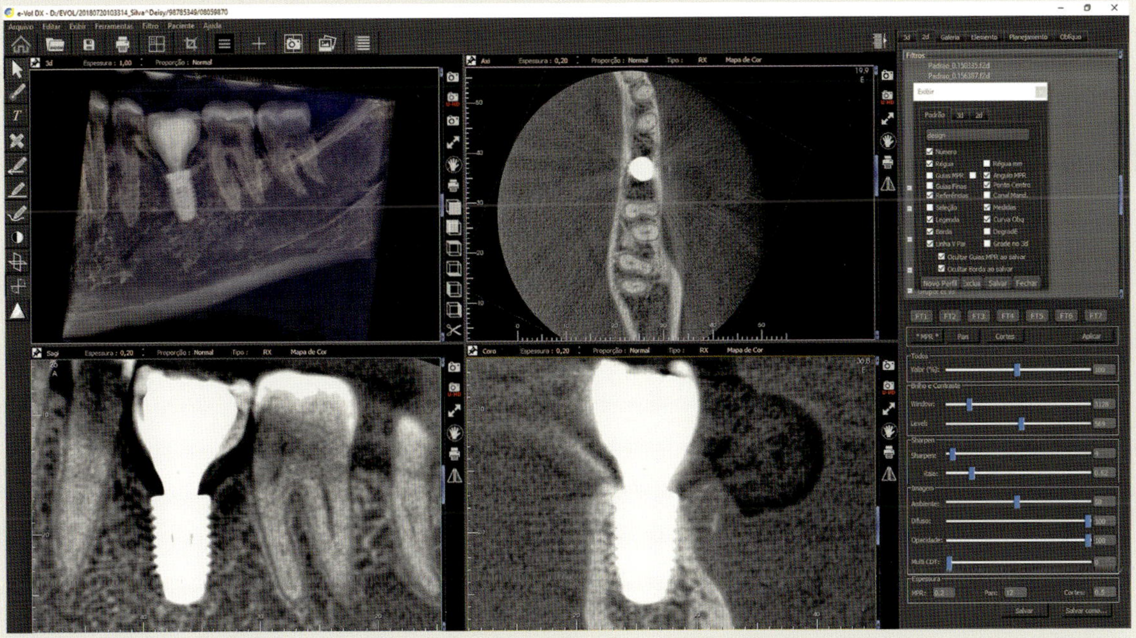

2.9 An average image with excessively radio-opaque implant processing in implantology. (Credits: courtesy of Dr. Mike Bueno, Evol-DX software by CDT.)

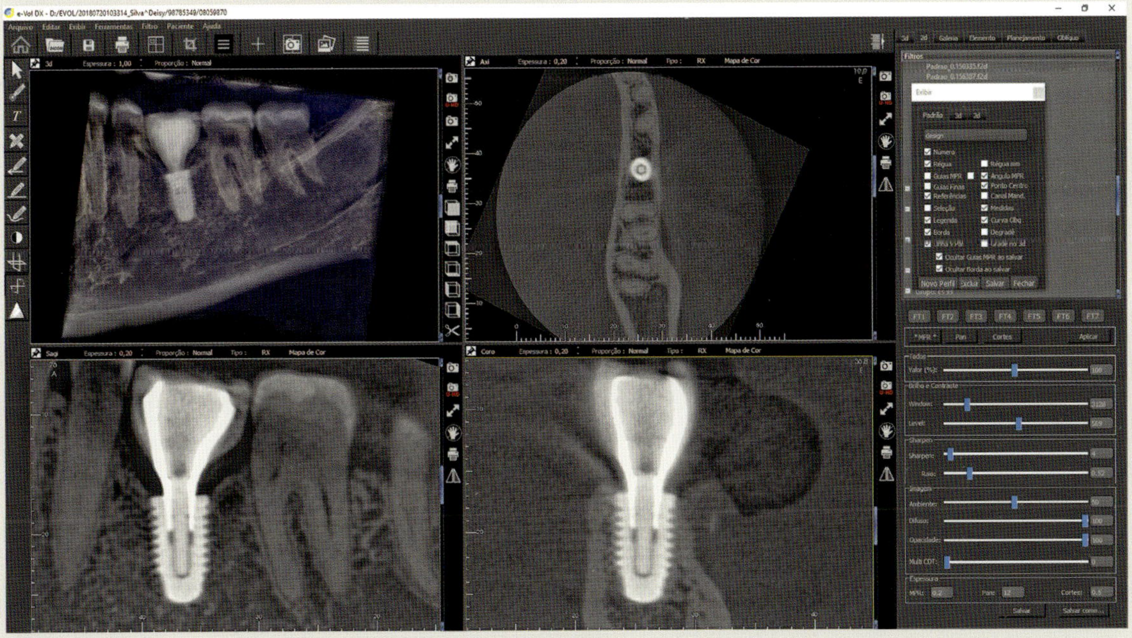

2.10 The same image as in Fig. 2.9, but with the appropriate filters, which make it possible to check all the details of its integration, as well as adaptation of the components, proper visualization of whites and blacks adapted to the purpose of the investigation. (Credits: courtesy of Dr. Mike Bueno, Evol-DX software by CDT.)

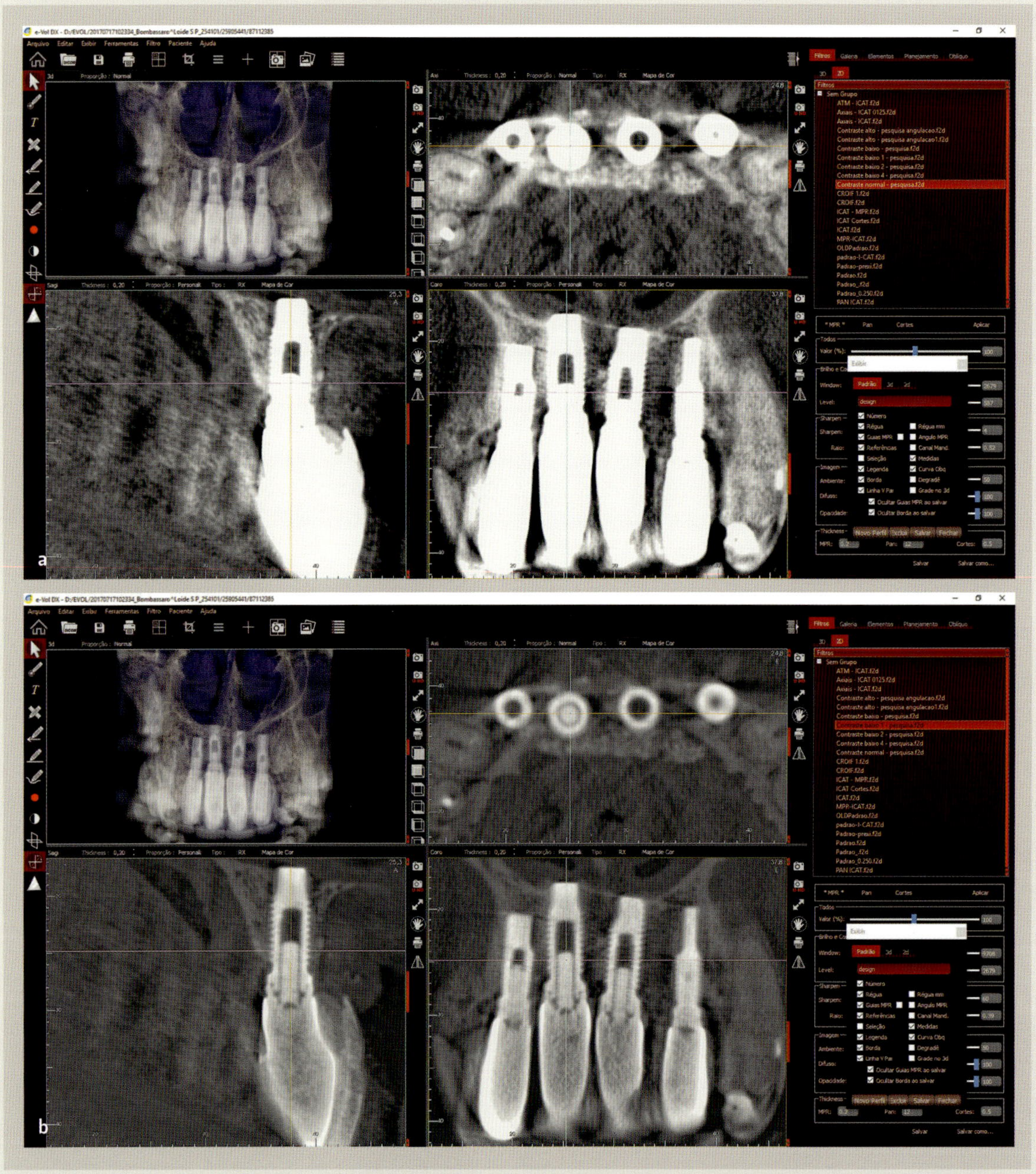

2.11 a,b) A still from a 3D video showing that we can also manipulate in 3D all the images with applied filters, which is a huge leap forward for diagnosis and planning, since we are able to filter and "clean" the DICOM file before combining it with an intraoral scan for greater accuracy in size. Many scientific papers have reported different measurements when unfiltered CBCT images were used: scattering and metal noise may lead to inaccurate measurements by the operator, and many article reviews have been carried out using this technology to "correct" the final values and to further reduce final errors. (Credits: courtesy of Dr. Mike Bueno, Evol-DX software by CDT.)

Appendix

In cases of total or partial edentulism with a lack of sufficient dental elements to be used as reference points, especially in the posterior region, matching up the cone beam examination and the optical impression can be challenging.

For this reason, we use adhesive radiopaque marks (2.12).

Before the radiographic examination, a sufficient quantity of marks are fixed on the adherent mucosa and balanced between the intraoral regions, ensuring they are applied in a stable area free from movement (2.13). The examination must be immediately followed in the same session by the optical impression (2.14 a,b). After the quality of the two exams has been verified (2.15) the marks can be removed.

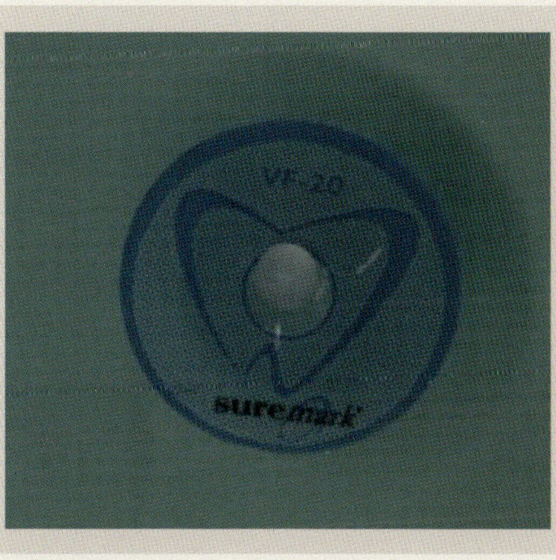

2.12 Adhesive radiopaque mark.

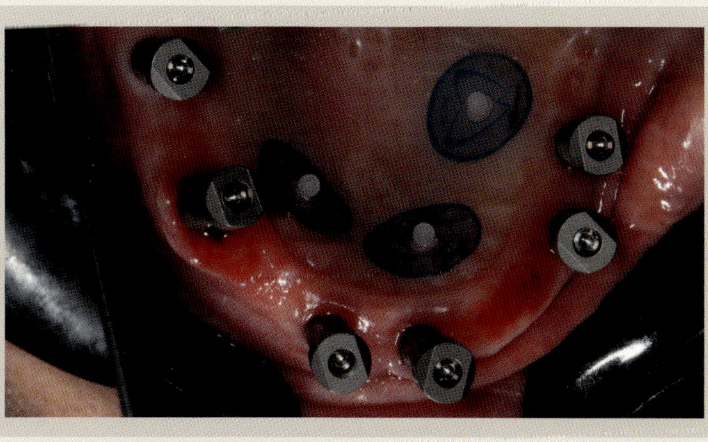

2.13 The marks applied in the mouth; they can also be used during the optical impression for the construction of the prosthesis.

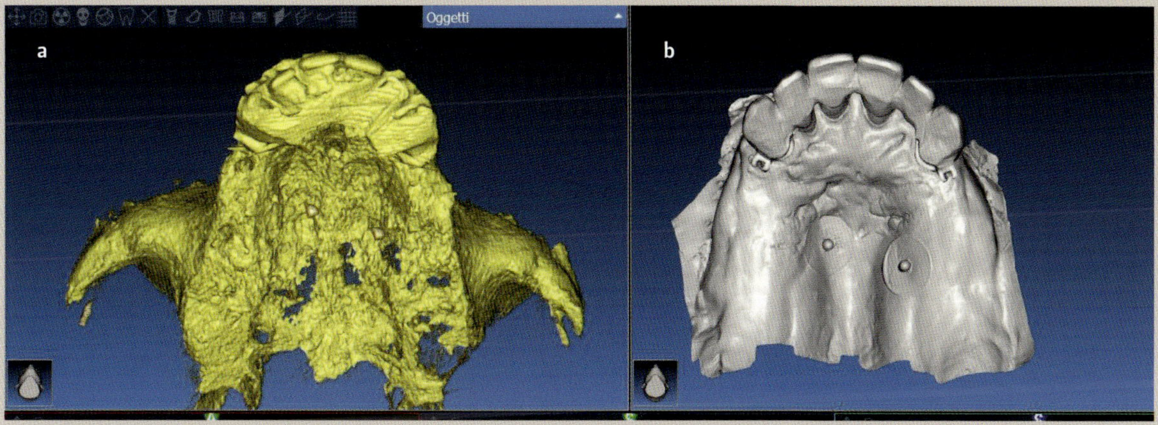

2.14 a,b) The marks are visible both in the cone-beam (a) and in the optical impression (b).

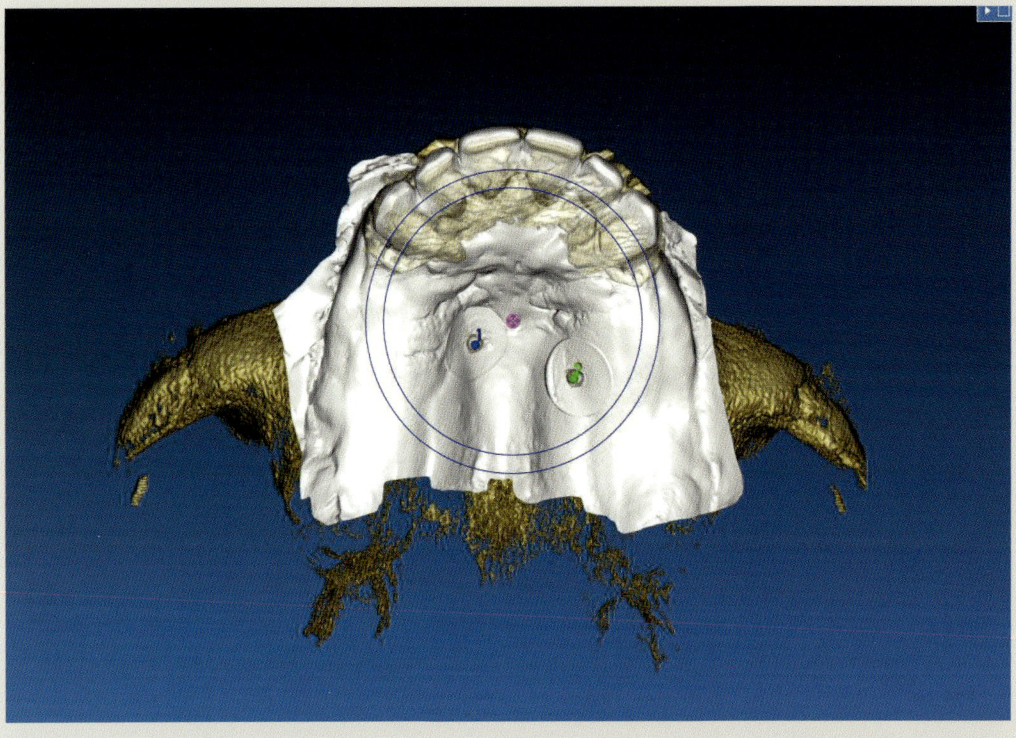

2.15 The Matching up the two files.

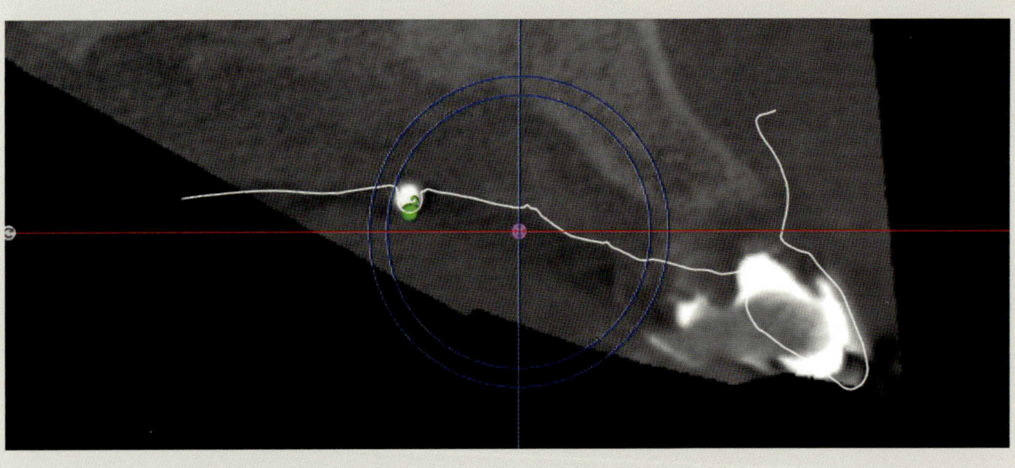

2.16 Verification of the accuracy.

REFERENCES

1. CASALINI ED. La tomografia computerizzata a tecnologia Cone Beam nell'imaging radiologico 3D. Implant Tribune Sept. 2007.
2. DUBRUL EL, SICHER H. Sicher and DuBrul's Oral anatomy. 8th ed. Ishiyaku EuroAmerica 1988; 257-68.

Digital instruments and techniques in implant surgery and CAD-CAM implant prosthodontics

Andrea Baruffaldi

CAD-CAM is the acronym of Computer Aided Design-Computer Aided Manufacturing; with this type of systems, design and manufacturing are assisted by computer. Over the last forty years, CAD-CAM has revolutionised the world of industry and that of medicine, by shortening processing time frames and improving quality performance.

The first uses of this technology, which has influenced industrial production procedures so much, date back to the early 1960s, with the introduction of the first graphic interface that made use of a tablet and light pen.

CAD-CAM was boosted and supported by automotive and aerospace companies, large groups that immediately understood the advantages brought by CAD-CAM in terms of automation. Since then, the use in the medical and dental sector has required approximately twenty years to start being competitive on the market and effective in terms of results.

The first application of CAD-CAM technology in the dental field was conceived by Francois Duret in the 1970s. In the following ten years, this technology and its application in dentistry were extensively researched, leading to the development of the first specific systems.

The very first was CEREC®, developed by Mörmann and Brandestini from the University of Zurich, in 1981. Four years later, in the same University, the first inlay was produced with this system and cemented.[1]

At the same time, a CAD-CAM system was also being developed in Sweden: the first titanium crown was produced in 1983, thanks to the work of two Swedish researchers. Over the years, the development of other laboratory CAD-CAM systems has considerably stepped up, as a consequence of the significant improvement in the performance of computers as well as application software. However, this new work method has really been taking hold in the dental sector only in recent years.

The CAD-CAM technology has been developed with the aim of designing and producing prosthetic structures with consistent quality features. Indeed, CAD-CAM makes it possible to use codified procedures that follow protocols, are controllable and above all repeatable.

CAD-CAM methods applied to dentistry are, from a technological point of view, the state-of-the-art of the tools currently available to technicians, to provide the clinician with prosthetic items of excellent quality. More than twenty-five years have elapsed since the first studies on CAD-CAM dental applications, and the progress made in modern scanning techniques have raised the level of applicability of this method. As a matter of fact, the current laser and optical technologies provide reliable data that, jointly with ever more sophisticated software, result in precise and accurate milling paths.

CAD-CAM technology has been able to establish itself as a valid alternative to conventional ceramic and metal-ceramic restoration methods, especially with the evolution of metal-free solutions. CAD-CAM machining ensures high quality products by using zirconium oxide, bio-titanium, cobalt-chrome and synthetic materials. These materials are biologically compatible and can easily be veneered.[2]

The machine is not taking the place of the professional, specifically the dental technician, but it is at the service of the professional, in order to increase their productivity, precision and manufacturing possibilities.

Operational features

With regard to the actual operational stage, the operator plans and models the prosthetic design with the computer, which will then be fabricated by machines guided by the same computer. The computer virtual world is accessed via a 3D scanner; indeed, the scanner reads the dental arches directly from the patient or from the model obtained from the impression provided by the dentist. After reading, the computer software processes the data and shows a version of the model on which the desired structure can be created, with appropriate software instruments (📷 3.1).

A file is obtained at the end of this step, containing the data to be sent to the machine tool (CAM), which can then machine the chosen material. After CAD-CAM machining is completed, the structure is delivered for try-in in the patient's mouth.

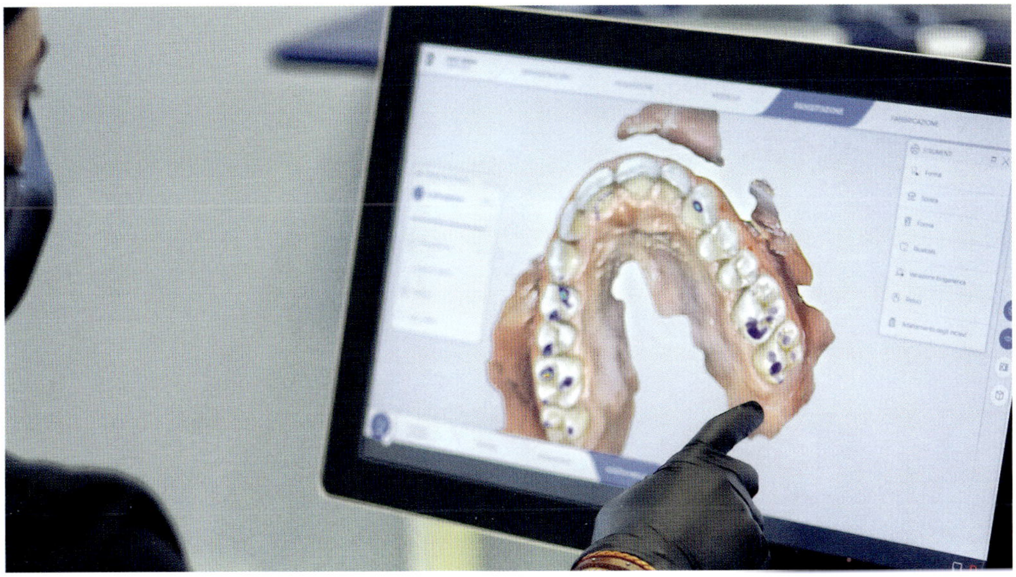

3.1 Thanks to intraoral scanning systems, a virtual model is immediately available.

The possibilities offered by this system include designing directly on a computer, then letting the computer itself translate the design into commands to be given to another machine, to fabricate the design either in part or completely.

The CAD-CAM technology features a number of advantages compared to conventional techniques.

The first advantage is certainly **precision**: a design made on the computer is more accurate than that made with manual systems; the clinician is able to zoom in on the design, to examine and fine tune the details.[3]

Rapidity should be taken into consideration: digital scanning has the potential of being faster than conventional impressions, because gypsum models, use of wax and traditional casts are limited. With the intraoral scanners of the leading manufacturers, impressions of half an arch require 40 seconds, while the full arch impression only takes two minutes. CAD-CAM makes both design and fabrication faster. Complete machining of a crown only takes a few minutes of milling (between 4 and 7 minutes).

Secondly, there is **reproducibility**: a design that has been digitized can be reproduced exactly at any time, not as a copy, which might be subject to degradation, but as an identical item to the previous one, because it derives from the same matrix. This also means being able to retouch or partly modify, with no need to entirely redesign the item.

And again, one should not overlook the extremely important advantage of having a 3D simulation that makes it possible to view, not in one's hands but on a screen, the three-dimensional image of the object one is designing, in order to be able to assess it from every angle.

CAD-CAM technology is able not only to create restorations by milling, but enables accurate quality control of dental devices, designing optimal shapes based on the features of the CAD material, preventing degradations, such as deformations that may occur with conventional techniques and finally, providing designs that can be reproduced an endless number of times.[4]

Furthermore, CAD-CAM restorations have a natural appearance, because porcelain blocks are available with varying degrees of translucency that mimic enamel and are available in a wide range of shades.

The time and work savings potentially reduce costs, and the promise of speed and quality may be attractive for patients.

There are a number of CAD-CAM systems available for dentistry today and some of them are especially reliable in terms of simplicity of use and, above all, accuracy of the results. In general, the procedure entails the steps seen above: scanning, design, milling, sintering and veneering, with a commercial diversification proposed by the manufacturing companies, which varies from complete management of the whole process by the laboratory, up to the one where the whole process is commissioned to specialized centres.

Scanning systems make it possible to automatically detect an unknown surface, thereby speeding up the acquisition process of the point coordinates, which as a whole describe a three-dimensional object (3.2).

These scanning systems can be classified into two main families:

- contact systems;
- non-contact systems.

Contact scanning systems were developed to meet industrial needs whereby, based on a master, the male and female parts of a mould needed to be obtained. They have started being used for other applications too only recently, thanks to the evolution of CAD systems.

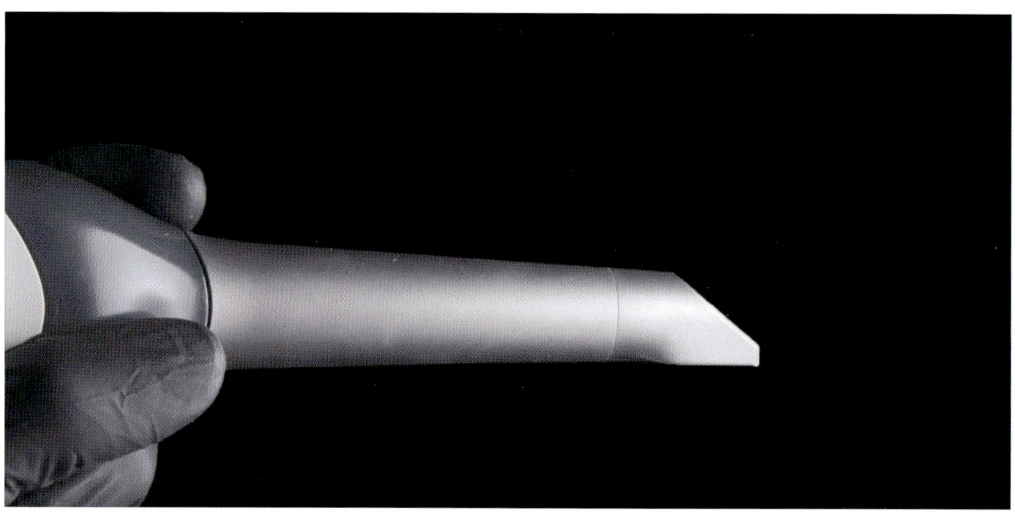

3.2 Scanning systems are continuously evolving.

They use an analogue probe of known diameter which, by moving on the surface of the part, acquires its points based on its deflection. Compared to non-contact systems, they feature certain advantages:

- no treatments are required on the surface of the part in order to prevent reflection;
- it is possible to scan vertical surfaces;
- the density of data is not fixed, but it varies according to the complexity of the surface;
- better precision and repeatability.

On the other hand, scanning time is longer and the application of a force on the surface may damage the object in the case of delicate materials (e.g. wax) or alter the detection, in the case of flexible materials (e.g. elastomers). They are portable devices and consist of a contact sensor, to be installed on the spindle of a numerical control milling machine or on the head of a measuring machine, and of a management software, which communicates automatically with the control unit of the machine. The tolerances and repeatability are less than 0.01 mm and the applied forces range from 100 to 300 g.

Non-contact scanning systems were developed specifically as an aid to design activities and make it possible to take points on the surfaces of the object without the need for physical contact; this advantage is combined with a higher scanning speed compared to contact systems. Precision and repeatability have considerably improved in recent years, to the point of differences being in the order of a handful of microns.

The principles applied in the development of scanning systems are as follows (Box 3.1):

- laser triangulation;
- moiré interferometry;
- photogrammetry;
- conoscopic holography;
- optical scanner;
- tcomputed tomography.

In the field of dentistry, among the various scanner technologies that have just been examined, the ones that are most commonly used in clinical practice are contact scanning systems and non-contact scanning systems, through the use of a laser light or an optical scanner. Whatever the system used for the surface survey stage, the result is a point cloud that is transferred to the CAD-CAM computer application, which may or may not be built into the scanning system. According to the need, the point cloud can be used to:

- generate the STL file for prototyping the copied component;
- establish the tool path for a numerical control machine;
- generate the three-dimensional mathematical model.

BOX 3.1

PRINCIPLES APPLIED IN THE DEVELOPMENT OF SCANNING SYSTEMS

Systems based on laser triangulation

In systems based on laser triangulation, the operating principle consists in reading the laser beam reflected by two sensors located on the sides of the laser emitter. These systems consist of a laser emitter, whose laser beam is turned by appropriate optics into a few tenths of a millimetre thick line; in addition, one or two cameras with solid state CCD sensor detect the position of the beam on the object.

The surfaces of the object to be replicated must ensure reflection of the laser beam; in some cases, treatment with opacifier sprays must be performed. A number of options are available on the market, which essentially differ by the dimensions of the working field, by precision and by installation type.

Systems based on moiré interferometry

In systems based on moiré interferometry, the operating principles exploits the mechanical interference of light that is generated when two angularly mismatched lattices made up of equally spaced light-dark lines are superposed. The so-called moiré fringes occur, whose property is to lay on surfaces and which allow, through sophisticated image processing, to determine the coordinates of the points on said surface. The advantage compared to laser scanning consists in the higher model digitization speed, since the entire visual field of the camera is available for processing.

Photogrammetry-based systems

Photogrammetry-based systems are extremely powerful optical techniques for three-dimensional image processing; the scenes or objects to be measured are recorded and analyzed in three dimensions. They are based on optical triangulation: photogrammetry uses the stereoscopic images obtained with different camera positions.

The sensor can cover measurement volumes ranging from a few square millimetres to a few square metres. System configurations with multiple-field sensors or colour cameras enable adaptive data acquisition in addition to the combination of 3D digitization with colour image processing.

Calibration devices and user-friendly software have been developed for integration on coordinate measuring machines and milling machines, which enable fast and reliable adaptation of the sensor coordinate systems with respect to the positioning system.

In the case of free sensors, adaptation and combination of partial views are achieved thanks to reference elements (typically integrating spheres) and measuring the position of the reference points with other types of metrology is not necessary.

Conoscopic holography-based systems

In conoscopic holography-based systems, the scanning system was initially applied as an instrument to measure dimensions, with high precision, for variable distances from 0.04 µm to several metres. Subsequently, some modules have been developed that allow the conoscopic method to be used in a wide range of industrial applications, including "reverse engineering". The key benefit of conoscopic holography is the independence from a coherent light source; this property exceeds the practical constraints of stability and sensitivity affecting conventional laser interferometric instruments. A further advantage is that these optical systems are intrinsically collinear, meaning relative immunity to mechanical vibrations, optical noise and temperature fluctuations. The physical basis is the optical interference produced by birefringent crystals, illuminated by converging rays of polarized light. An incoherent monochromatic point-like light beam strikes a uniaxial (birefringent) crystal; within that, the ray is split into two separate rays (ordinary and extraordinary), which propagate at different speeds along identical geometric paths. The two rays feature separate wave fronts, which emerge from the crystal with different polarization and phase angles. These magnitudes are determined by the angle of incidence of the individual ray with respect to the crystal. The use of polarizing filters enables alignment of the directions of the electrical components of the rays, which are subsequently split and recombined to generate an interference fringe on output. As in classic interferometry, the spacing of the fringes is proportional to the distance from the reflection point.

Optical scanner

The optical scanner is also referred to as the internal geometry capture system: indeed, jointly with tomography, it allows to survey the internal parts of the physical model. Therefore, the system performs simultaneous scanning of the internal and external surface of the object. Compared to tomographs, it is more precise in terms of dimensional tolerances.

Computed tomography

As seen previously, in computed tomography, a rotating device projects an X-ray through the object and detects its structure through a sequence of parallel planes, which also contain the internal geometry of the solid. On output, the result is a set of greyscale images, which represent the various sections taken. A three-dimensional mathematical model can be traced through specific software suites. In view of the high investment costs required, CT is especially used in the medical sector, as a diagnostic tool and to plan surgical procedures.[5]

The actual three-dimensional model is achieved through a process consisting of the following steps:

- filtering the point cloud to eliminate redundant information;
- recognition of edges, curves and surfaces by means of primitive extraction algorithms. The primitives used normally belong to the typical database of solid modelling systems;
- check and any modification of the generated solid, paying special attention to the connection areas between the various surfaces.

Currently, all scanning systems provide an ordered point cloud already processed and filtered by the software supplied with the machine. Once the 3D virtual model has been defined, it is possible to export to other CAD-CAM systems or rapid prototyping machines.[6] The virtual 3D model thus obtained can also be modified or used as a basis for designing and fabricating other structures directly in the CAD environment.

This, in a nutshell, is what happens in the dental sector; specific software receives information from the device that scanned the model, processes it and provides a virtual 3D rendering. The technician will fabricate the desired structure starting from this condition, and by using the appropriate instruments provided by the software suite. This is the most critical stage of reverse engineering, since, unlike the digitization or scanning stage, it entails a greater commitment of resources in terms of time and actual human skills - intellectual, professional, creative, as well as manual skills. The whole creative process is managed with clicks of the mouse, but as is the case when using other software applications such as CAD, photo editing or pictorial graphic design, also in this case the use of a graphics tablet may be useful and more convenient.

In 3D computer graphics, files can be saved in different formats. Often, when certain applications are used, the resulting file is a specific, proprietary file, which can only be managed through that specific software program (for example, the .3dm file of RHINOCEROS or the .max file of 3D STUDIO MAX). However, there are also standard formats, such as the STL format, the IGES format (Initial Graphics Exchange Specification), the STEP format (Standard Exchange Product Model Data) and the DXF format (Drawing Exchange Format), developed by Autodesk as a solution to exchange data between the AutoCAD program and other programs. In the field of dentistry, the software used as interface between the real and virtual worlds is able to generate all the types of file formats mentioned above: it all depends on the type of system in use and on the commercial policy adopted by the company that offers that specific system.

Therefore, in the field of CAD-CAM systems aimed at the dental market, one may identify two opposite commercial trends, which lead to the definition of two types of systems: closed ones and open ones.

In the former case, the software used generates a file in a proprietary format, which can only be read and used by the type of system it was created with. On the contrary, in the latter case, the software generates a file in standard format, which can be read by various 3D software applications and can be used with various pieces of CAM equipment. That is what happens if an open system is used, such as the one offered by 3 Shape Dental Designer – the software suite generates a file in standard format, named STL format.

STL is the acronym of Standard Triangulation Language. In computer science, it defines the file extension that is the current standard, accepted by nearly all rapid prototyping systems on the market. The STL file is a description of the object through the surfaces it consists of. In essence, the surfaces of the piece are translated into a set of triangular elements – the more one intends to approximate the surface, the higher the number of these triangles (3.3).

STL files are managed in CAD environment with the aid of more specific or less specific software (Box 3.2)

As mentioned before, the item can be fabricated by following entirely different methods. On one hand, the file can be sent to a numerical control milling machine, which machines the item starting from a suitable shape of raw material; on the other hand, the item can be fabricated according to the "Layer by Layer" prototype construction philosophy, which entails depositing the material in layers, until achieving the end result.

Based on this operating philosophy, in the industrial sector, a prototype can be made with a variety of prototyping techniques and with different materials.

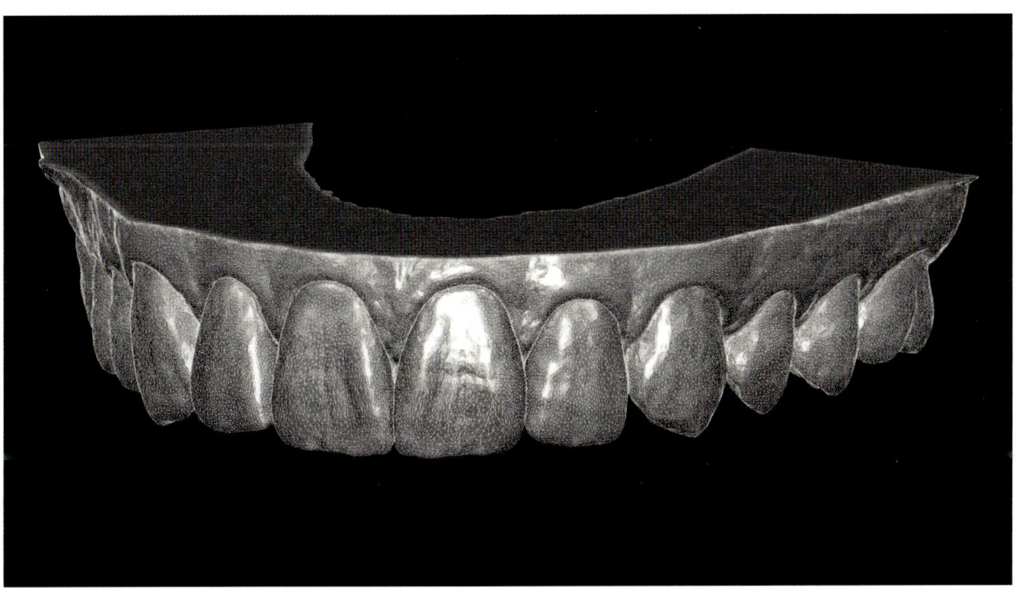

3.3 The higher the number of triangles, the greater the resolution of the STL file.

BOX 3.2

PROTOTYPING TECHNIQUES

STL file generation may take place in two different ways:

1. by means of the integral use of CAD software. In this case, the designer makes the mathematical model, only working in a CAD environment;
2. by means of re-engineering techniques. In this case, appropriate instruments scan the surface of the object, for which a CAD model is required. These acquire a given number of points belonging to the scanned surfaces - referred to as a "point cloud". The cloud is processed via CAD or specific software to obtain the three-dimensional mathematical model.

The first method is followed when an item is made from scratch, or when an existing product needs to be modified, and its mathematical model has already been acquired. The second method is indicated when a three-dimensional shape needs to be transferred into a CAD environment, thus creating its mathematical model. This is done via reverse engineering techniques, or when a 3D scanner is used in dentistry. The design of the end item to be fabricated will be created on the mathematical model thus obtained. The design will be carried out in the CAD environment, according to the first method described above. Also in this case, the result will be an STL file. The next step will consist in sending the STL file to the machine for the design to be finalized, and the item to be made from a three-dimensional point of view.

The main techniques are set out below:

- **SLA (StereoLitographic Apparatus)** Stereolithography was the first technique to be developed. It is based on polymerisation of a liquid by effect of a laser beam. In the first stage, the piece to be fabricated is placed on a workstation and supports are made, if required. The laser is focused on the worktop by means of optical systems and light cures the first section of the prototype. Subsequently, the top is lowered and the process continues by light-curing the next layer- To reduce processing times, the laser cures only the external contours of the surfaces and connects them with a honeycomb structure, so at the end of the fabrication stage, the piece must be exposed to UV rays, using special curing lights, for a time sufficient to achieve complete polymerisation.
- **PolyJET** The process is based on laying successive layers of liquid photopolymers sensitive to UV light. At the same time, two powerful UV lights cure - i.e. solidify - the layers. Once the photopolymer layer, which is a few microns thick, has been laid and exposed to UV radiation, the top is lowered as required and the procedure is repeated, until complete fabrication of the prototype.

- **Multi Jet Modeling (MJM)** This method is similar to how an ink jet printer works. The thermoplastic resin stored in the head is applied on the working table to form a slice. Subsequently, the table is lowered and the resin adheres to the previous slice (3.4).

- **Drop on Demand** This method is similar to MJM; the material of the model and that of the support are laid in sequence to form the first slice, then the next slice and so on, until completion of the prototype. The support material is removed in the post-processing stage.

- **Laser Sintering** Once called Selective Laser Sintering (SLS), laser sintering makes use of powders (thermoplastic, metal, silica) and uses laser to sinter the materials used to fabricate the prototype. A thin layer of powder is laid on a platform by means of specific equipment, which the laser sinters selectively. Then, the platform is lowered as required, another layer of powder is laid, and the process is repeated. The advantages of this technique are the use of various types of powders and the absence of supports, since the upper layers are supported by the non-sintered powder itself. At the end of the process, the prototype obtained must be cleaned up from the excess powder. If metal or ceramic powders have been used, a thermal treatment may be required, to improve their features.

- **Fused Deposition Modelling (FDM)** It is a technique that uses wires and bars of thermoplastic material, which are laid on a work surface by a head that moves along three axes. The production process is fully automated, as is the fabrication of any support structures. The finished prototype does not require further treatments.

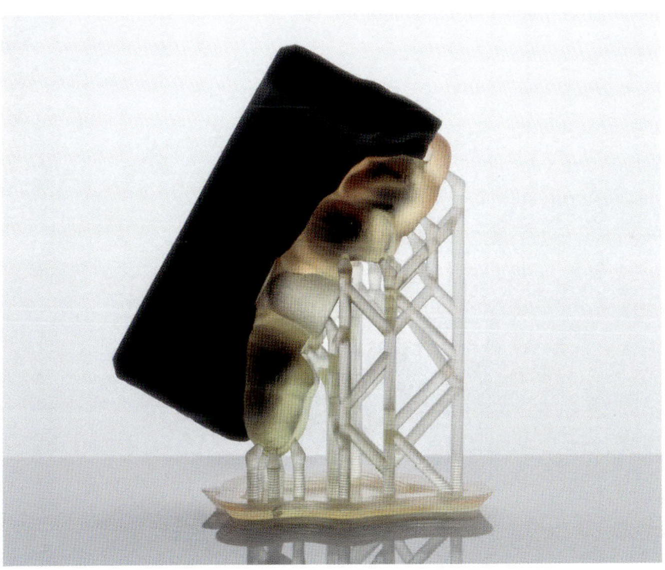

3.4 An example of 3D printed surgical stent.

- **Laminated Object Manufactoring (LOM)** Also called sheet lamination, the LOM technique uses special sheets of various materials, cut according to the size of the desired slice and then superposed and glued. The resulting prototype has an appearance reminiscent of plywood, therefore it must be finished with sandpaper, to remove excesses and prevent the risk of the layers peeling off. Furthermore, a waterproofing treatment is carried out, to prevent moisture absorption.
- **3D Printing** This method is similar to SLS – in this case, however, the powders are not sintered, but are held together thanks to an adhesive sprayed by a head, a bit like those of inkjet printers. The adhesive is dried quickly and the resulting prototype undergoes a heat treatment to improve its features.
- **Selective Laser Melting (SLM)** Very similar to SLS, this method differs in the use of wholly metal powders, that is, without the aid of low melt, so that an inert atmosphere is created in the working chamber. Furthermore, a powerful laser is used and in the end, a prototype is obtained that is wholly similar to serial production and does not require special surface finishes. The item may undergo conventional machining without any issues.
- **Electron Beam Melting (fusione da fascio elettronico)** Similar to the SLM technique, this method requires the creation of a vacuum in the work chamber, so as to allow the electron beam to properly focus on the work surface. This is in order to prevent the formation of metal oxides in the powders. The electron beam is able to melt high-melting metal powders such as titanium, concentrating a higher spot power than laser. A particular application of this technique is in the production of biomedical titanium prostheses, fabricated using highly biocompatible titanium powders.

In the field of dentistry, subtractive systems are used, as well as systems that work in the opposite way, i.e. additive systems.

- Blocks of zirconia or alumina, sintered or pre-sintered, are processed by *subtraction* by means of rotary systems consisting of dedicated numerical control milling machines. Titanium is also machined in the same way.
- On the contrary, products that use rapid prototyping or laser sintering systems are processed by *addition*.

Particular attention is paid here to laser sintering, which deserves further analysis, owing to the fact that this technology recently applied to the dental sector, offers additional potentials to the technician, as an alternative to metal structures obtained with traditional lost-wax casting or by electrodeposition. Laser sintering is a rapid prototyping technique that allows to fabricate an item using a metal powder, laid in successive layers and then sintered by a laser beam that reproduces, layer by layer, the sections obtained from the 3D CAD model.

The laser beam, controlled by specific software, is focused through an appropriate optical system on the surface of a powder bed.

The heat from laser sinters the powder, creating a solid body. This microthermal laser beam joins, by microfusion, perfectly spherical metal particles, having microscopic dimensions (from 0.5 to 20μ). Subsequently, the platform is lowered by the thickness of the layer; a powder distribution mechanism then covers the already sintered layer with another layer of molten powder, which is in its turn solidified and joined to the previous layer. All that takes place under a controlled atmosphere, preventing any form of oxidisation.[7]

This system prevents the phase transformations typical of casting (solid-liquid-solid) and all the typical micro-tensions when material must be removed by milling. The direct transition from powder to structure completely prevents any contamination (carbon, polluted burs, coatings); in addition to that, the possibility of always having new metal is a further guarantee for the patient.

The structure obtained by laser sintering ensures optimal retention for cement: in this regard, the inner surface of the crowns has been covered by a number of studies and analyses. This new technology makes it possible to fabricate even highly complex structures. The advantages of laser sintering may be summed up as follows:

- constant precision;
- use of ever new metal;
- computed design;
- absence of issues due to coatings and/or lost-wax casting procedures;
- no undesired casting residues;
- absence of porosity or imprecision.

Benefits and comfort for the patient in using the CAD-CAM technology

The absence of the discomfort caused by the conventional impression taking procedure, with a tray, is one of the main benefits linked to the use of the CAD-CAM technique. The advent of the optical impression, which does not require the use of opacifier powder, has completely eliminated the discomfort resulting from this procedure. What is more, virtual design of the prosthesis may involve the patient, who can see the design and proposed restoration in real time. The shorter time frames required by the CAM phase allow the patient to receive the finished prosthesis in few sessions, if not even in the same session.

Components of the CAD-CAM system

The main components are:

- CAD unit consisting of a PC, the software and a high definition 3D intraoral scanner;
- CAM unit consisting in a numerical control milling machine, directly connected to the design software or otherwise.[8]

Thanks to the intraoral camera, the graphic capture of the implant site or the tooth to be restored can be obtained in a matter of seconds. The acquired scan will be subsequently processed in the design stage.
By optimizing the shooting procedure, the intraoral scanner captures very sharp images, with an exceptional depth of field. Optical impression taking is guided by the "search mode" procedure, which is activated by a foot switch or one placed directly on the scanner handpiece. The image is captured in approximately 500 milliseconds and the quality of the scan can be evaluated before being stored.[9]

If required, the surface of the prepared area to be acquired with the scanner can be treated; this is because the different depths of preparation and the discrepancy in the quality of the surfaces may result in intensities that are too high to be detected by the sensor, to the point that the steepness of the walls is rendered as a black area; the cusps on the other hand, which reflect incident light in a mirror-like manner, tend to shine, generating an effect similar to that which occurs in the human retina when one looks directly at a light source. On the other hand, tooth enamel is translucent, so it absorbs at least partly the impression projected onto its surface. To eliminate these problems, a thin layer of titanium dioxide-based opacifier powder should be spread on the tooth surface and on the entire region to be shot.

Today, the evolution of intraoral scanners allows the scanning of the natural surfaces of teeth and gums without using any opacifier powders. The scanner just needs to be placed on the area of interest, and it starts capturing automatically. Doing away with the powder coating makes the scanning process easier to learn and more comfortable for the patient. The virtual 3D model in natural colours is generated by moving the camera at a maximum distance of 15 mm from the surface of the teeth, in a single scanning procedure. From a clinical point of view, it is possible to clearly distinguish the gingiva from the preparation margin. In the preliminary consultancy stage, it is possible to record videos to be shown directly to the patient. The realistic visualization and rendering of teeth and gums help convince the patient of the actual need for the treatment, so that they can assess and accept the therapeutic proposal in a more informed manner. The software renders the preparation model, design proposals and antagonists three-dimensionally. The preparation margin is highlighted with just a few clicks, and the software takes care of the rest, by automatically recognizing the type of work to be carried out and creating a design proposal.

The software shows a finished restoration, with adequate contact points at occlusal and proximal level. This is made possible by making use of several databases. In particular, if a bite registration was taken previously, the occlusal surface will be automatically adapted to the antagonist teeth.

At this stage, the operator is required to modify or perfect the virtual restoration. The possibility of designing freely in a "three-dimensional environment" makes the design operation simple and fun, yet precise. There are various options to modify and customize the design automatically created by the software, which are easy to understand and use. The so-called design "tools" are used (3.1), that is, a set of virtual instruments that enable to modify the restoration in the design stage, allowing the operator to view the image generated in real time (3.5).

3.1 Main design tools [10]

Zoom	To magnify the image of the restoration or individual details up to 20 times (20x).
Trim	To cut the item in order to separate it from the rest of the arch and be able to rotate it by 360°.
Finish line search	This takes place automatically, but it can be edited by the operator. This feature makes it possible to achieve a high level of marginal precision.
Contact points	The automatic thermographic analysis of contact points allows the contact points to be highlighted directly on the screen at the level of the proximal and occlusal surfaces. It also makes it possible to highlight the extent of the contacts directly on the screen, through a colour scheme: · Green: 0–50 µm, optimal contact; · Yellow: 50-100 µm, minimal reduction of contacts is required; · Red: contact greater than 100 µm, significant reduction of contacts is required.
Edit	To edit all design lines.
Form	To increase or decrease the occlusal or proximal contact area.
Drop	It enables three-dimensional modelling of ceramic, immediately displaying the result of the operation on the screen.
Shape	To modify the occlusal surface.
Position	To change the height and angle of the restoration.
Rotate	To rotate the item on its axis or in the mesio-distal or vestibular-lingual direction, allowing the operator to observe specific areas of interest.
Minimal thickness check	To check for areas where the thickness of the material is insufficient.
Quadrant	Once restoration modelling has been completed, to view the way in which the restoration is integrated within the arch and the relationships with the adjacent teeth.
Virtual grinding	Provides an actual selective grinding, thanks to a set of specific instruments.

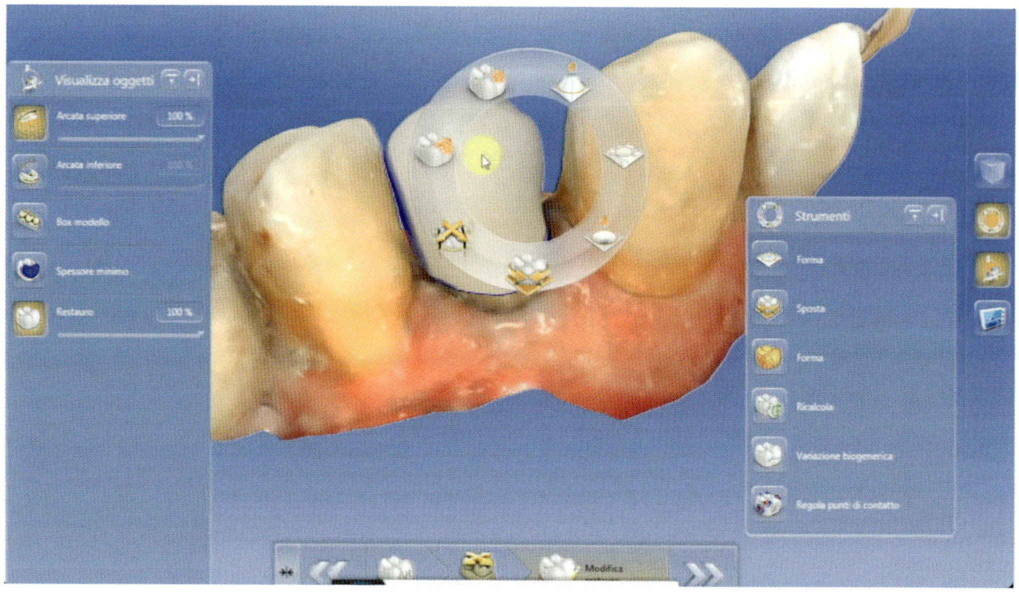

3.5 There are a number of available instruments for virtual modeling.

Before the prosthetic item is fabricated, the operational method for the restoration must be indicated, by selecting from three options:

1. Database with antagonist;
2. Correlation;
3. Replication.

In the **Database with antagonist**, in addition to the type of tooth (incisor, canine, premolar, molar), it is also possible to choose the most appropriate morphology and size according to the patient's age, gender and face type.

By using the **Correlation** mode, a copy of the pre-existing occlusal surface can be made. Therefore, the images of the tooth must be acquired before preparing it, so that by means of virtual modelling, the software is able to render an occlusal morphology that is wholly identical to that of the natural tooth.

The **Replication** mode is based on the mirroring effect: the morphology of the tooth can be reconstructed by using the exact mirror copy of the contralateral counterpart.

Once the design has been completed, the grinding process can begin, by using blocks of material supplied by manufacturers.

For the milling phase, it is possible to choose between the milling machine communicating directly with the cad software, or it receiving the STL file of the project to be milled through a CAM software.

A wide variety of materials can be processed with milling machines (zirconium oxide, aluminium oxide, infiltration ceramics, feldspar porcelain, lithium disilicate ceramics, glass ceramics, residue-free combustible synthetic materials, non-precious metal alloys, polymeric materials for long-lasting provisional crowns), indicated for the fabrication of copings for crowns, frameworks for bridges, monolithic ceramic full crowns without frameworks, inlays, onlays, veneers, surgical stents, mesostructures for implant abutments made in zirconium oxide or titanium, provisional crowns and wax-ups (3.6 and 3.7).

Milling units consist in a numerical control milling machines, containing diamond and tungsten carbide burs. The differences between the various milling machines consist mainly in the number of machining axes, in the number of burs that can be used simultaneously and in the possibility of dry or wet working.

During milling, multi-bur systems produce more precise results compared to systems consisting of a single bur, while reducing the time needed to complete the process. Milling time depends on the dimensions of the restoration to be fabricated.[11]

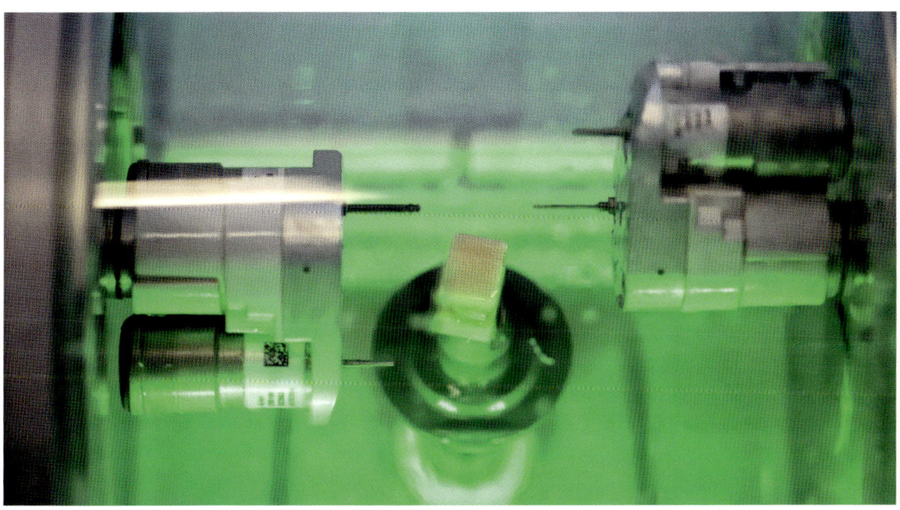

3.6 4-axis milling machine with 4 fixed cutters.

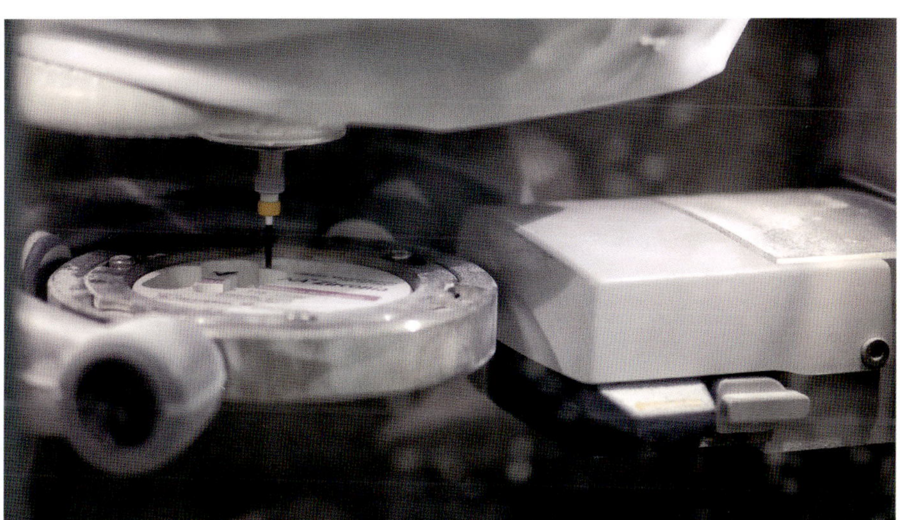

3.7 5-axis milling machine with the option of using a number of cutters during processing.

To avoid overheating of burs and material, milling machines are equipped with a cooling system that works with distilled water, whose function is also to protect the material and remove the dust and debris produced by milling. The system can be integrated with a sintering furnace, so the process can be completed with glazing or crystallization process, by means of specific furnaces.

Materials for CAD-CAM systems

The launch onto the dental market of CAD-CAM systems has made it possible to produce indirect restorations with a high esthetic value, directly chairside and in a single appointment, seeking to reduce the use of metal materials and to meet the requests of patients.

The materials used are diverse and include titanium, different types of all-ceramic (alumina, zirconia, spinel, yttria-stabilized zirconia) and modern second-generation micro-hybrid composites (3.8).

The CAD-CAM system has been developed to produce ceramic restorations from blocks of various sizes and a variety of colour shades. Feldspar ceramics are normally used, leucitic or lithium disilicate based.[12] The common ceramic materials previously used for CAD-CAM restorations were machinable glass ceramics, such as Dicor (Dentsply Caulk, Milford, DE 19963) and Vita Mark II (Vident, Bera, CA 92821). Although monochromatic, these materials provide excellent esthetic qualities, biocompatibility, colour stability, low thermal conductivity and excellent wear resistance. These have been used for inlays, onlays, veneers and crowns. However, it has been observed that Dicor and Vita Mark II are not very good at withstanding the occlusal load, if used for posterior crowns. That is why materials in alumina and zirconia are now widely used for dental restorations.[13]

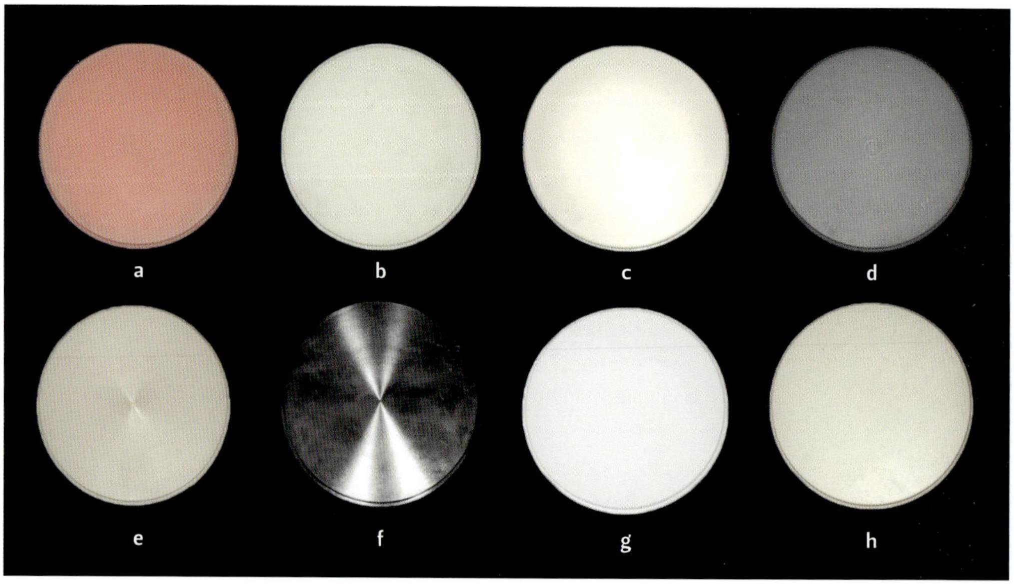

3.8 The advent of CAD-CAM has led to the development of a number of materials. From left to right: **a)** pink acrylic resin, **b)** glass fiber in resin matrix, **c)** polyetherketoneketone, **d)** cobalt-chrome, **e)** PEEK, **f)** titanium, **g)** zirconia, **h)** composite.

These materials might not be appropriate without the aid of the CAD-CAM technology: for instance, the In-Ceram system, initially described by Degrange and Sadoun, has been shown to have good bending resistance and excellent clinical performance. However, fabrication of a conventional In-Ceram restoration requires 14 hours, while milling pre-sintered alumina or zirconia blocks only takes 20 minutes; the glass infiltration time is reduced from 4 hours to 40 minutes and thanks to CAD-CAM systems the fabrication time is reduced by approximately 90%.[14]

Therefore, CAD-CAM systems nowadays are based on machinable blocks or discs in zirconia, pre-sintered alumina, lithium disilicate and metal, which meet most demands. The variety of materials in blocks meets most needs (3.9).

Aluminium oxide, or alumina, is the ceramic oxide of aluminium, having chemical formula Al_2O_3. It has interesting properties in the industrial field, such as acid resistance and thermal conductivity; it is an electrical insulator. At room temperature, it appears as a white and odourless solid. The stable form of alumina, α alumina, is an extremely hard and refractory material. In its mineral form, it is known as corundum and, among precious stones, as sapphire. Alumina is commonly obtained from the bauxite mineral through the Bayer process. The main features of alumina[15] are:

- good thermal stability;
- excellent corrosion resistance;
- material not subject to oxidization phenomena;
- excellent wear resistance;
- excellent biocompatibility;
- bending resistance: 487-699 Mpa;
- toughness: 4.48-6 MPa.

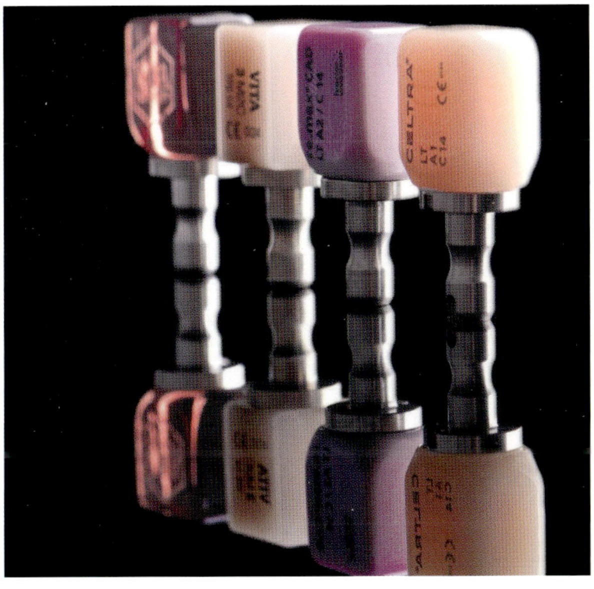

3.9 The variety of materials in blocks meets most needs.

The Procera system (Nobel Biocare), which uses alumina as core for the fabrication of crowns, was introduced in 1994. It was the first system on the market to fabricate crowns with a CAD-CAM technique. The material used is a dense lattice of 99.5% pure α alumina with 400-600 ppm in magnesium oxide, fully sintered. Alumina is highly appreciated for its high translucency, which makes it extremely suited for esthetic restorations in anterior regions (3.10).

Lithium disilicate is also a high-performance material from a functional as well as esthetic point of view, managing to combine high resistance (about 500 MPa) with varying degrees of translucency - a property that makes it particularly versatile. Lithium disilicate is only partially crystallized, so that it can be milled when it is blue, hence still soft. Subsequently, this material requires crystallization to be completed by means of a specific furnace (3.11 and 3.12). The market also offers formulations that combine lithium silicate crystals and zirconia, within a glass matrix, and which do not necessarily require crystallization after milling, being pre-crystallized (3.13).

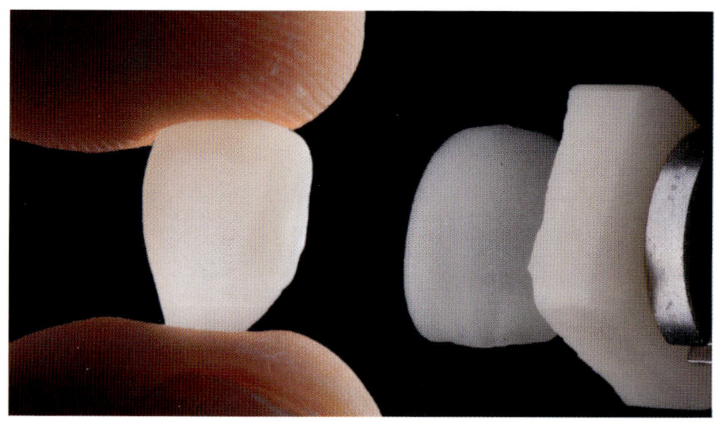

3.10 Aluminous porcelain makes it possible to work in minimal thickness.

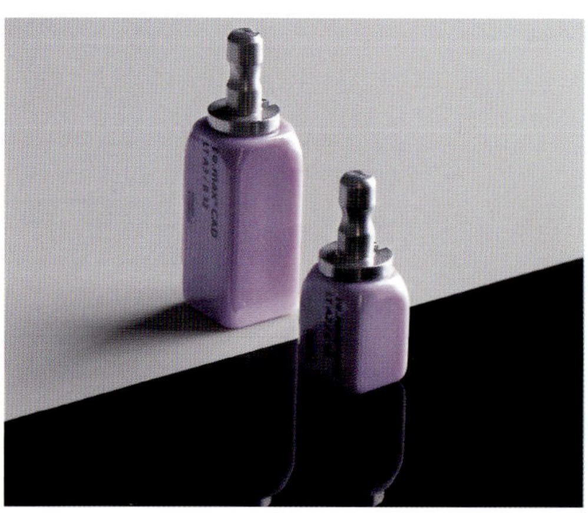

3.11 Lithium disilicate blocks ready for processing.

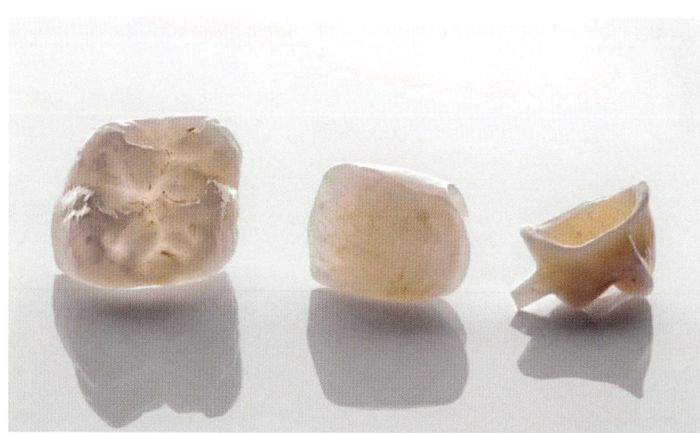

3.12 The features of lithium disilicate make it a highly versatile material.

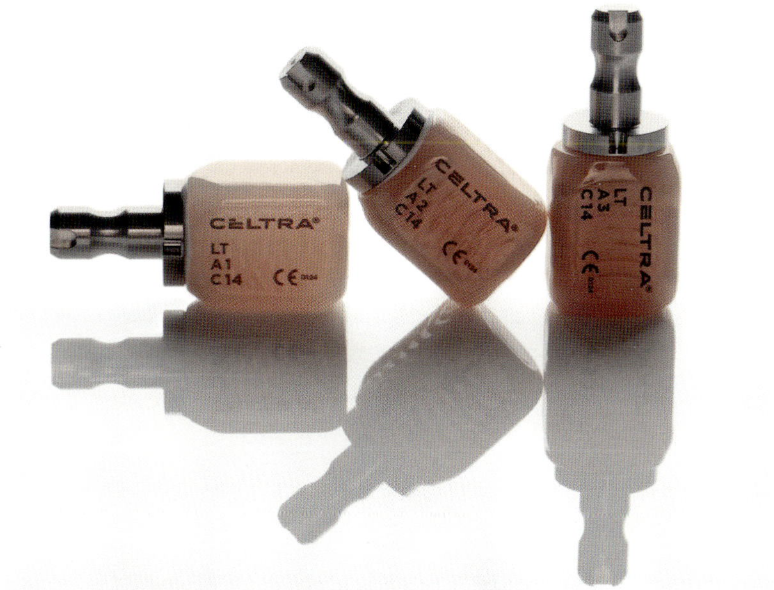

3.13 Lithium silicate and zirconia blocks.

Zirconium is a hard, white-grey coloured transition metal whose appearance resembles titanium. Zirconium is not used as a pure element in dentistry, but in the form of zirconium dioxide or zirconia, the formula of which is ZrO_2. Zirconia is no longer a transition metal, but a ceramic oxide; it holds a prominent place among ceramic oxides, thanks to its excellent mechanical properties. At ambient pressure, pure zirconia may take on three crystalline structures, depending on temperature:

- at room temperature up to 1170 °C, the structure is monoclinic (m);
- from 1170 °C to 2370 °C, the structure is tetragonal (t), useful for frameworks in dentistry;
- over 2370 °C, the structure is cubic, up to the melting temperature, which is 2720 °C.

The various crystalline forms are not stable, but may change as the temperature changes. While cooling, the inverse transformation, from the tetragonal to the monoclinic form, begins at ~950° C and is a displacive martensitic transformation: the atoms rearrange cooperatively, in a new crystalline structure, without changing the chemical composition of the starting phase. This transformation goes hand in hand with a 4.5% increase in volume, capable of leading to complete failures. By adding stabilizing oxides to zirconia, such as yttrium oxide (Y_2O_3), the tetragonal shape is maintained even at room temperature: in this way, by controlling the stress induced by the t - m transformation, the propagation of fractures is stopped and resistance is increased. This type of zirconia is commonly referred to with the acronym Y-TZP, which stands for yttrium cation-doped tetragonal zirconia polycrystals.[16]

This is the type of zirconia in use today in dentistry as support material for crowns or bridges: no applications have been found for another type of zirconia, partially stabilized zirconia, i.e. having the three structural forms (monoclinic, tetragonal and cubic) present simultaneously, due to its high porosity and the large size of its granules (30-60 μm) (3.14).

The appearance of zirconia-based ceramics on the market has sparked huge interest and significant changes in the dental world. The mechanical properties of zirconia are the highest ever achieved with dental ceramics; it is indeed the most resistant of all ceramic materials (bending strength 900-1200 MPa). These properties make it possible to fabricate fixed prostheses in the posterior quadrants, with a substantial reduction in framework dimensions compared to the previous, non-metal systems. These features are very interesting in prosthodontics, where esthetics and resistance are extremely important.

The mechanical properties of zirconia are decidedly affected by the size of its granules. Above a given critical granule size, zirconia is structurally less stable and may more easily undergo spontaneous t-m transformations, while a smaller granule size (<1 μm) is associated to a lower transformation index. Granule size is also affected by temperature and sintering time: high temperatures and longer sintering times lead to the formation of larger granules, hence lower resistance. Zirconia frameworks are only fabricated through CAD-CAM system.

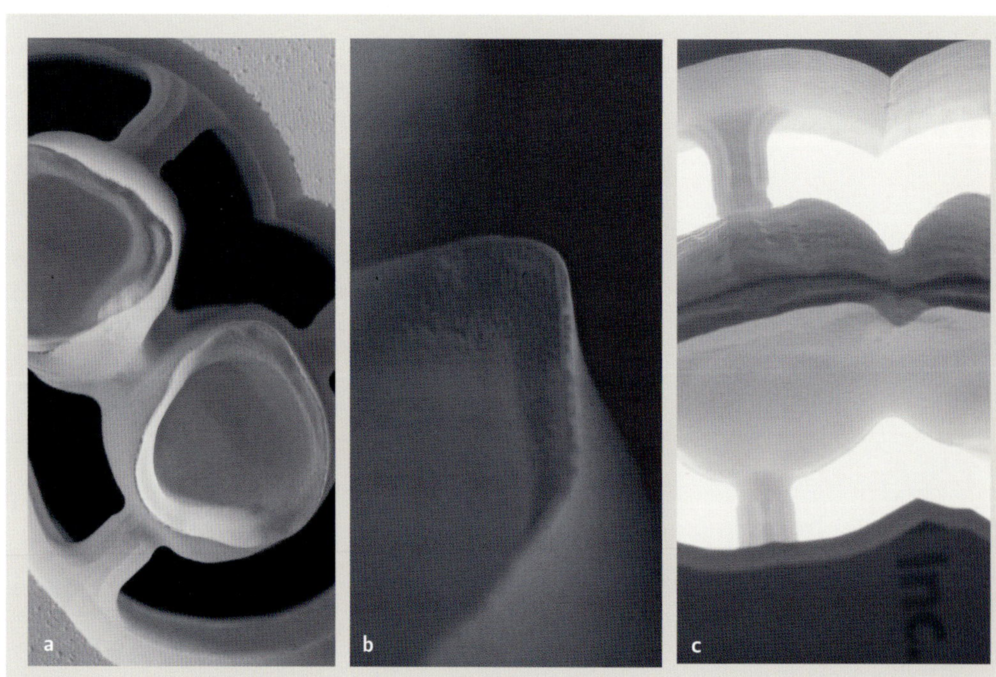

3.14 Zirconia is "soft" machined.

Machining can be performed by soft milling of a pre-sintered block, followed by complete high-temperature sintering, or by hard milling on fully sintered blocks.

Soft milling and subsequent sintering should be preferred, as they seem to produce less stress, and the surface of the pieces machined in this way is free from areas with monoclinic phase.

Currently, zirconia-based ceramics with different degrees of translucency are available, which make it possible to achieve truly appreciable esthetic results (3.15).

With the current CAD-CAM systems and sintering furnaces, zirconia can be considered a material compatible with chair-side techniques, as a single item only requires 90 minutes for machining. In summary, the factors that affect the mechanical properties of zirconia and which concern the manufacturer are as follows:[17]

- composition;
- purity of the raw materials;
- granule size;
- production processes.

The items made of crystalline ceramics, zirconia and alumina can be cemented with traditional cements, such as glass ionomer cements, or with an adhesive technique, after appropriate surface treatment.

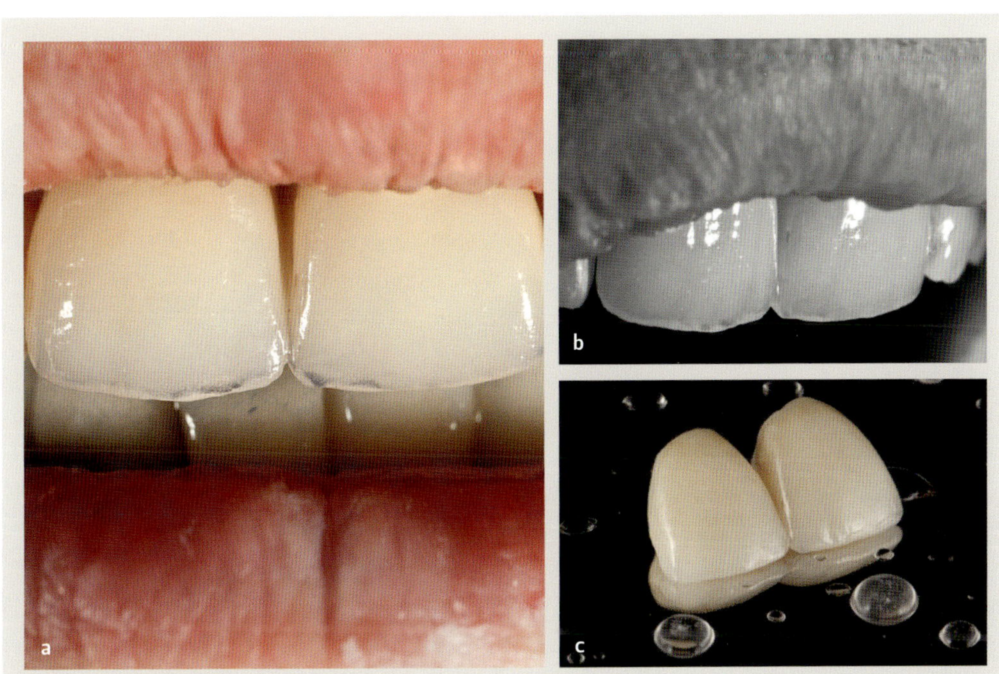

3.15 The current features of zirconia make it an esthetic material.

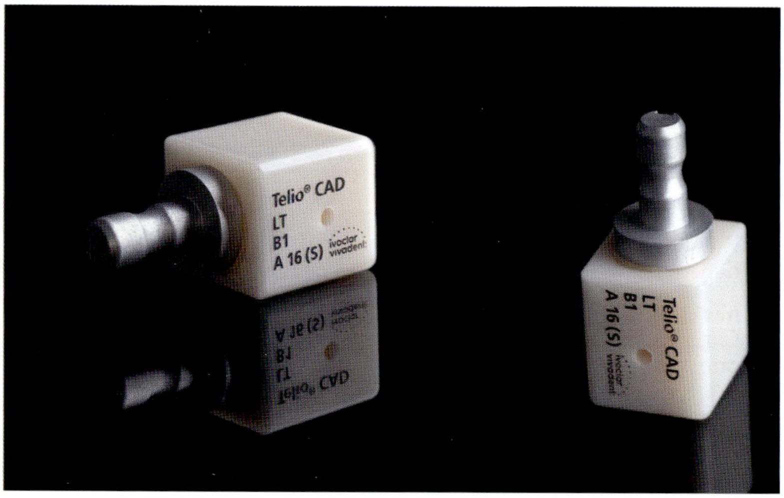

3.16 Pre-holed PMMA blocks for prostheses on implants.

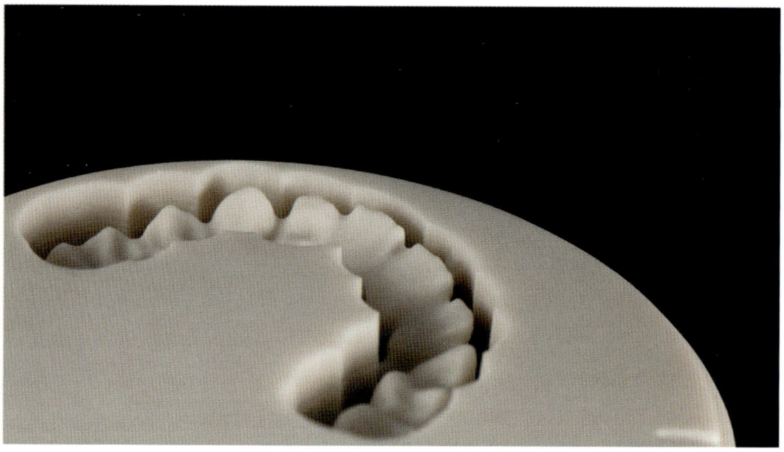

3.17 Polyetherketoneketone structure after milling.

CAD-CAM-specific polymers are a recently developed class of materials. An example is PMMA (polymethylmethacrylate), a very useful material especially for making temporary structures (3.16).

The so called "high performance" polymers, such as PEKK (polyetherketoneketone), belong to the same family (3.17).

This material offers a range of benefits, such as a Young modulus of 5.1 Gpa and hardness of 252 MPa. It is a radiotransparent and light material, when compared to materials such as titanium or zirconia. It can be used for permanent substructures, which are veneered with composites or on which superstructures in ceramic materials are cemented.

In conclusion, the availability of a variety of materials for fabricating a restoration expands the possible therapeutic solutions. Thus, the clinician is faced with the choice of the most suitable material, according to the type of restoration, the tooth involved and further essential parameters, in order to achieve an end result that is satisfactory from all points of view.

REFERENCES

1. **Mörmann WH, Brandestini M.** The CEREC Computer Reconstruction Inlays, Onlays und Veneers. Berlin: Quintessence, 1989.
2. **Johnson AE. E.** Spin-Images: A Representation for 3D surface Matching. Ph. D. Thesis, Carnegie Mellon University, Pittsburgh, August 1997.
3. **Palacci F, Nowzari H.** Soft tissue enhancement around dental implants. Periodontol 2000 2008;47:113-32.
4. **Mörmann WH, Brandestini M, Lutz F.** The Cerec system. Computer- assisted preparation of direct ceramic inlays in one setting. Quintessenz 1987;38(3): 457-70.
5. **Casalini ED.** La tomografia computerizzata a tecnologia Cone Beam nell'imaging radiologico 3D. Implant Tribune 2007.
6. INFODENT, **2008;** 3:33-34.
7. **Esposito M, Hirsch JM, Lekholm U et al.** Biological factors contributing to failures of osseointegrated oral implants. (I). Success criteria and epidemiology. Eur J Oral Sci. 1998 Feb;106(1):527-51.
8. **W.H. Mörmann, M. Brandestini, F. Lutz et al.** Chairside computer-aided direct ceramic inlays. Quintessence Int 1989; vol 20: 329-339.
9. **Allen KL, Schenkel AB, Estefan D.** An overview of the Cerec 3D CAD-CAM system. Gen Dent 2004;52(3):234-5.
10. **Touchstone A.** Simplifying CAD/CAM Dentistry: The fast track to CEREC excellence. Dental Products Report (Supp 1) Nov 2005; 1-7.
11. **Mörmann WH, Bindl A.** Milling quality of Cerec 2 and Cerec 3 CAD- CAM crowns. A SEM investigation. The Editorial Council of the Acta Stomatologica Naissi 2004.
12. **Giordano R.** Materials for chairside CAD-CAM - produced restorations. J Am Dent Assoc 2006;137Suppl:14S-21S.
13. **Rekow DE.** A 20-year success story. J Am Dent Assoc 2006;137 Suppl:5S-6S.
14. **Tinschert J, Natt G, Hassenpflug S. et al.** Status of current CAD/CAM technology in dental medicine. International Journal of Computerized Dentistry2004;7(1): 25-45.
15. **Valbonesi S.** Ceramiche metal free: indicazioni cliniche e possibilità tecniche. Associazione Amici di Brugg 2009, Quaderno n. 26.
16. **Giordano R.** Materials for chairside CAD-CAM - produced restorations. J Am Dent Assoc 2006;137Suppl:14S-21S.
17. **Ironside JG, Swain MV.** Ceramics in dental restorations - a review and critical issues. J Australasian Ceram Soc 1998;34:78-91.

Guided implant surgery

Martino Baruffaldi

Introduction to the digital world: the CAD-CAM computerized production process

The acronym CAD-CAM (Computer-Aided Design/Computer-Aided Manufacturing) identifies a set of methodologies, processes and instruments used for designing and manufacturing a product with the aid of a computerized system.

The prefix CA (Computer-Aided) indicates that the workflow for manufacturing the product is carried out by means of software and hardware.

A CAD-CAM technological system consists of:

- at least one computer, equipped with CAD software and CAM software;
- a computerized numerical control (CNC) machine tool (for example, a milling machine).

The term Reverse Engineering (RE) identifies all techniques and technologies that, starting from a real object, make it possible to obtain the same object in a virtual environment.

RE techniques include methods as well as software and hardware systems, used with the aim of reconstructing the virtual model, or CAD model, of an existing object. In the dental sector, these techniques are applied to import the patient's anatomy into a virtual environment.

The systems used in RE are the scanner, as a digitization tool, and the software applications for processing digitized point clouds (Standard Triangulation Language - STL file) and CAD modelling.

These systems are suited to the design of models with a high degree of detail. The high precision of these digital instruments enables to use 3D models, obtained via RE, also for the final engineering of the design and fabrication of accurate prototypes or moulds.

CAD is the whole set of software and hardware systems that support the design stage of a product, in which its geometry is precisely defined and the dimensions of every detail are established.

The concrete result deriving from the use of CAD systems, therefore, is the transformation of a product into a virtual object, which is the digital model of the product.

CAM is a software instrument, through which the information required for processing the product with programmable numerical control machines is generated. The CAD file of the product is transferred to a second graphic environment, CAM, which enables programming of the machining movements, starting from the CAD information, taking into account the raw volume, the kinematic structure of the machine tool and other elements, until a text document is created, which contains the instructions to be sent to the computerized numerical control (CNC) machine tool.

CNC machines, which belong to subtractive systems (milling machines), make it possible to fabricate a product, even with complex geometry, starting from a wafer of raw material. The movements of the cutter that “sculpts” the designed product are executed on the basis of the instructions that indicate the trajectories to be followed and the characteristic kinematic parameters of the trajectories (acceleration and speed).

Additive manufacturing systems, which we will deal with below, manufacture the product – always designed using CAD – with additive techniques, using rapid, flexible and automated processes, regardless of shape and geometric complexity.

Selective laser sintering-melting and stereolithography belong to these systems.

CAD design software

The CAD design software is the program with which the acquired data can be viewed in three dimensions, processed, planned and designed for a 3D dental restoration.

The scans can be transformed into various file formats, according to whether the system is open or closed.

In open systems, the STL format (Standard Triangulation Language) allows to freely choose various CAM systems, whereas closed scanning systems generate encrypted files, with a specific and different format for each manufacturer.

Sometimes, it is possible to purchase an evaluation key from the system manufacturer that can decrypt the proprietary file and transform it into the STL format.

The main features of the CAD design software, now present in all systems on the market, are: archive, customized parameters, modeling and library.

- The **archive** is used to store the data of each individual process. This feature makes it possible to repeat a job and always obtain a perfect copy, which is useful in the case of follow-ups or prosthetic remaking.
- The **customized parameters** are used to customize the thickness of the supporting structure, the dimensions of the connector between intermediate elements, the cervical contour, height and shape, the thickness of the esthetic veneer, to define the axis of prosthetic insertion and to blockout any undercuts (4.1).
- **Modeling** is the main feature of this kind of software. It makes it possible to mould the tooth directly on the computer, modifying the dental shape with the mouse, in the same way as the dental technician would do with wax and a spatula (4.1). Every CAD modeling system has a library.
- The **library** is a catalogue, in which pre-designed and predefined dental shapes are available, which can be edited at will, as well implant abutments, through which customized, perfectly parallel posts can be created, with the advantage of being able to use precision machining.

In this connection, the manufacturers of dental implants very often have appropriate libraries covering the virtual components of their implants.

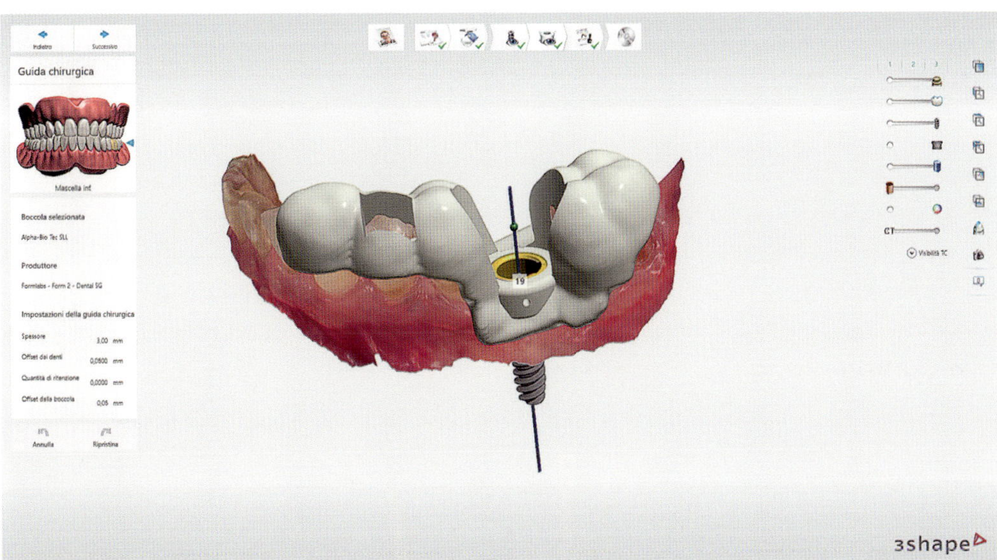

4.1 Design of a surgical guide for implant placement in position 3.6.

CAM fabrication systems

CAM fabrication systems have evolved in step with CAD systems, opening up new scenarios in the field of the production of prosthetic items. CAM systems can be broken down into two main categories:

- Subtractive Manufacturing
- Additive Manufacturing.

Numerical control machine tools (Subtractive Manufacturing) with chip removal mainly differ in the number of axes controlled by the CNC (Numerical Control Machining Centres, machine tools with computer-controlled movement of the axes).

The minimum number of axes to make objects in space is 3: this means that the tool (the revolving cutter) is positioned in space according to the 3 coordinates controlled by the CNC.

The other CAM systems, as an alternative to CNC machines, are identified as Additive Manufacturing systems.

The Additive Manufacturing technique (AM) differs from the Subtractive Manufacturing technique in the fact that the latter works by removing material, whereas AM techniques work by adding material. The first AM machine was SLA-1 (StereoLithographic Apparatus). Subsequently, technological progress led to other techniques such as LOM (Laminated Object Manufacturing), SLS (Selective Laser Sintering), FDM (Fused Deposition Modeling). Manufacturers provide a range of materials in the form of blocks, with regard to Subtractive Manufacturing techniques, and materials in the form of powder, liquid or solid for Additive Manufacturing techniques (4.2).

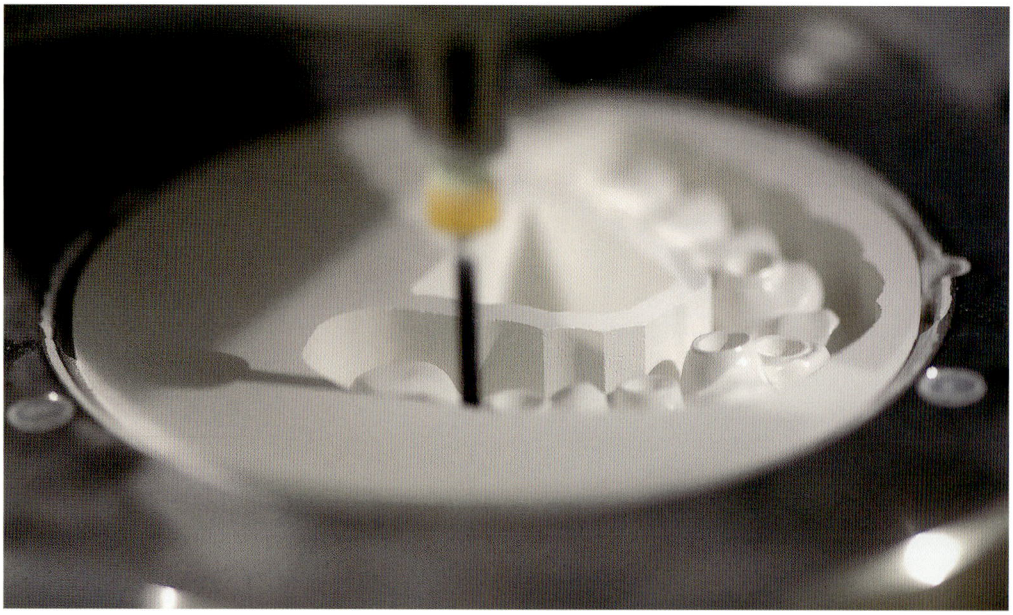

4.2 Milling process of a full-arch implant-supported FPD from a zirconia wafer.

The manufacturing technology of most prosthetic products made with CAD-CAM technology is based on the Subtractive Manufacturing technique, whereby machine tools fitted with cutters are used to sculpt blocks of sintered or pre-sintered materials, into the desired geometry. However, the Subtractive Manufacturing technique results in significant waste of material and energy for the fabrication of the prosthetic item. In view of that, manufacturers focused on developing alternative fabrication techniques, such as AM (4.3).

Also in the AM technique, the first step is the creation of an STL file, which may be generated in two clearly distinct ways, and precisely:

1. through the integral use of CAD software;
2. by using Reverse Engineering techniques.

In implantology, the first workflow is the one most commonly used. The dental technician models a prosthetic device virtually on the computer, using specific and appropriate CAD design software. The second workflow can be used when a mathematical model is unavailable and reverse engineering techniques (RE) are used, i.e. an object is scanned and then imported into a CAD environment.

The scan results in a given number of points, referred to as "point cloud", corresponding to the scanned surfaces. The cloud is processed via CAD or specific software to obtain the three-dimensional mathematical model.

In guided surgery procedures, it is essential never to lose information and being able to transfer it at the various stages of the procedure.

Very often, not only do CAD-CAM procedures make it possible to design and execute the immediate loading surgical stage, but the immediate provisional crown can also be transformed into the definitive item thanks to the digital technique.

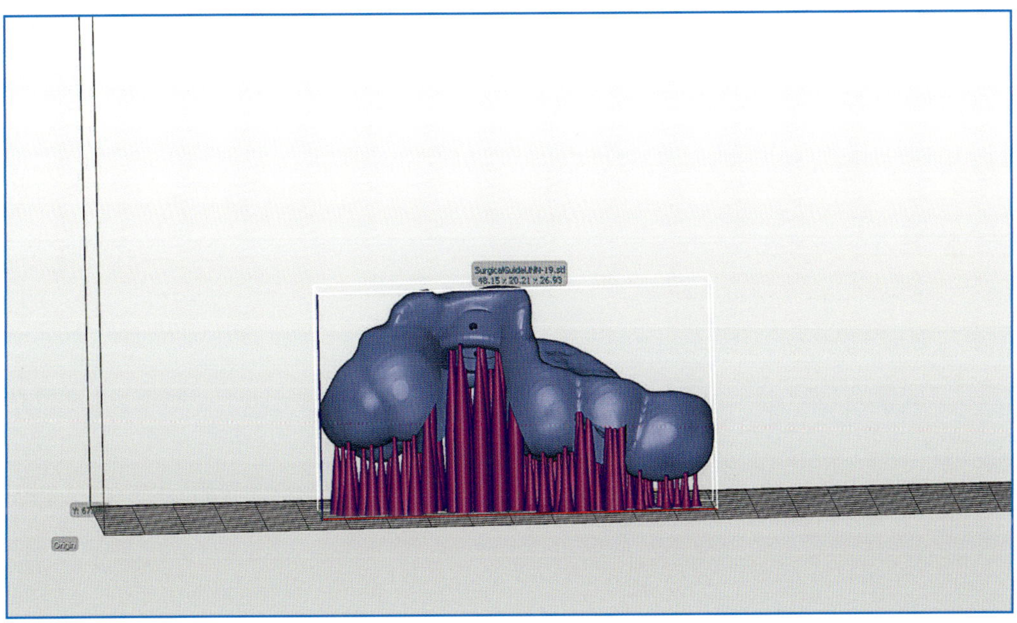

4.3 Fabrication of a surgical guide through a 3D printing method.

This allows the clinician to reproduce all the esthetic and functional features of a provisional crown in the final prosthetic item, following the steps of the procedure:

1. the clinician can scan the provisional crown with an intra-oral scanner, or take an alginate impression, from which the gypsum model can be obtained, which can be scanned with the laboratory scanner (4.4);
2. starting from the CAD mathematical model, the file with STL extension is obtained by means of appropriate exporting utilities or directly from CAD, if this utility is built-in; as an alternative, the design may first be saved in an intermediate format, then the STL file is generated with specific software (4.5);
3. production of the device consists in sending the STL file to the machine operating with AM technology, which then deposits the material layer by layer, until the end object is obtained;

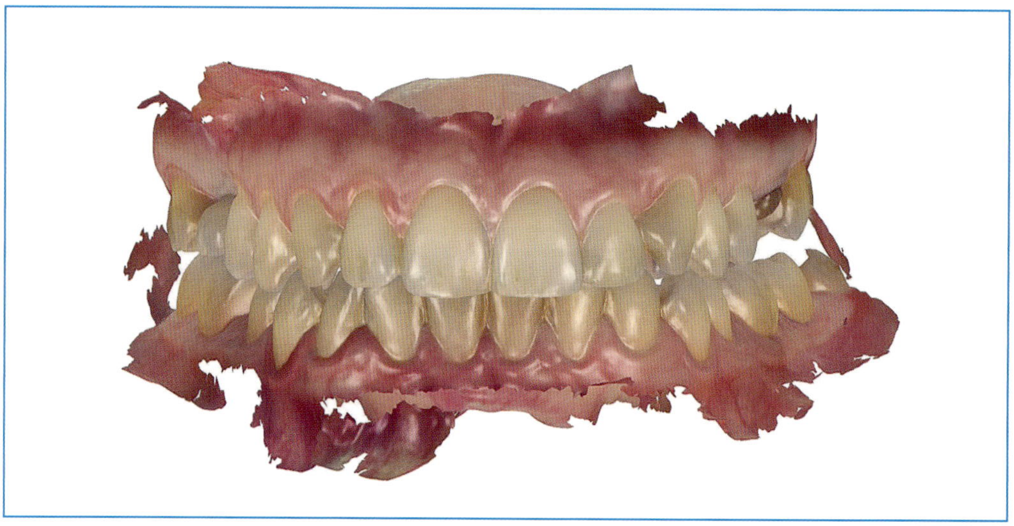

4.4 Example of digital impression of both arches for diagnostic purposes.

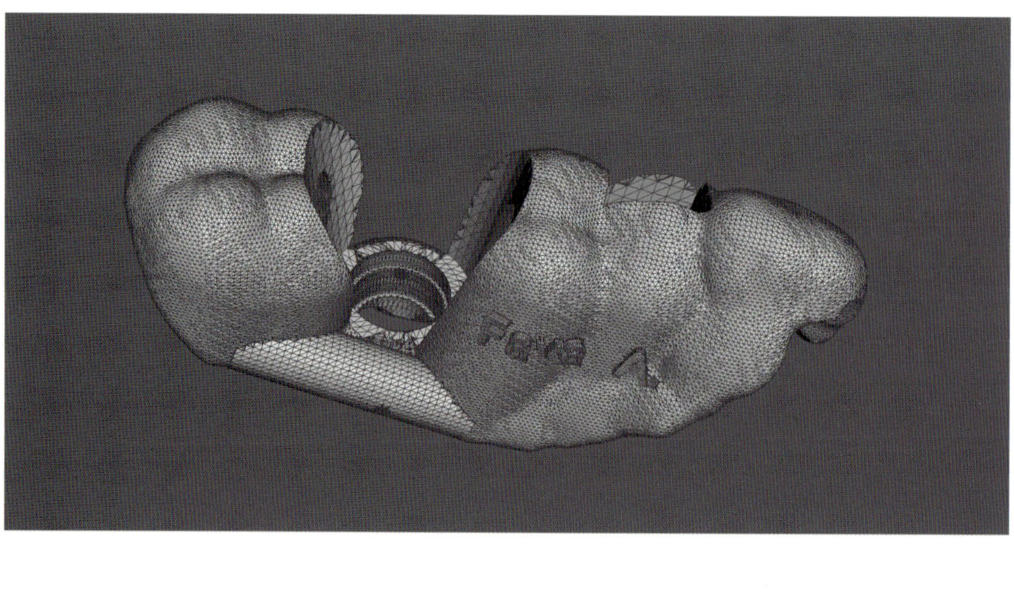

4.5 File in STL format of a surgical guide ready for the production stage.

4 manually performed post-treatments are required for finalizing the object, which consist in polishing and finishing the material.

One ought to remember that the resolution of a 3D printer is the minimum thickness of the material it uses to produce an object. Usually, this dimension is expressed in microns and may vary from 100 to 300 µm for a common 3D printer; therefore, the lower the resolution value, the thinner the layer of material deposited and consequently, the more defined the object (the layers are so thin that the object seems to have a particularly smooth surface) (4.6-4.8). However, longer processing times are required to achieve high resolution.[1]

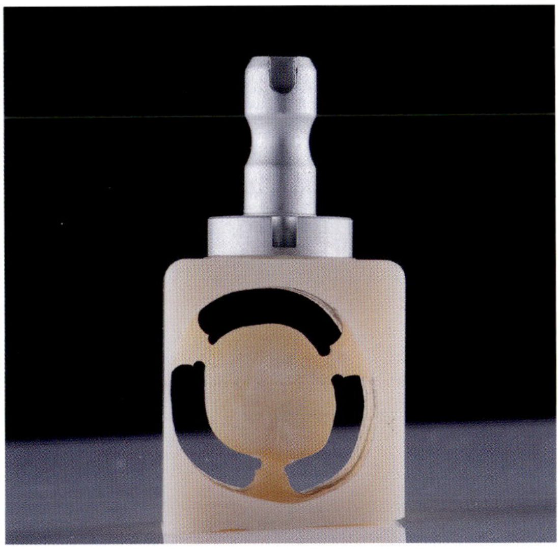

4.6 Provisional PMMA crown fresh out of the milling machine.

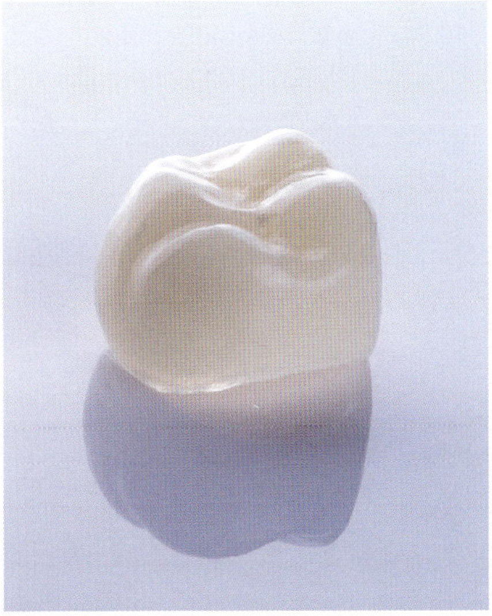

4.7 The same crown following finishing and polishing, ready for delivery.

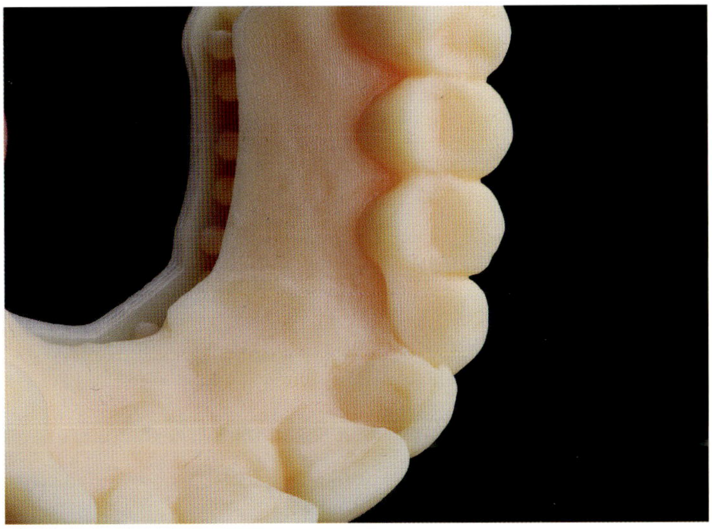

4.8 Detail of the layers through which the 3D printing process takes place.

Computer-guided implant surgery

Computer-guided surgery is a technique that, by exploiting three-dimensional radiology and complex programming software, makes it possible to plan the surgery down to the smallest detail. Based on volumetric radiographic investigations, and by using specific software, the clinician is able to plan implant placement in a precise manner and without being subject to the stress and constraint of the surgical procedure.

In the field of dentistry, it was only introduced very recently, first as an aid in gnathology and, only later, in the surgical field, for implantology, for osteogenic distraction procedures, for the study of osteotomic lines for reconstructive purposes, and for the removal of foreign bodies.

Two types of guided surgery can be distinguished:

1. **static computer-guided surgery**: it entails the use of a static surgical guide, which reproduces the previously planned virtual position of implants, through computerized stages; this method does not allow for intra-operative modifications;
2. **dynamic computer-guided surgery**: it entails the use of a surgical navigation system, which reproduces in real time the position of the drills in three dimensions on a screen, allowing for intra-operative modifications.

The two systems have different production processes, with certain similarities. For instance, both go through computerized planning of implant placement, but have entirely different diagnostic and surgical guides:

- static surgery enables the production of radiographic stents, which duplicate the patient's future dentition and allow the CT to be viewed on a computer. Based on planning, rigid surgical guides are produced, generally in plastic material, which are placed in the patient's mouth (4.9). Surgery uses metal sleeves inside the guide; thanks to diameter reducers, drills of different diameter can be used, with or without depth stop. Surgery the-

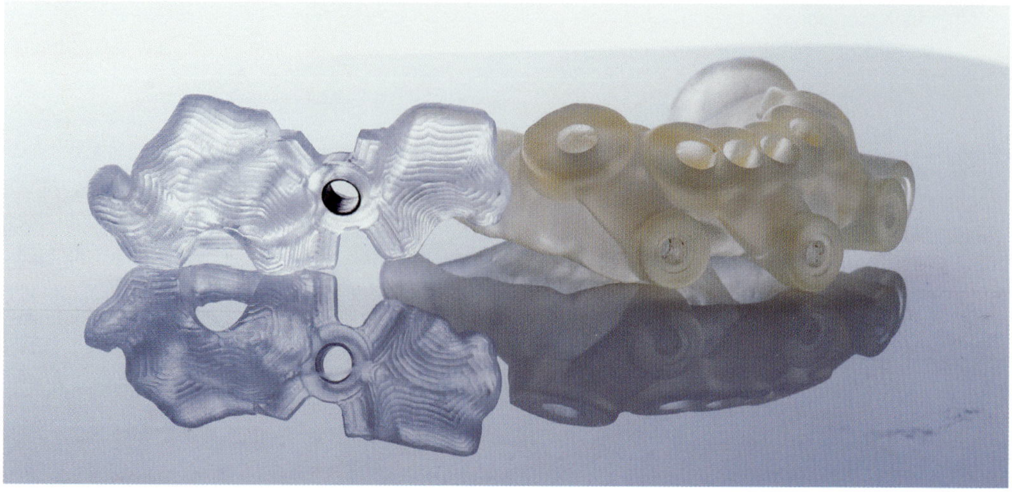

4.9 Surgical guides for implant placement: milled (left) and 3D printed (right).

refore takes place according to the plan prepared blindly, which cannot be changed, unless one leaves guided surgery and proceeds with conventional surgery

- On the contrary, dynamic surgery is based on a more advanced process. The patient undergoes the CT with a special diagnostic index and with extraoral cranial landmarks fitted with infrared sensors. Implant planning is performed in a similar manner to the software used for the static version. On the contrary, surgery is based on complex machinery, fitted with infrared cameras, that not only reads the patient's cranial landmarks, but also landmarks fitted on the surgical handpiece. Thanks to this complex system, the live position of the drill with respect to the alveolar crest can be seen on the screen. No static surgical guides are used, but the patient's CT scan and the position of the osteotomy drill are displayed live on the screen, in order to guide the clinician in performing the surgery with precision (4.10). This system entails the option of making intra-operative modifications, precisely thanks to the possibilities offered by live viewing. In this case, surgery is not executed blindly, but the exact position of the drill in the three dimensions of space is also displayed, allowing the clinician to optimize implant position and avoid anatomically significant structures.

In order to perform reliable and predictable implantology, the clinician must frequently subject the patient to first and, often, second level radiographic examinations.

The clinician needs the following radiographic information:

- bone height and thickness;
- bone quality;
- any pathological condition of the residual teeth, in the case of partial edentulism;
- position of anatomical structures, such as vessels and nerves, that might be damaged during the surgical procedures.

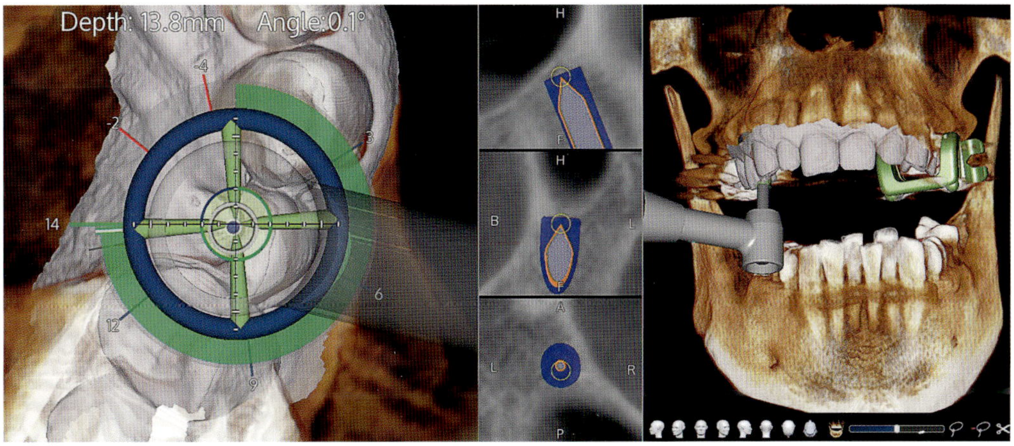

4.10 How guided navigation works for inserting an implant in position 1.4.

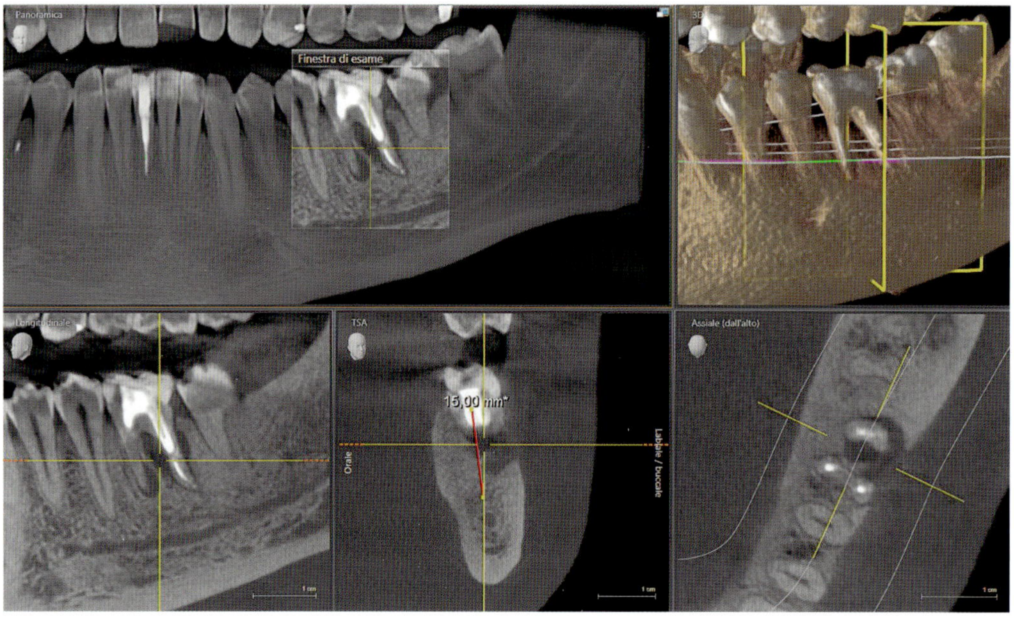

4.11 First step in the implant position planning, based on the CBCT examination performed during the first appointment.

In order to carry out this careful assessment, the clinician can make use of a number of radiographic instrumental examinations (4.11).

Design

The design of guided surgery implant cases is carried out through a series of steps, illustrated below. Each step must be performed properly and checked several times, since small errors in the planning stage, if added one over another, can turn into severe surgical mistakes

CHOICE OF THE COMPUTER SOFTWARE

Several implant planning software programs have been produced over the years.

Implant companies have developed or implemented some software programs.

These software programs are often closed, that is, they only support the manufacturer's implants. On the contrary, independent companies have developed software programs that are open towards other implant companies, so as to support the placement of any implant with the same software.

Another important aspect to be considered is the production process of indexes, which are fabricated by means of CAD-CAM systems, by milling, rapid prototyping, stereolithography or 3D printing.

MATCHING

The matching stage in guided surgery is essential to coordinate the patient's clinical data with those deriving from the three-dimensional radiographic investigation (DICOM). Indeed, it is necessary to transfer the spatial coordinates onto the patient, in relation to the future implant position.

At the moment, there are actually three procedures that enable this superposition: DICOM-model, DICOM-DICOM (or double scan) and DICOM-STL.

1. *DICOM-model matching.* This procedure entails using a gypsum model of the patient to fabricate a radiographic stent, with radiopaque landmarks. The model is calibrated on a precision dental surveyor, so that the landmarks are located on a reference plane, in relation to the surveyor. These landmarks are then recognized within the DICOM file by the programming software which can then relate them to the plane of the model and generate the necessary superposition. This procedure is often followed by a fabrication process of the surgical guide directly in the laboratory, by means of a surveyor or other instruments, suited to replicating on the model the implant coordinates generated by the software.
2. *DICOM-DICOM matching.* Also referred to as "double scanning", this procedure actually allows the use of a radiographic template (or the patient's denture, appropriately modified with radiopaque landmarks), as calibration parameter. Two DICOM radiographic volumes will be generated: the first relating to the patient, who wears the radiographic template (or prosthesis with markers) and the second of the template only. Subsequently, the software interfaces the radiopaque markers between the two DICOM files and generates the superposition of the two volumes. The DICOM file of the radiographic template will also be used to produce the surgical guide, transforming the DICOM data into STL data, which will enable fabrication with CAD-CAM methods and 3D printing. Once planning is executed on the software, the coordinates of the implants are correlated to the radiographic template, which is then transformed into a surgical guide.
3. *DICOM-STL matching.* This procedure is more recent and is based on matching STL data, that is, a digital impression. The files relating to the three-dimensional images of surfaces are saved in the STL format, which is considered the international standard for digital impressions, whether obtained from intraoral scans or gypsum model scans. Some guided surgery software programs do not support universal files such as STL, but closed files, generated by specific intraoral or laboratory scanners, however, without changing the matching rationale or logic. This process is based on superposing the STL data on the patient's DICOM data: therefore ,visible areas must be superposed simultaneously, in the impression as well as in the radiograph. The oral mucosa is not sufficiently radiopaque under the radiographic investigation to be able to exactly establish shape and volume. Therefore, this matching is based on the superposition of dental hard tissues: in cases of total edentulism, reference is made to the

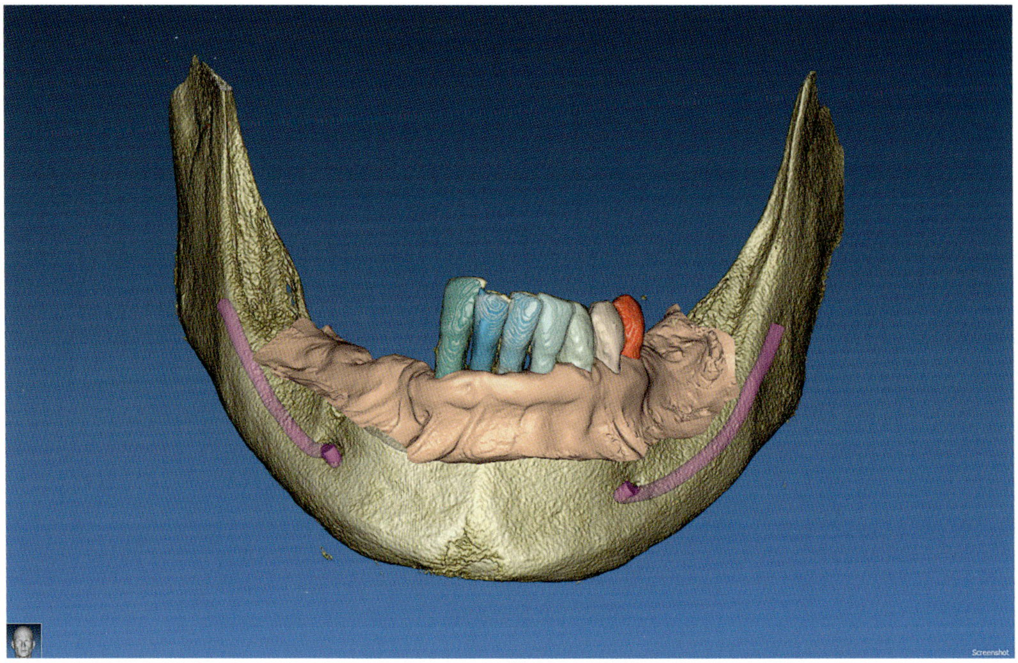

4.12 Matching the optical impression and CBCT in the implant planning software.

superposition of landmarks, which are radiopaque (for the DICOM image) and at the same time have a shape detectable by the scanner (for the STL image). That is why gutta-percha points inserted in a denture cannot be used. The generation of the surgical guide no longer takes place by transforming the DICOM data of the radiological template (as is the case in the DICOM-DICOM or double scan), but by drawing a mucosa- and/or teeth-supported guide via CAD software, in relation to the patient's surgical needs (4.12).

The advantages of these procedures are different, but the main ones consist in giving greater evidence to soft tissues, especially in cases of partial edentulism, and in enabling virtual diagnostic wax-ups, by means of CAD/CAM software.[2,3]

Solutions for simple cases

In the following case, it is possible to observe how guided surgery can be applied also in simple cases such as replacement of this 4.6. It would certainly be possible to place the implant freehand, but the option of being absolutely faithful to the digital design makes it possible to fabricate the future restoration with an ideal emergence profile while respecting the correct distances from the mesial and distal teeth as well as from the vestibular cortical bone (4.13-4.26).

4.13 Pre-operative CBCT showing single edentulism in position 4.6.

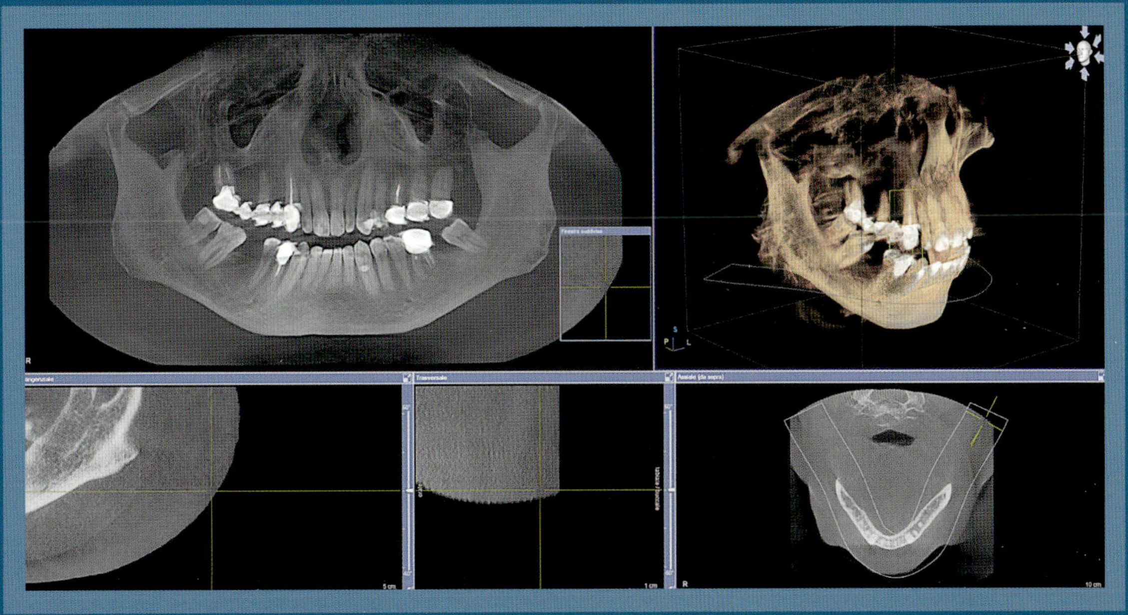

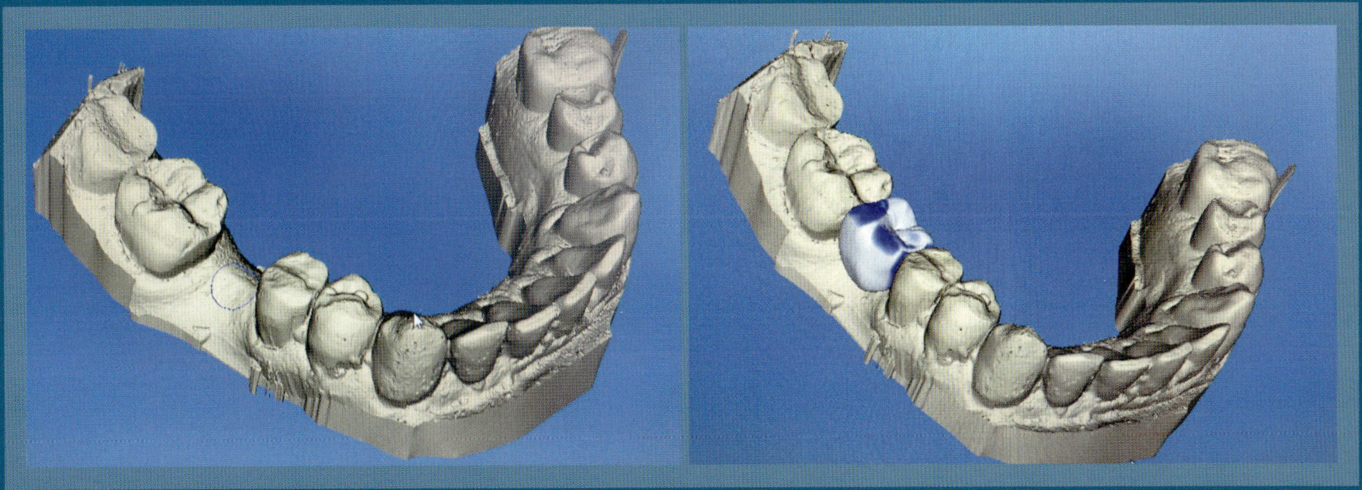

4.14 An optical impression is taken to perform the prosthetic planning that will guide the implant position.

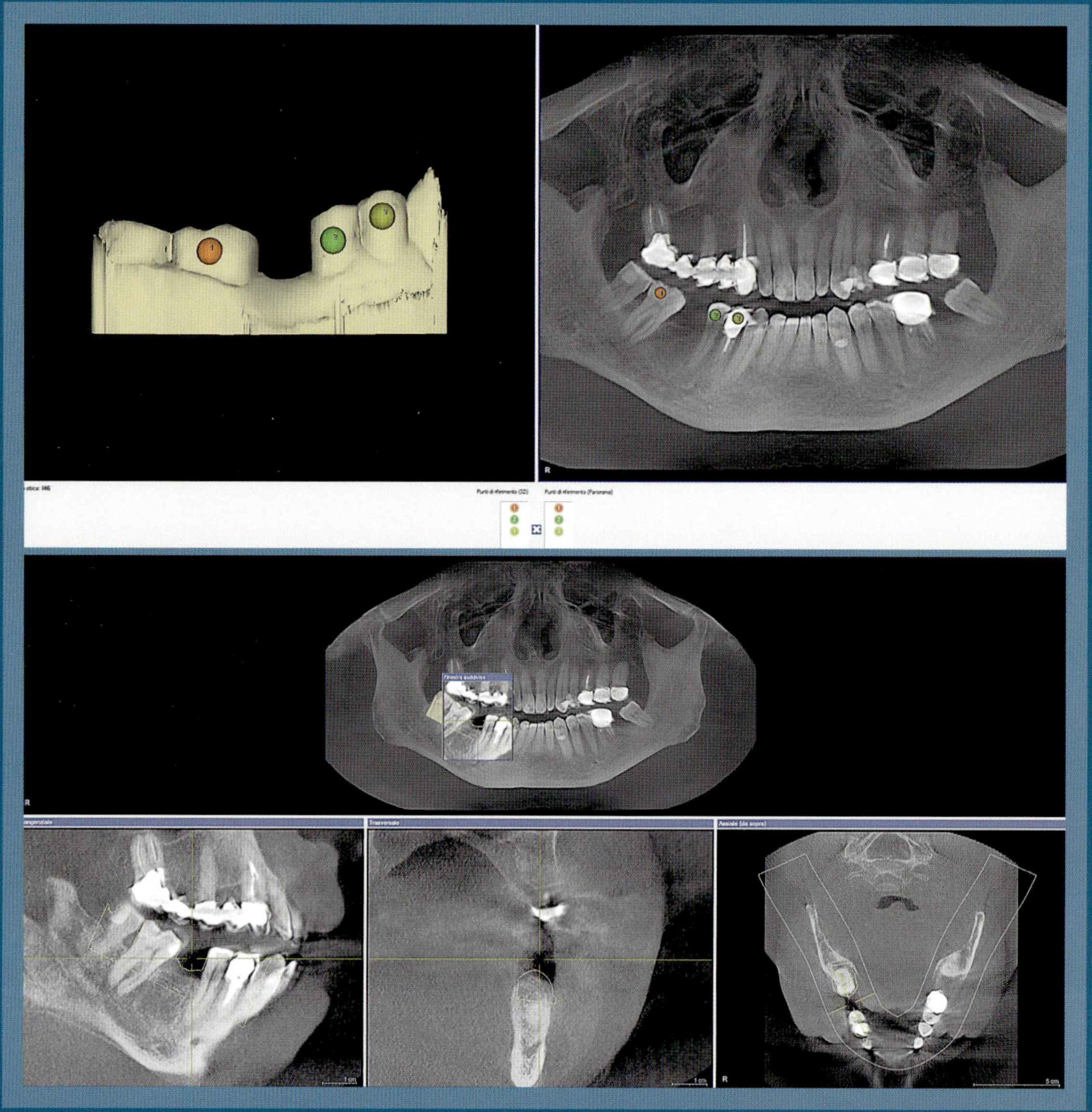

4.15 The radiographic examination is matched with the optical impression.

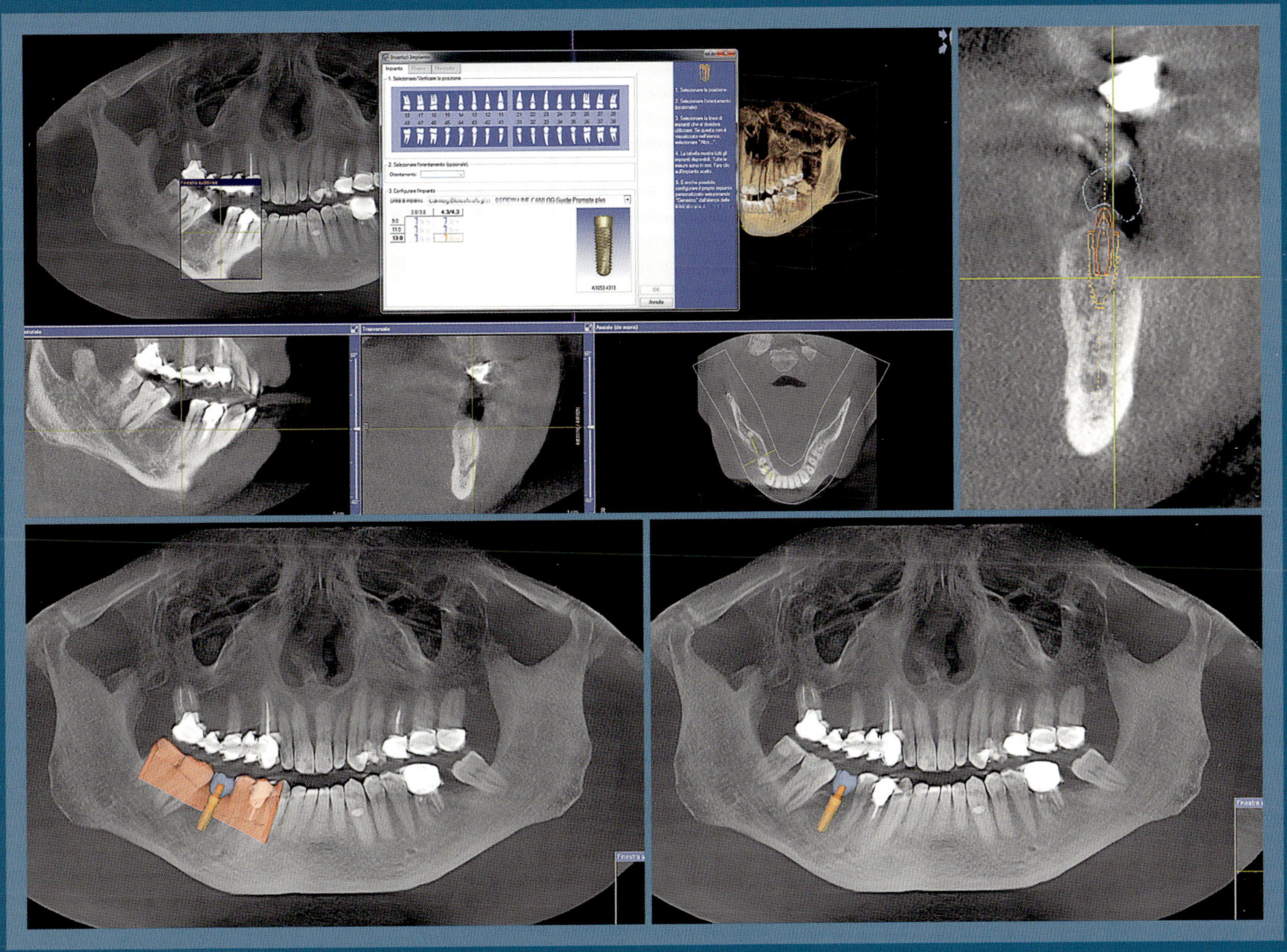

4.16 The position of the implant is planned on the basis of the prosthetic design.

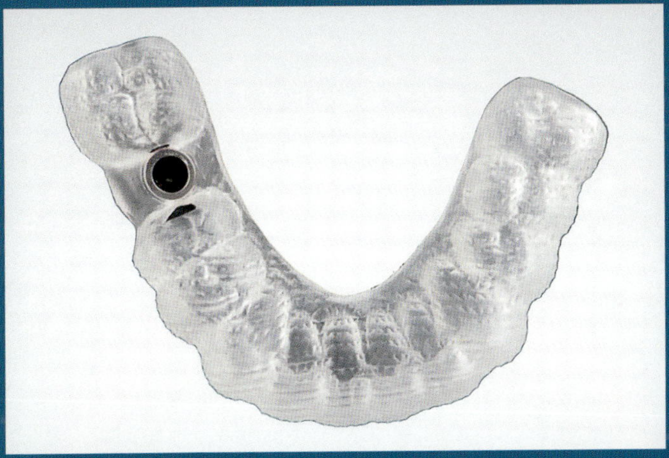

4.17 A surgical guide is fabricated by 3D printing or milling, then the sleeve corresponding to the selected implant is inserted.

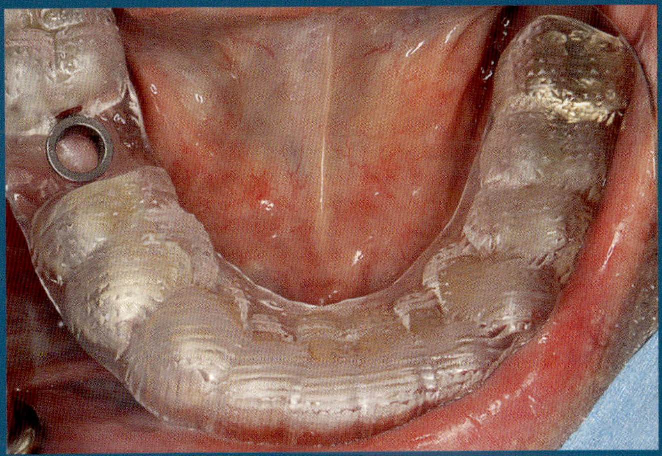

4.18 The surgical guide is tested in the patient's mouth, to ensure there is no discrepancy with the dentition.

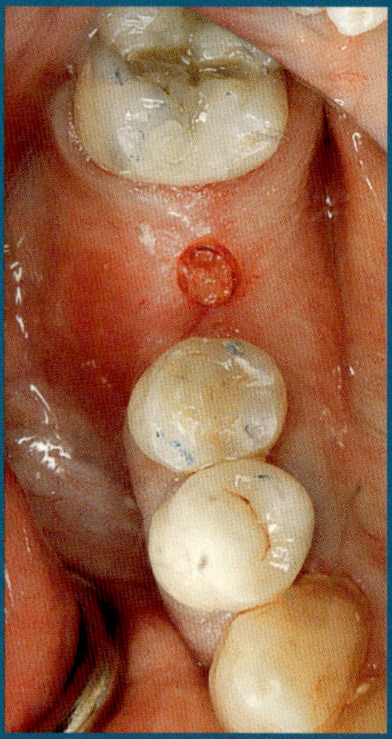

4.19 First step with the mucotome.

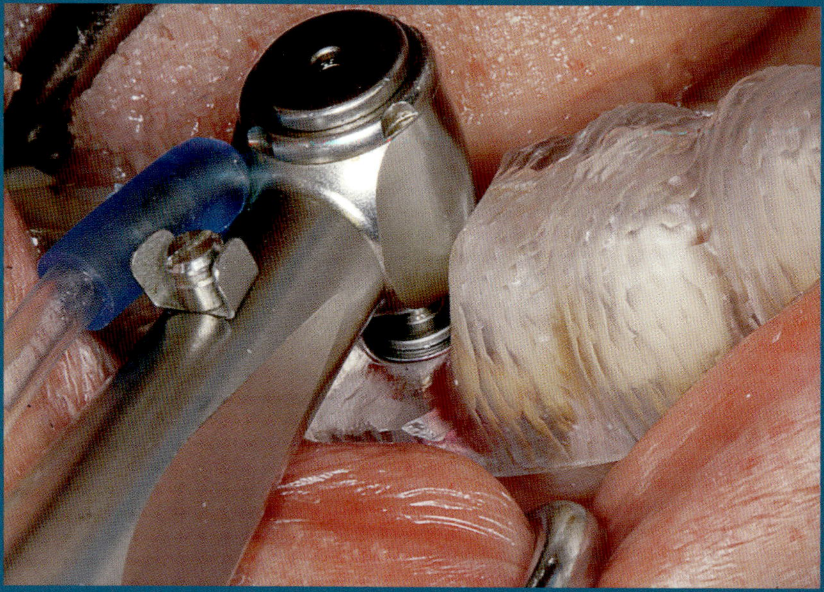

4.20 The implant site is prepared with the appropriate drills, guided in their direction by the titanium sleeve.

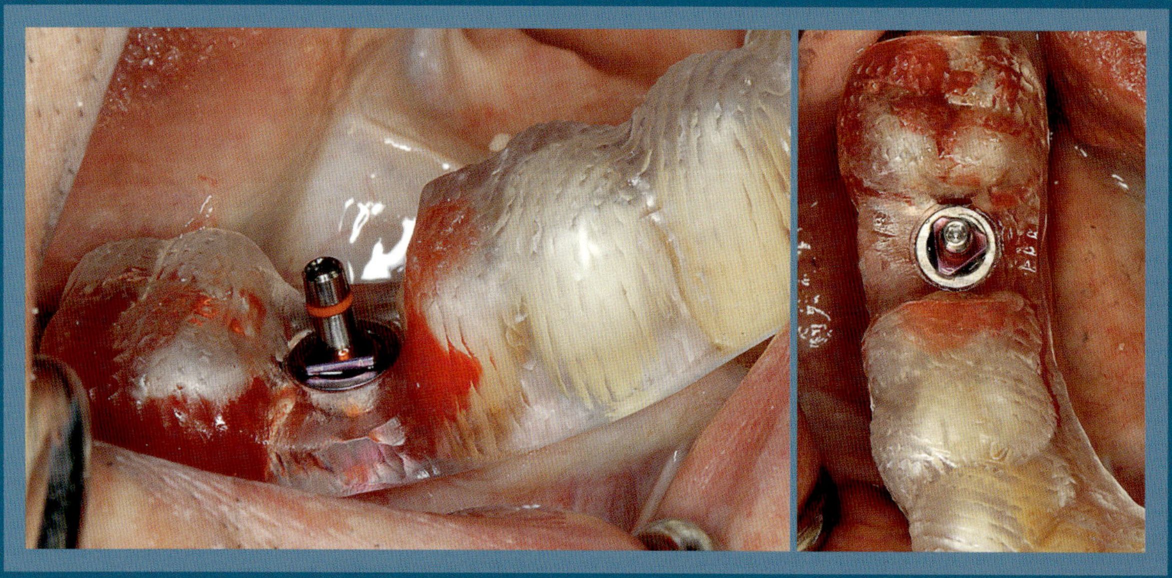

4.21 The implant is inserted. The contact between mounter and sleeve provides a depth stop.

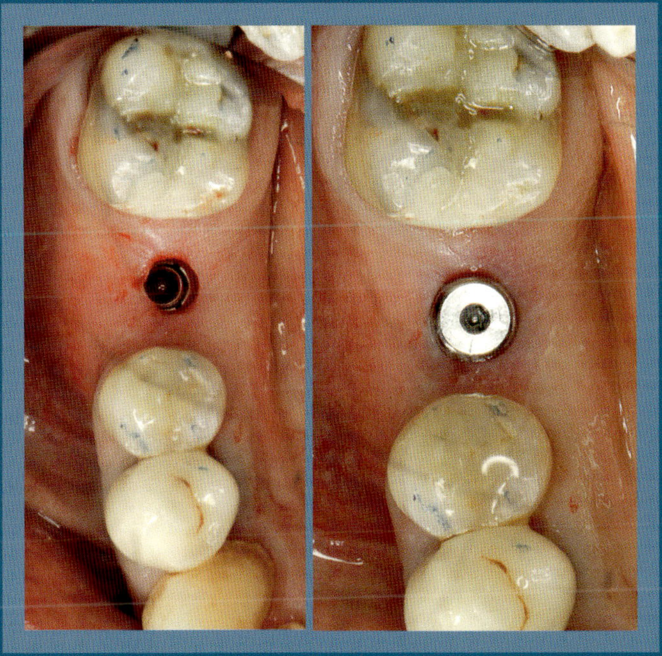

4.22 Removal of the index and placement of the transmucosal healing screw.

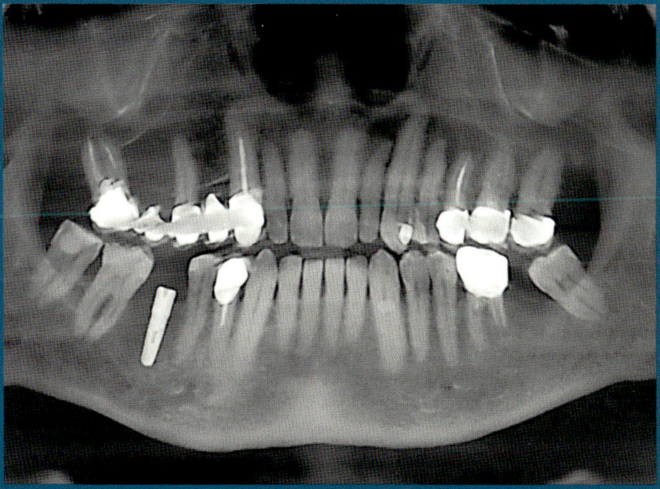

4.23 Post-operative radiographic examination.

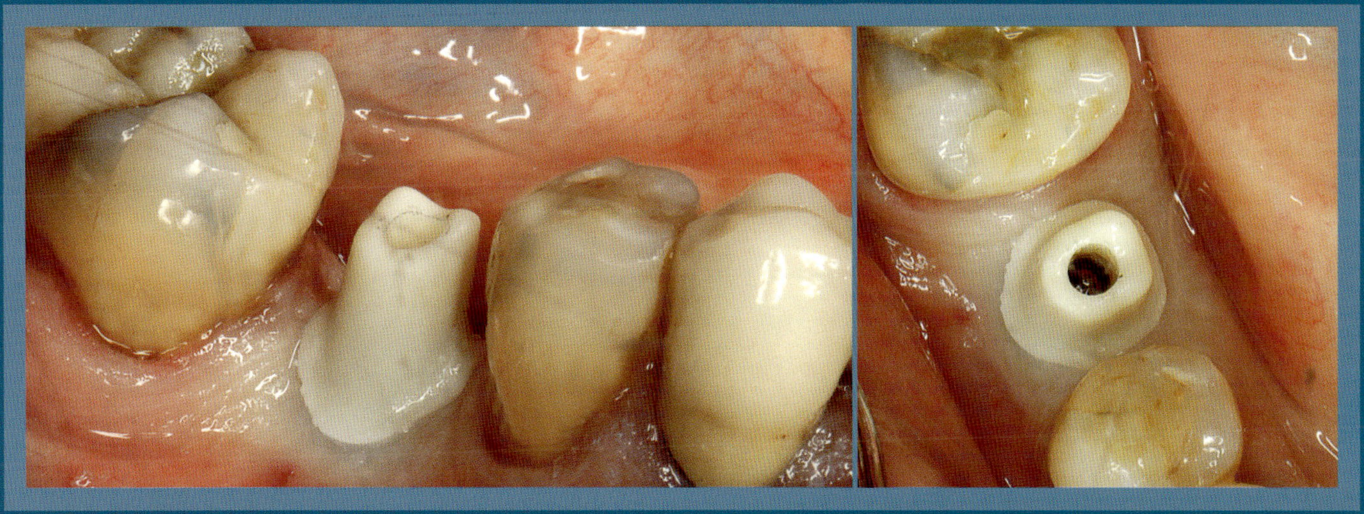

4.24 Placement of a custom zirconia abutment.

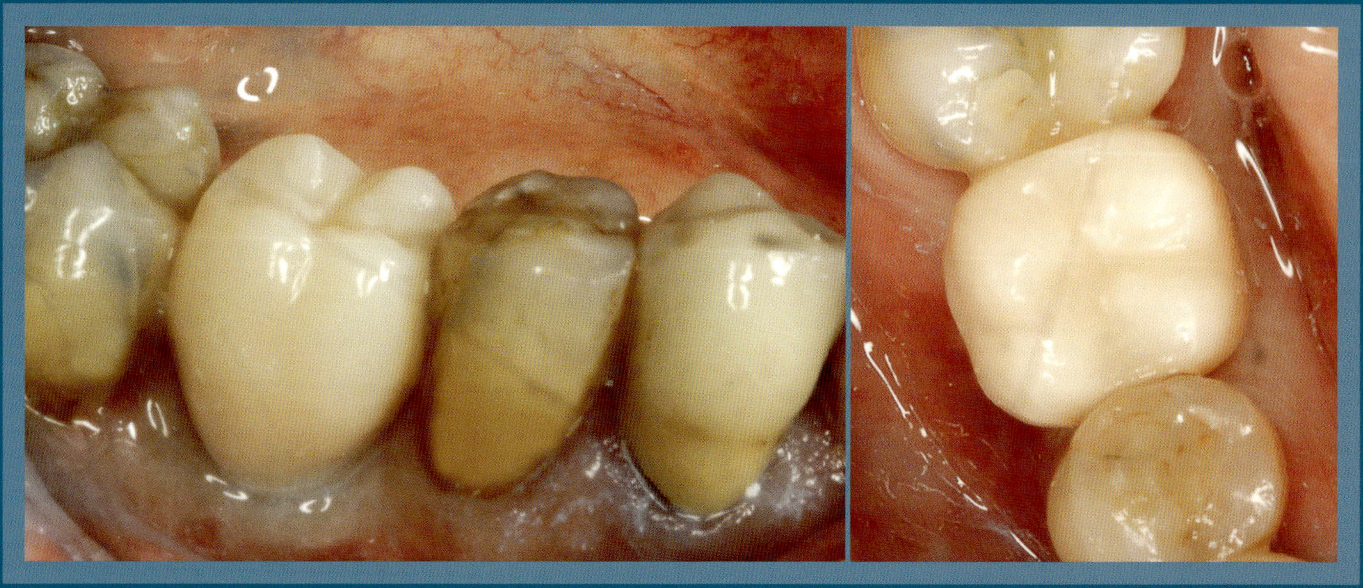

4.25 A PMMA provisional crown where a juxtapositional margin was cemented.

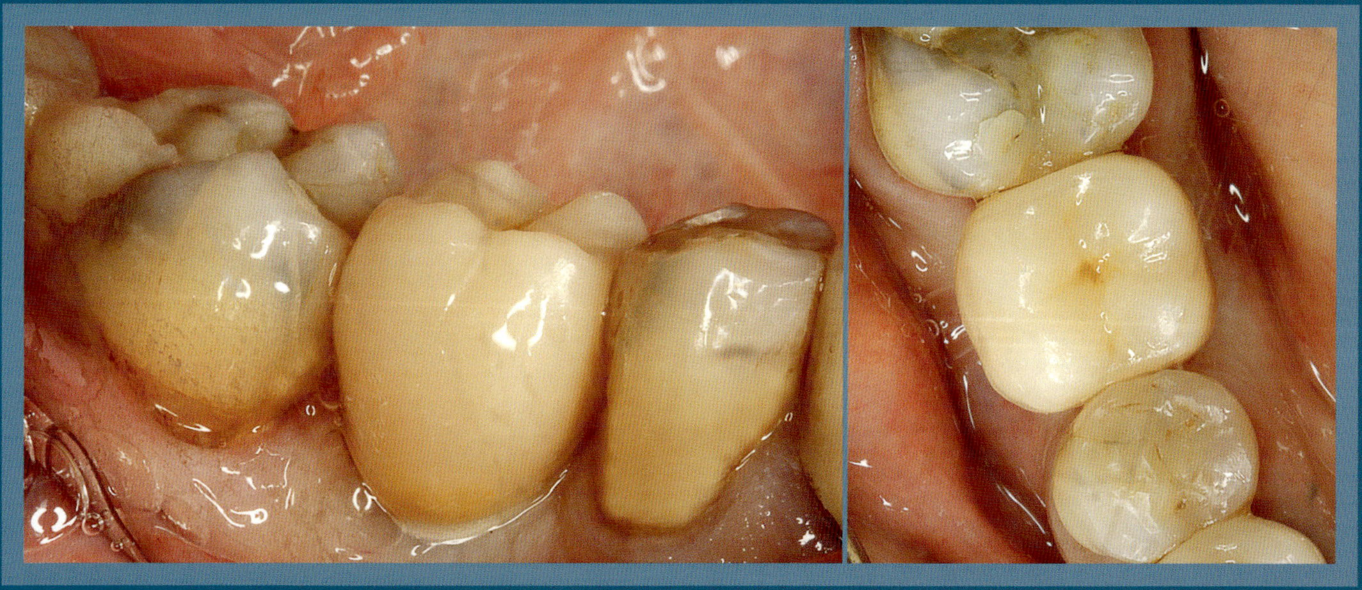

4.26 The final lithium disilicate crown is cemented.

Solutions for complex cases

In some cases, it might be necessary to apply expansion techniques of the residual crest and/or bone regeneration, which must always be guided by the position of the future prosthetic work. Here, it is of the utmost importance that the guide ensures absolute precision in implant placement. In the case illustrated below, the patient was requesting to rehabilitate with a fixed prosthesis the anterior region, where a severe resorption of bone volumes can be observed (4.27–4.43).

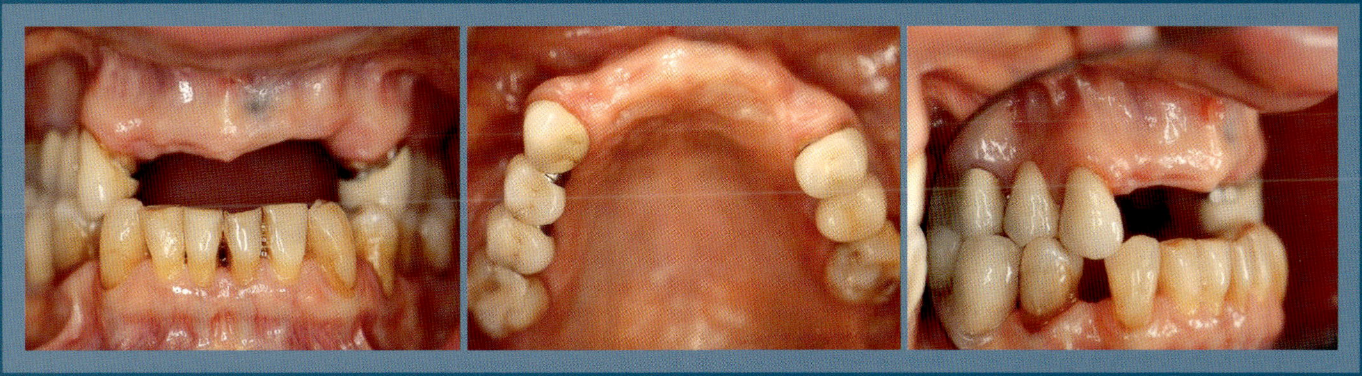

4.27 On the first visit, edentulism in the anterior region with severe resorption of the bone crest is observed.

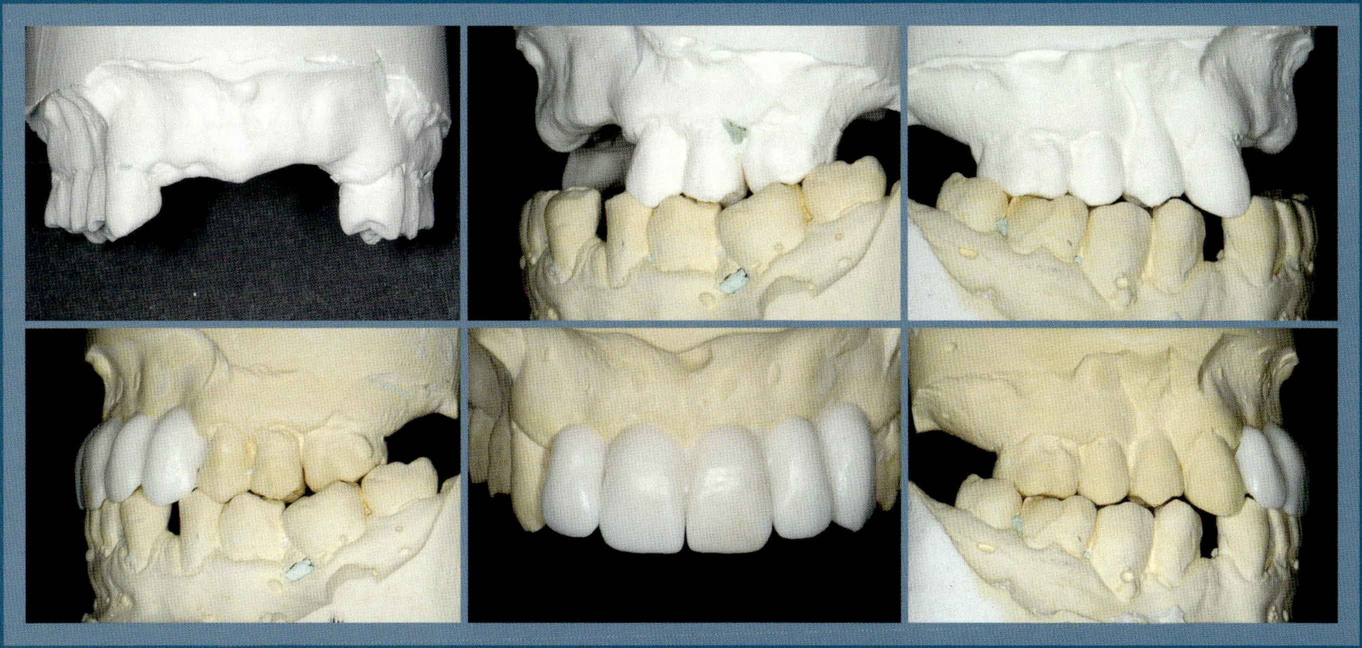

4.28 A gypsum model is cast, on which a wax-up of the missing teeth is performed. Unlike this case, which was treated a few years ago, nowadays this procedure is wholly carried out with digital techniques.

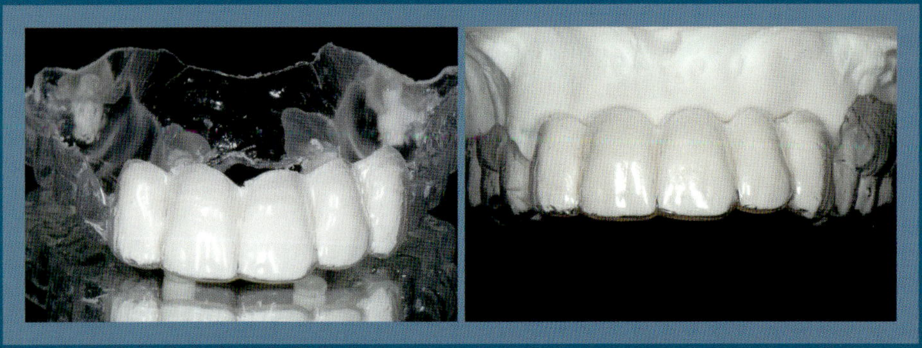

4.29 A radiological template is made, which simulates the position of future implant-supported crowns. The missing teeth are coated with barium.

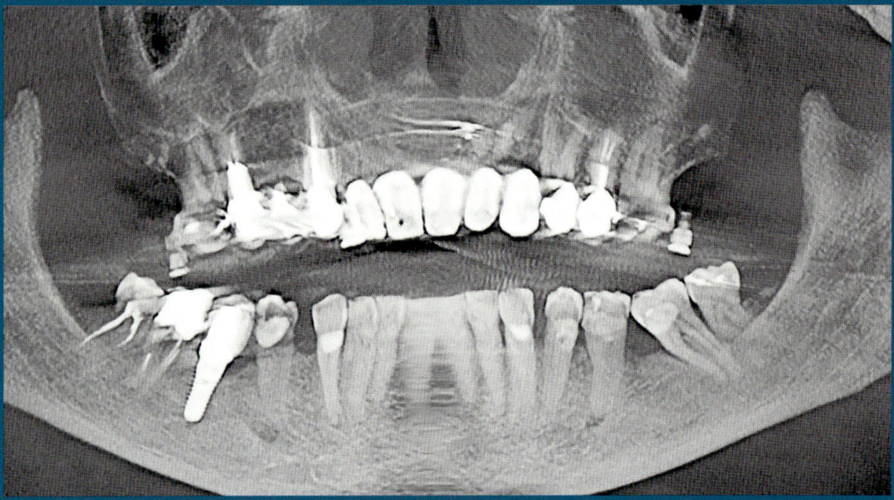

4.30 A CBCT scan is performed, which makes it possible to identify the position of the future restorations thanks to their radiopacity.

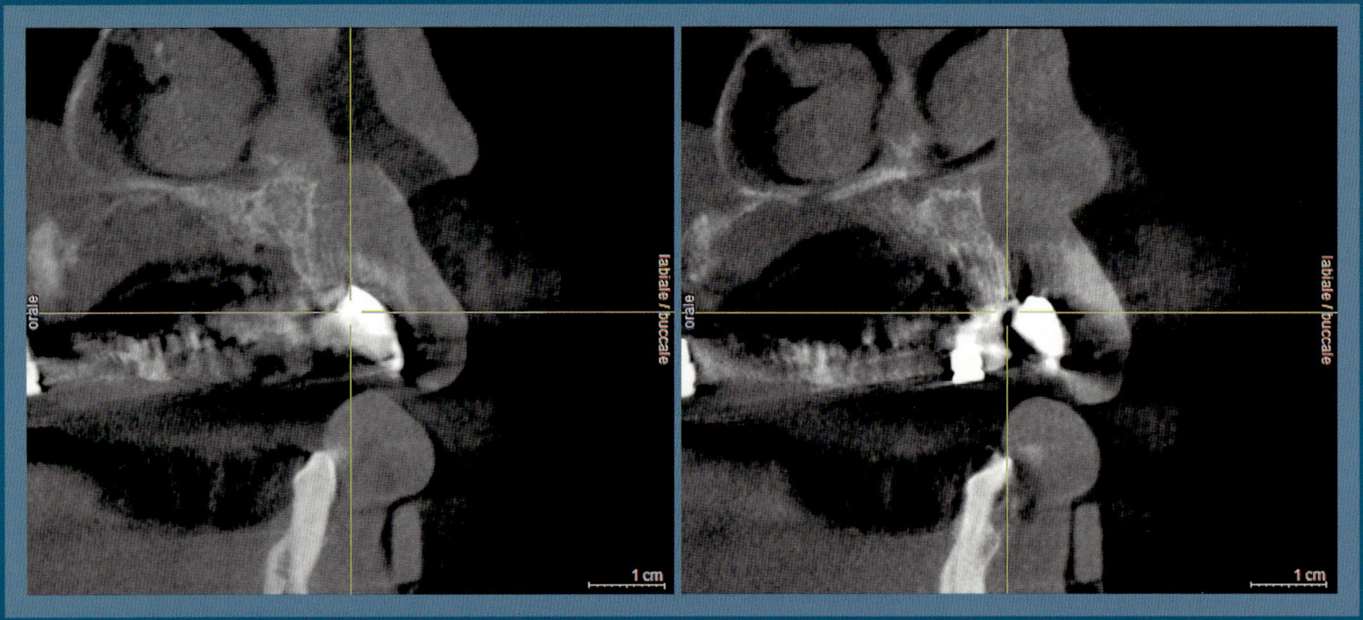

4.31 It is evident how the position of the restorations is completely outside the bone contour.

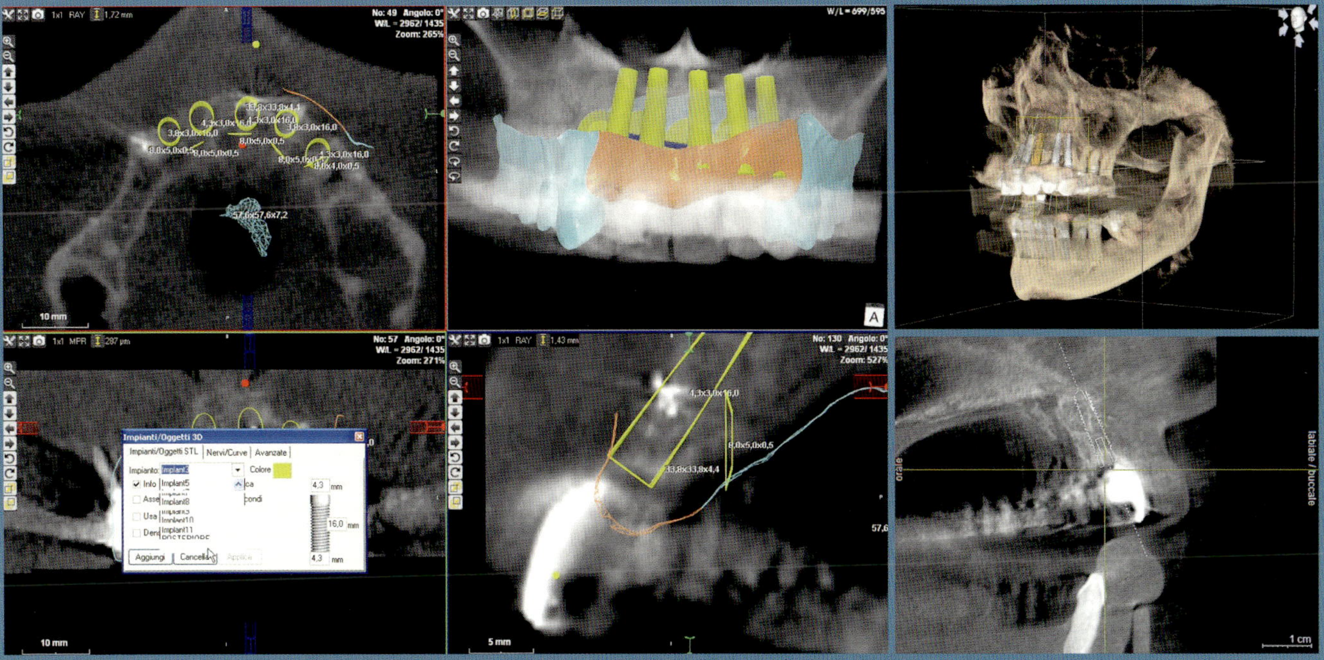

4.32 The position of the implants is planned, based on the prosthesis and not based on the available bone, already taking into account the need to resort to crest expansion procedures.

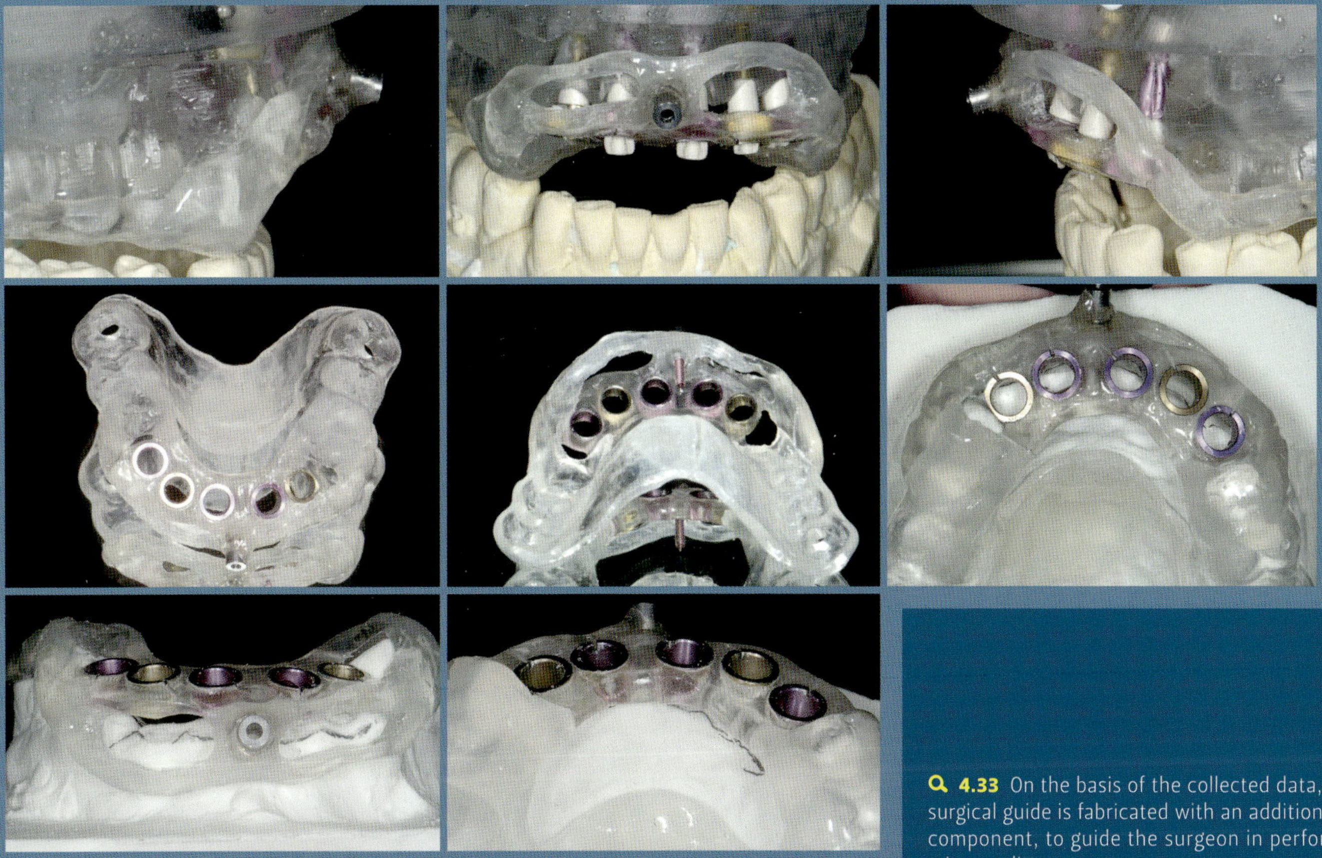

4.33 On the basis of the collected data, a surgical guide is fabricated with an additional component, to guide the surgeon in performing a split crest.

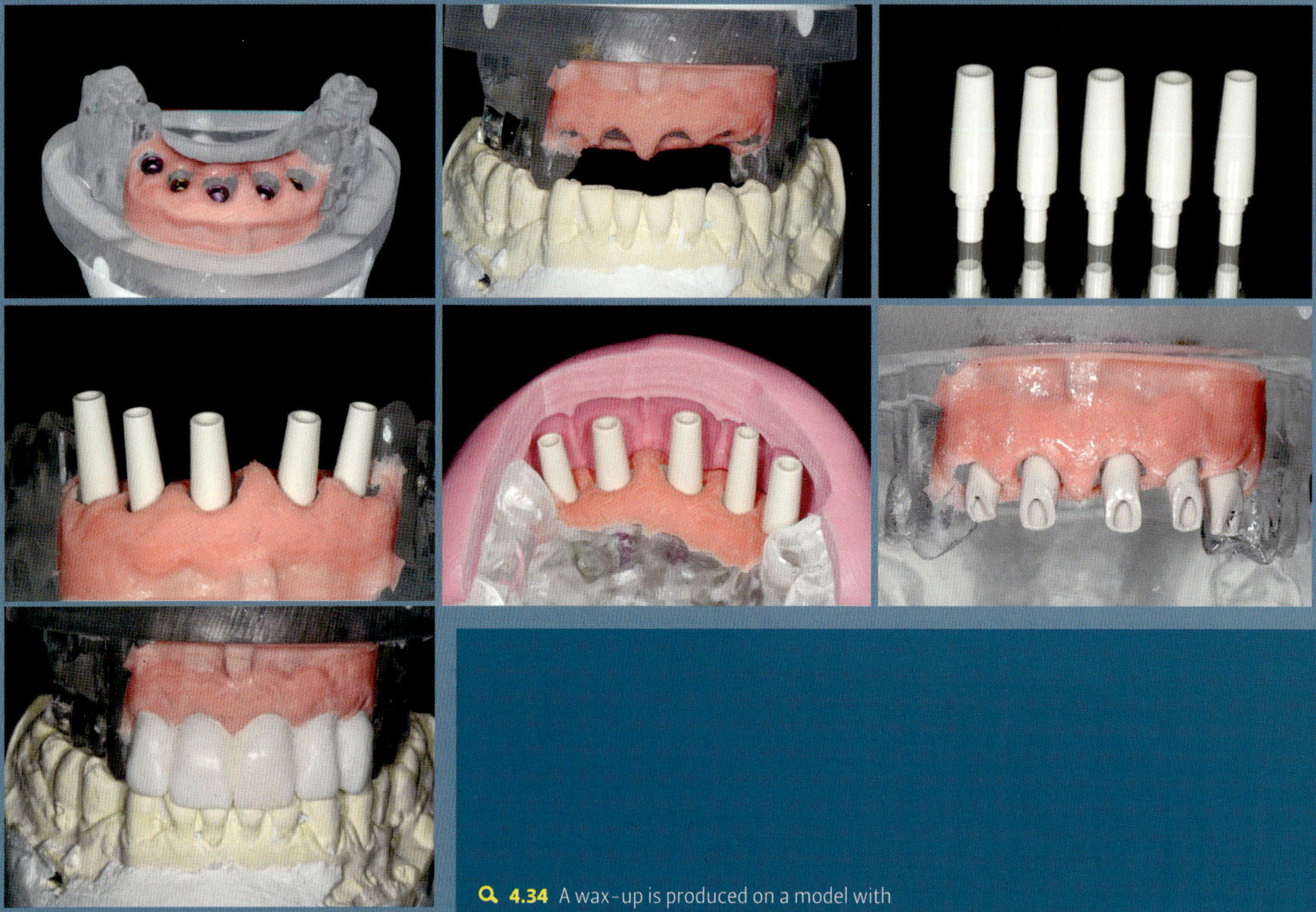

4.34 A wax-up is produced on a model with silicone gingiva, using PEEK abutments.

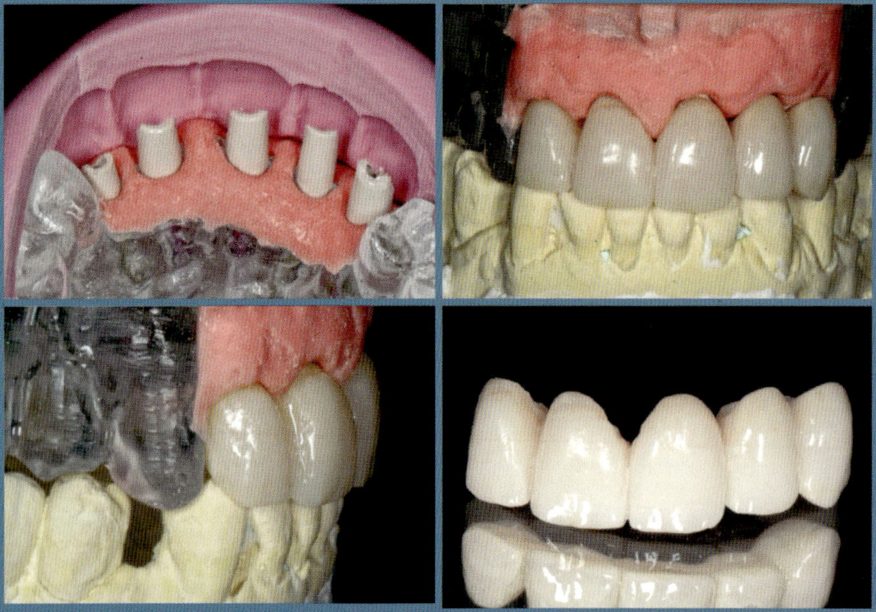

4.35 Even before surgery, the laboratory makes a provisional bridge with correct occlusion, which only needs to be relined on the abutments once the implants have been inserted.

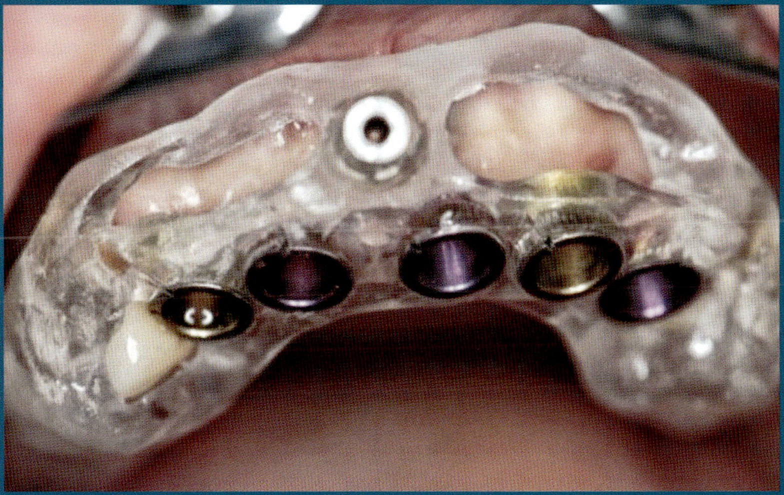

4.36 The index is secured in the patient's mouth by means of the appropriate pins.

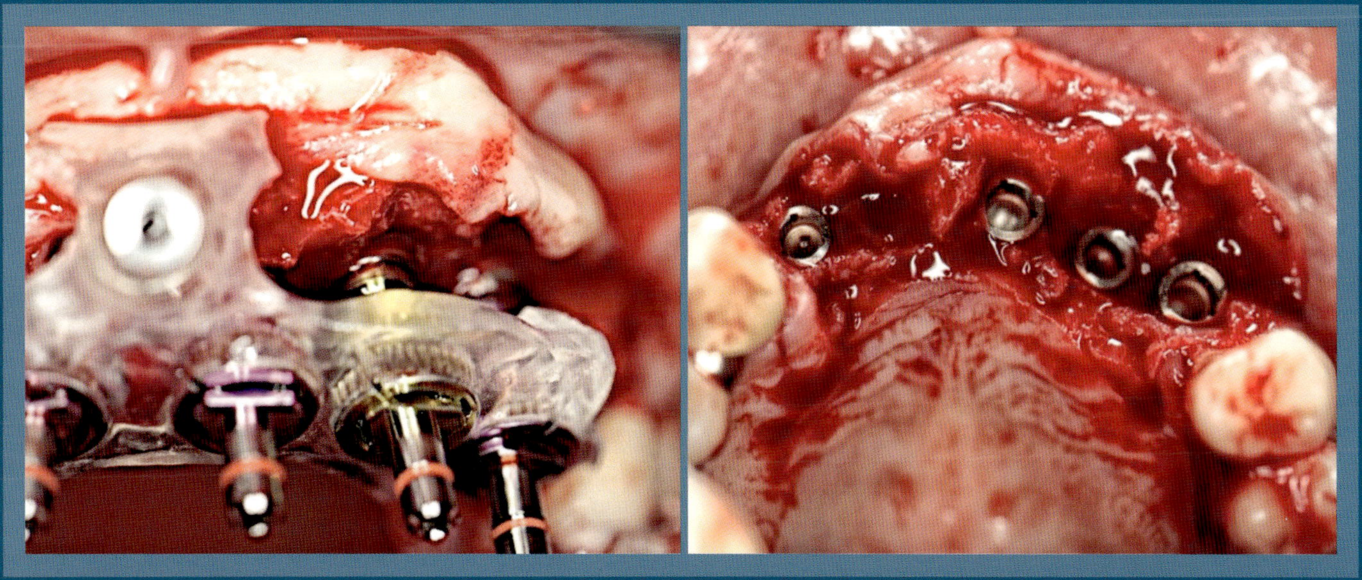

4.37 Once bone distraction has been executed, the implants are inserted, achieving an adequate torque for immediate loading.

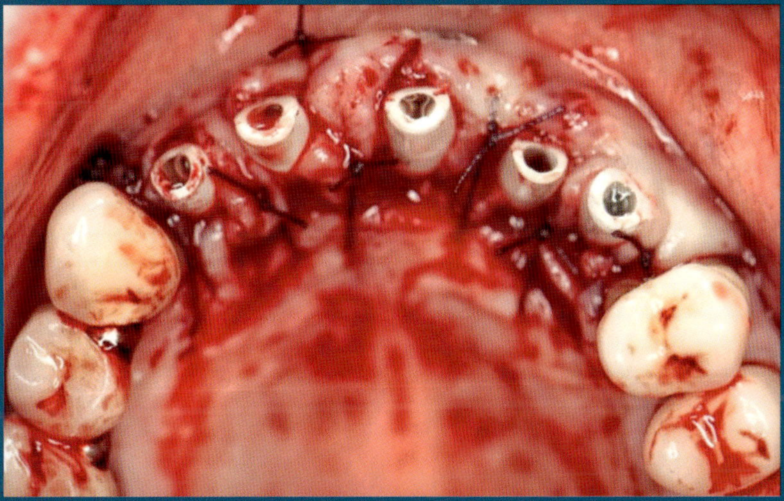

4.38 The provisional abutments are screwed onto the implants.

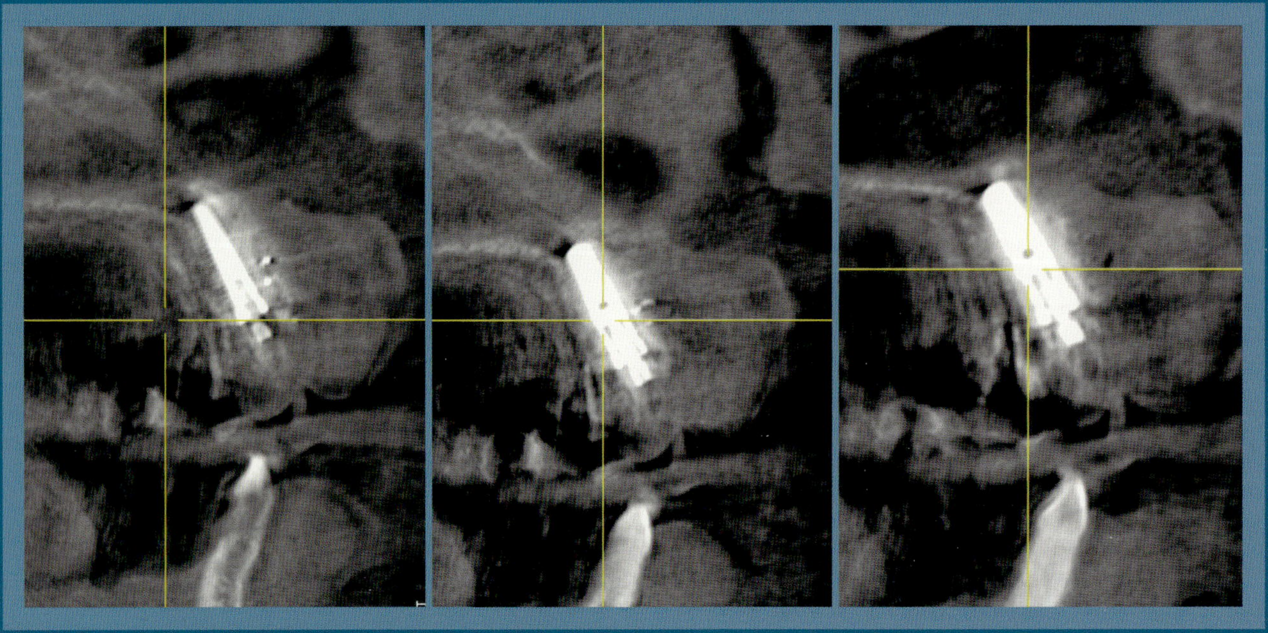

4.39 The post-operative CBCT shows how the implants are now entirely included in the bone volume.

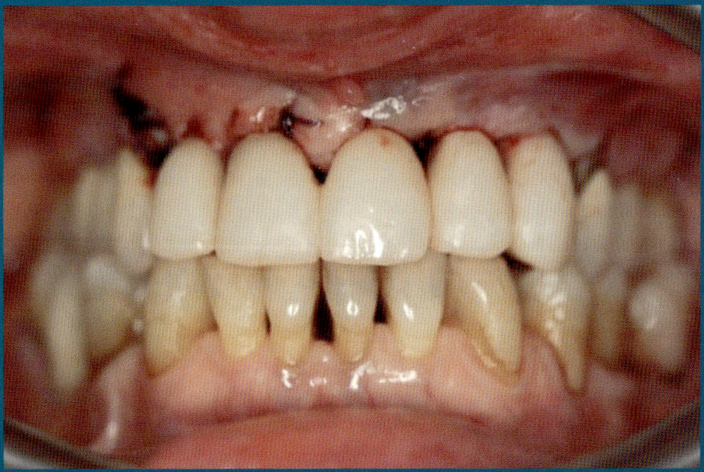

4.40 The provisional bridge is relined, finished and cemented.

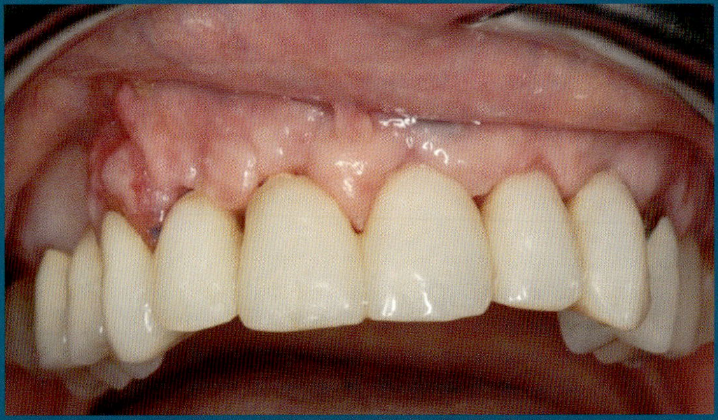

4.41 The 14-day follow-up for removal of the sutures already shows good restoration of soft tissue volume.

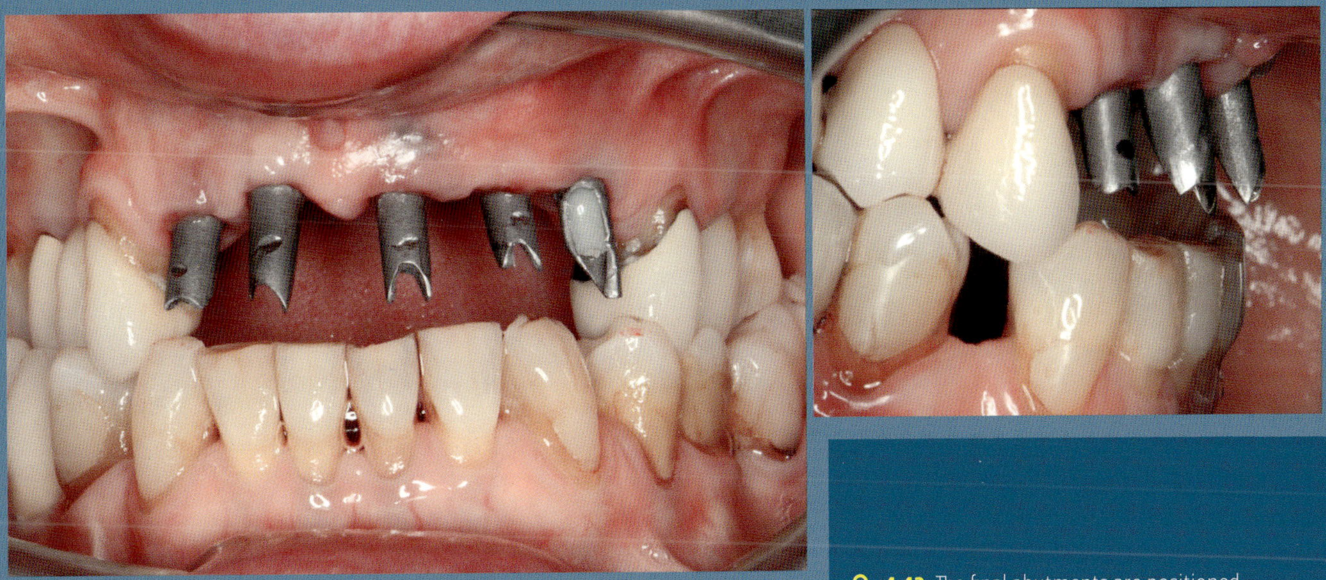

4.42 The final abutments are positioned.

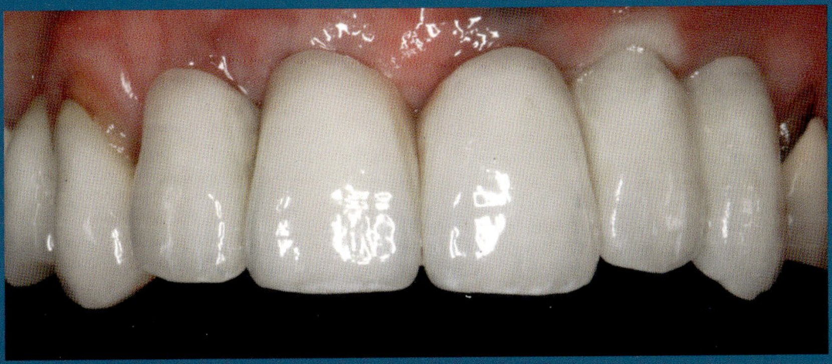

4.43 Case finalization with the definitive prosthesis.

REFERENCES

1. DAVIDOWITZ G, KOTICK PG. The Use of CAD/CAM in Dentistry. Dental Clinics of North America 2011; 55(3): 559-70.
2. BARUFFALDI A, POLI PP, BARUFFALDI A ET AL. Computer-aided flapless implant surgery and immediate loading. A technical note. Oral and Maxillofacial Surgery 2016; 20(3): 313-9.
3. D'HAESE J, ACKHURST J, WISMEIJER D ET AL. Current state of the art of computer-guided implant surgery. Periodontology 2000 2016; 73(1): 121-33.

DIGIT technique

Alfonso Baruffaldi

This chapter describes the DIGIT (Dental Implant Guided Immediate Therapy) technique developed by the Authors, which is mainly used for fixed full arch rehabilitations by means of prostheses supported by six implants with a flapless surgical procedure.

The Toronto-type prosthesis (5.1) has become very popular in recent years,[1] largely because the immediate loading technique has shown success rates equaling that of delayed loading, in which the implants are allowed to heal without being subjected to stress due to loading immediately after insertion.

Although the one-year survival rate of implants placed by guided surgery ranges from 89% to 100%, the corresponding prostheses have demonstrated a survival rate between 62% and 100%.[2] This may be due to a number of factors which could be classified as postoperative complications, such as, for example, prosthesis fracture, screws loosening, poor precision when connecting to the superstructure, or the need to perform extensive occlusal adjustments.

A possible explanation may be the difficulty in correctly placing the prosthesis during rebasing procedures. Indeed, provisional prostheses either wholly made of resin, or including metal reinforcement structures, are traditionally delivered to the patient immediately after the procedure. The unavoidable slight inaccuracy between the position of the implant in pre-surgical planning and the actual position, is offset by a small space between the abutments and the prosthesis, which will then be filled during the rebasing stage.

However, in cases in which partial edentulism turns into total edentulism, following the extraction of teeth and/or implants, all the reference points taken in the design stage are lost as a result of the changes that occur in hard and soft tissues.

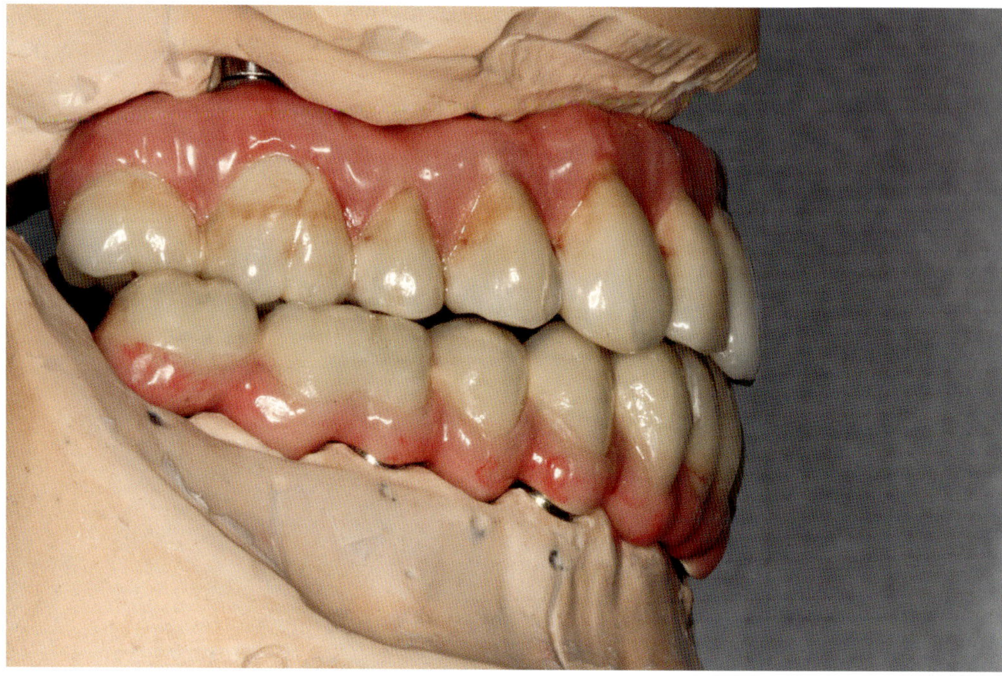

5.1 Example of lower and upper "Toronto" prostheses: the fixed prostheses are supported by implants.

Specifically, it can be difficult to establish the proper vertical dimension and balancing of occlusion during the rebasing procedures of the provisional prosthesis.

Another factor to be taken into account is the likelihood of the patient not being fully cooperative owing to possible sedation and anesthesia.

There are no publications in the literature concerning the precision of the transferring process from the models in the articulator to the intraoral final position of the prosthesis, neither with regard to the designed VDO, nor to proper occlusion.

The Authors sought to address this issue with a first working hypothesis described in our publication,[3] by using the same pins used to stabilize the guide in the surgical stage, to secure the prosthesis in a certain position during procedures for rebasing and cementing the retentive conometric copings in the structure. An incorrect placement of the prosthesis might well lead to the build-up of torsional moment and high load stress, which cause multiple complications of a prosthetic as well as biological nature (bone remodeling, micro-fractures, loss of osseointegration), and could explain the high rate of failures. [4]

The DIGIT technique has been developed with the aim of maintaining the points of reference that are normally lost in the transition from the surgical guide stent to placement of the provisional prosthesis.[5] Unlike previous techniques, this method allows the operator to switch, with the same degree of precision, from surgical guide placement to the provisional fixed prosthesis, without ever changing the existing references. This not only makes it possible to minimize complications,[6,7] but also to limit the components of the procedure and of the post-surgery stages that are still operator-dependent.

The purpose is therefore to reduce prosthetic inaccuracies and the likelihood of the onset of complications, thus increasing the predictability of the restoration.[8]

Obviously, this surgical technique can only be applied to patients who have adequate dimensions of the residual bone crest, in order to keep at least 1 mm of bone around the implants, both on their vestibular and lingual/palatal sides. Specifically, the minimum recommended dimensions for the interforaminal region in the mandible are at least 4 mm in bucco-lingual direction and more than 8 mm in the apico-coronal direction. With regard to the anterior (canine to canine) maxilla, however, the minimum thickness in the bucco-palatal direction is also 4 mm, whereas in the apical-coronal direction it is equal to 10 mm. Soft tissues must also be properly present, with a band of keratinized gingiva of at least 3 mm, circumferential to the surgical site. Prior to surgery, it is essential that good hygienic maintenance is ensured both by the clinician, through preliminary periodontal debridement and a recall every four months, and also – and above all – by the patient themselves, who must be educated on oral hygiene procedures to be implemented in the healing period as well as thereafter.

The DIGIT technique for Toronto Bridges

Based on the initial situation, three types of workflow can be described which will then converge into a common pathway after the first data collection stages:

1. complete edentulism;
2. partial edentulism with presence of metal restorations;
3. partial edentulism.

WORKFLOW FOR COMPLETE EDENTULISM

The first step consists of taking a first optical impression of the two full arches, using an intra-oral scanner (5.2), registering the VDO and the occlusion. At this stage, great attention must be paid so that the impres-

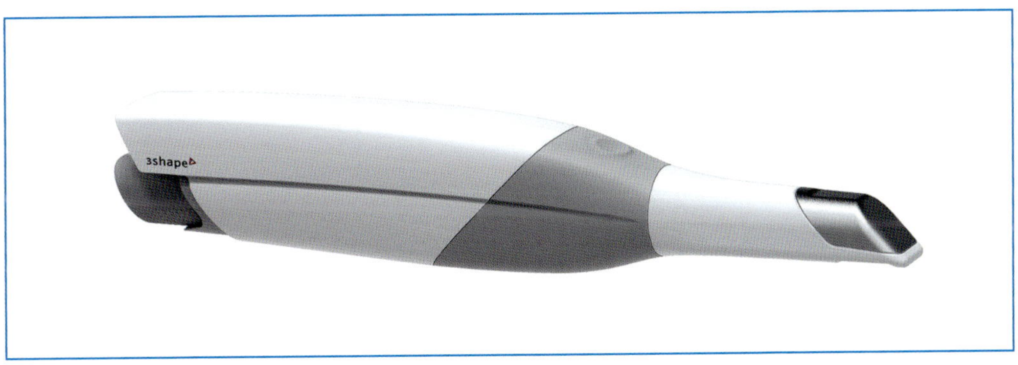

5.2 Intraoral scanner.

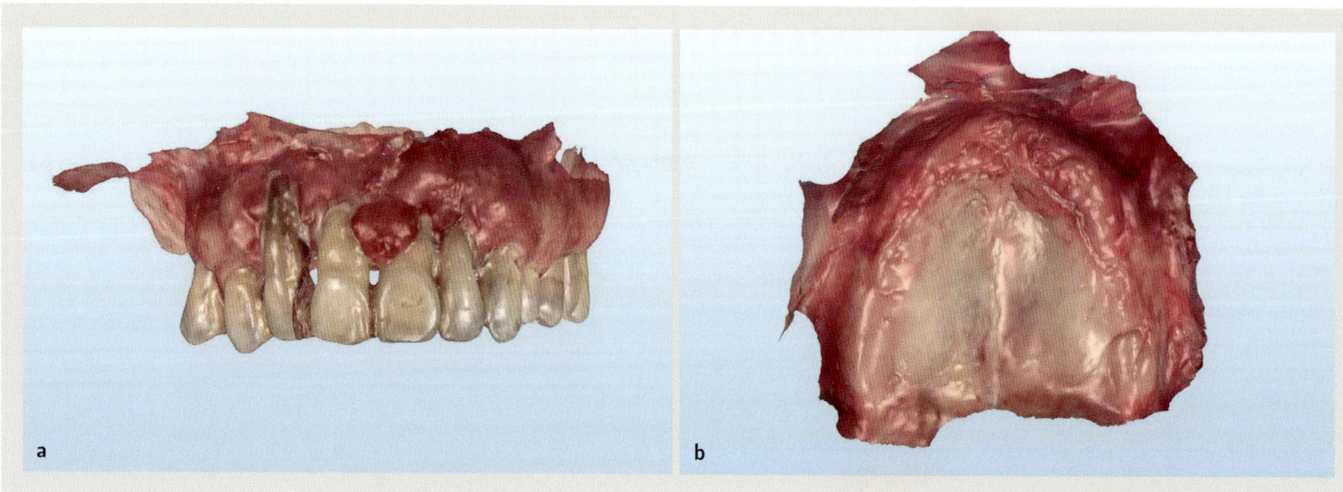

5.3 **a,b)** Optical impression with an adequate presence of soft tissues.

sion includes as much as possible the soft tissues (vestibule, palate and lingual or palatal aspect of the alveolar ridges) (5.3 a,b).

The study models are imported into CAD software, such as 3Shape or Exocad, placed in the virtual articulator and studied by the clinician to first produce a digital wax-up (see 5.4), which is an exact replica of the final prosthesis and which may be shown to the patient, so as to integrate functional and esthetic demands. The wax-up is fabricated according to the indications of the Skyn Concept technique, to be described later. Furthermore, in the case of edentulous patients, proper spaces are included in the wax-up to house radiopaque markers, which are applied once the piece is produced with a 3D printer, again using appropriate software (5.5 and 5.6).

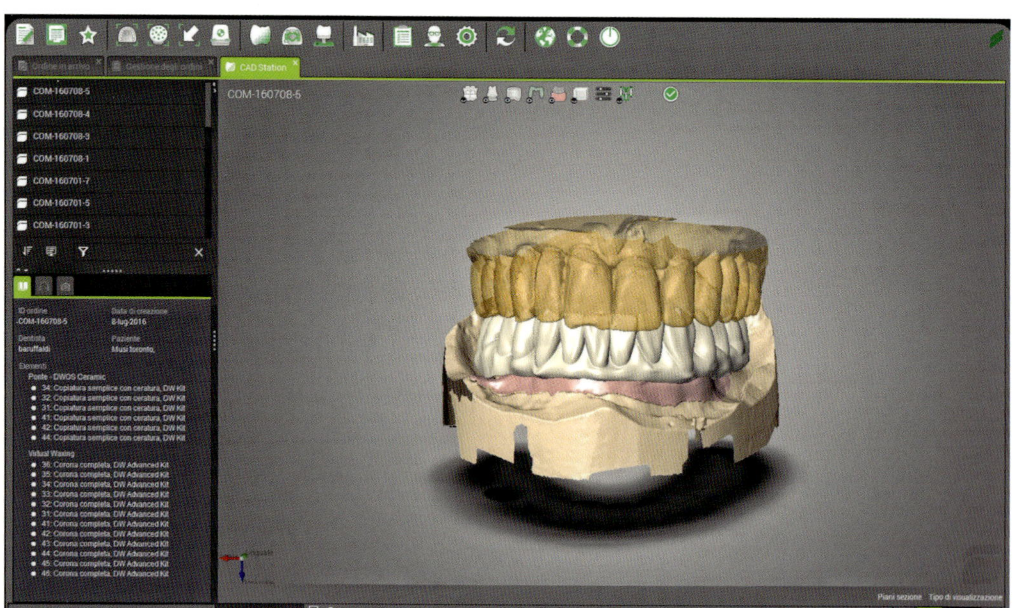

5.4 Wax-up created virtually with CAD software.

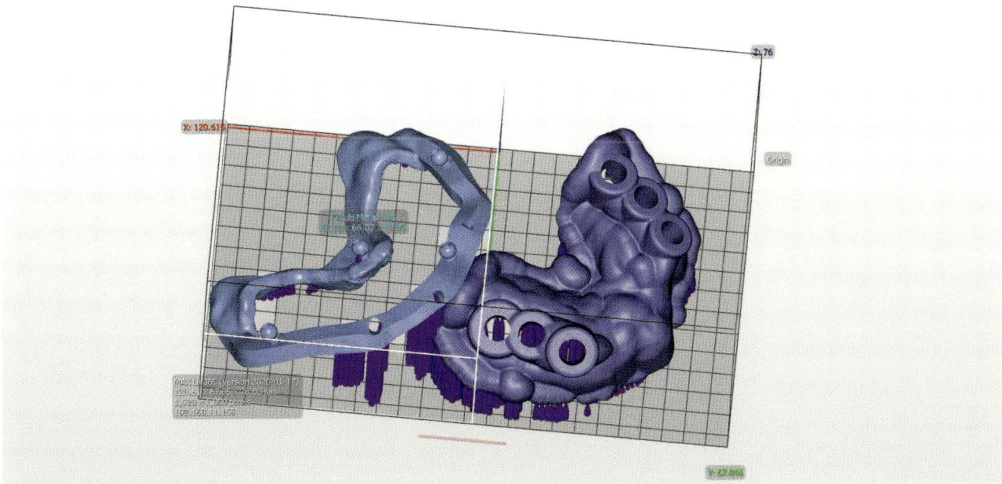

5.5 The STL file of the diagnostic index is imported into a suitable software, in order to be printed with a 3D printer.

To complete this stage, the models (arch to be rehabilitated, antagonist and occlusion) are exported in STL format as separate files in a single folder, to be used later in the digital workflow.
The second stage is the radiographic investigation. A transparent resin radiographic template replicating the wax-up, as described above, is used.

While performing the X-ray examination, the index (5.7) fitted with radiopaque markers – required for matching the intraoral scans with the radiographic examination – is kept in occlusion with the antagonist, to replicate as

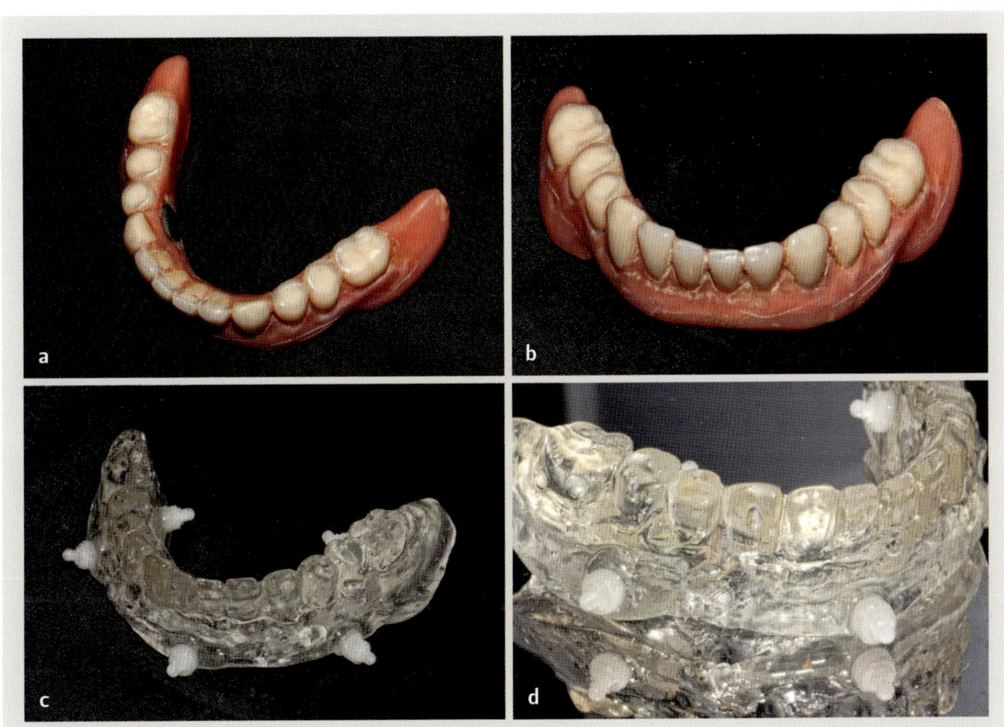

5.6 Index with landmarks printed by duplicating the existing complete denture.

faithfully as possible the compression that the surgical index, locked by the intra-bony pins, will exert on them during the procedure (5.8).

An existing denture can be used as guide to manufacture the Toronto prosthesis, so a duplicate is made in clear resin. This procedure entails a scan of the prosthesis, which is also transformed into an STL file (see 5.6). The choice not to directly use an index with barium teeth as landmarks, which might provide indications for the proper design of the implant position starting from the prosthetic design, is due to the fact that this would pose a constraint when designing a proper and modifiable mock-up, built with the appropriate software. As shown in (5.9), the landmarks must be outside the prosthesis in order to replicate the position also on our scan, to be able to match it seamlessly to the DICOM data.

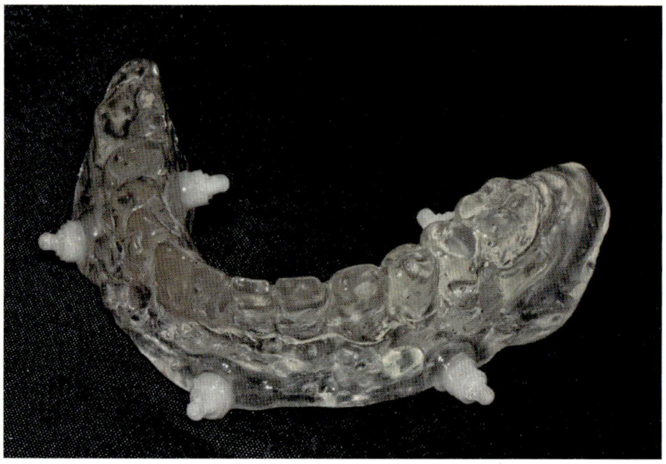

5.7 Radiographic template with radiopaque markers.

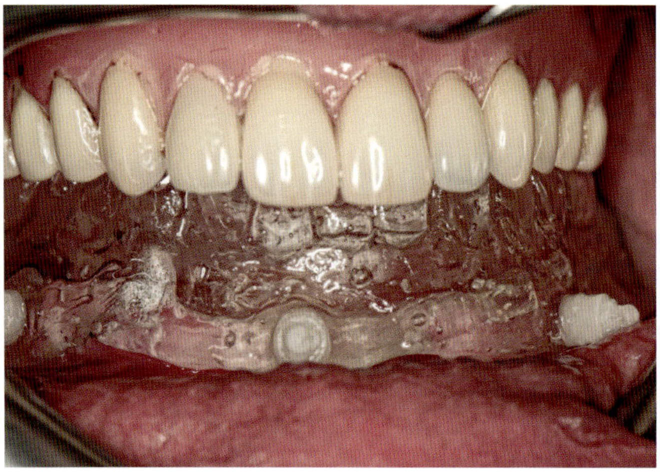

5.8 Radiographic template placed in the patient's mouth ready to undergo X-ray examination and stabilized by means of occlusion with the antagonist. In this case, it is a replica in clear resin of the existing denture, fitted with radiopaque landmarks.

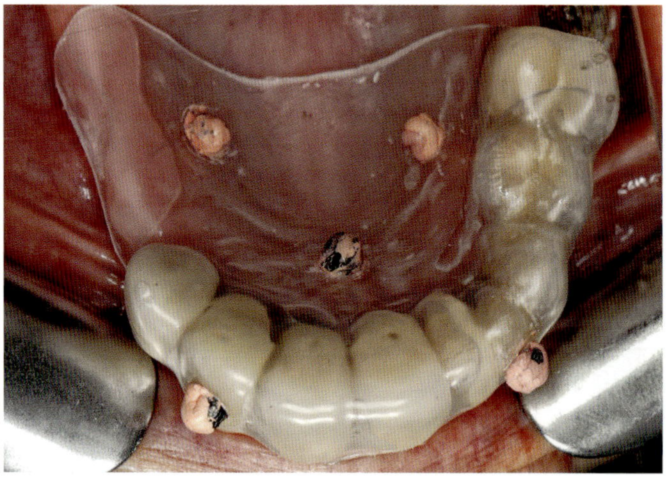

5.9 Transparent template with landmarks, which may be, as in this case, spheres of gutta-percha, a radiopaque material.

A CBCT scan of the patient's arch is then performed; at this stage, the clinician must ensure that:

- the FOV (Field Of View) is sufficiently wide to allow the radiographic data to be matched to the models generated in STL format, therefore also including the radiopaque markers (5.10);
- the radiographic template index exerts the same pressure on soft tissues as the surgical guide to be fabricated.

Once the CBCT examination is performed (5.10), in order to match the 3D radiographic examination to the STL file - containing the patient's anatomy - and the mock-up, the radiographic template must be captured, by means of intraoral or laboratory scanner (5.11). Thanks to the presence of landmarks in both files, matching will be straightforward.
To sum up, the scans must produce files in STL format including the following:

- arch to be rehabilitated with landmarks (teeth or radiopaque landmarks), displayed in two files, one for hard tissues and the second for soft tissues;
- antagonist arch;
- occlusion (5.12);
- any biocopy (if there is a situation to be replicated prior to extractions) or mock-up (5.13).

The file exported in STL format is assembled with the radiographic images deriving from the CBCT examination, in DICOM format, in the software chosen for design and fabrication - for instance, 3Shape Implant Studio, coDiagnosticX (Dentalwings) or Realguide (3Diemme) (5.13).

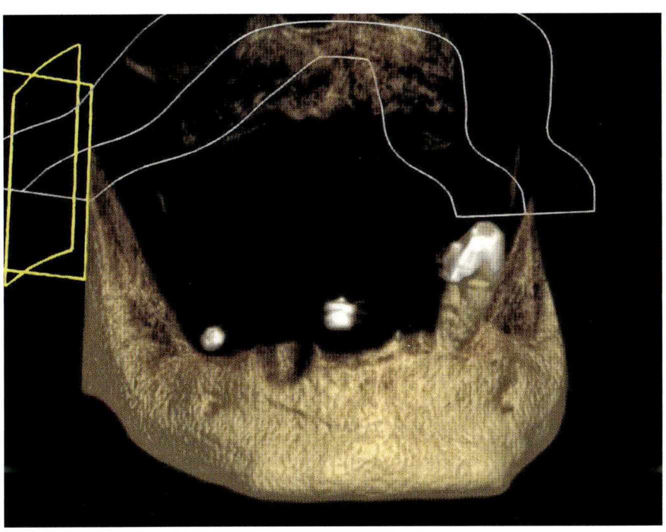

5.10 CBCT including the landmarks.

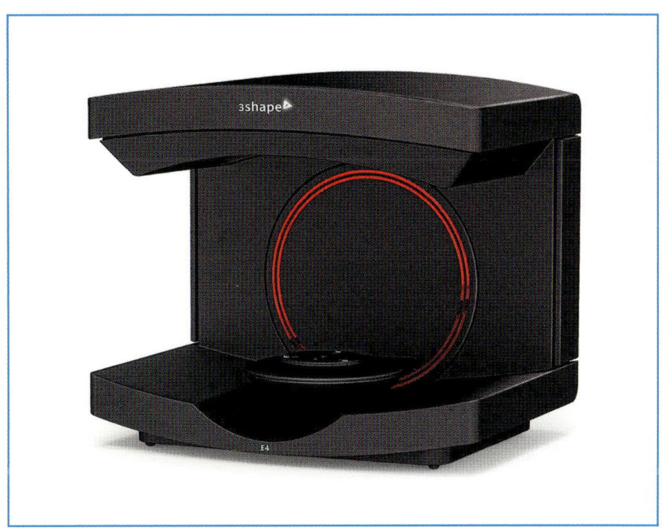

5.11 Laboratory scanner.

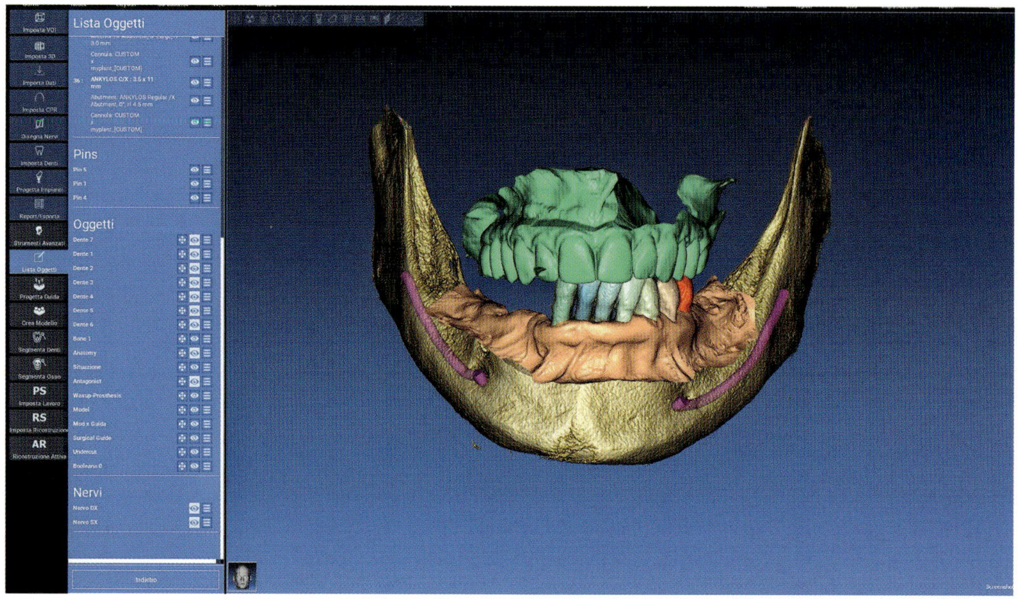

5.12 Matched STL files: arch to be rehabilitated, soft tissues, antagonist, occlusion.

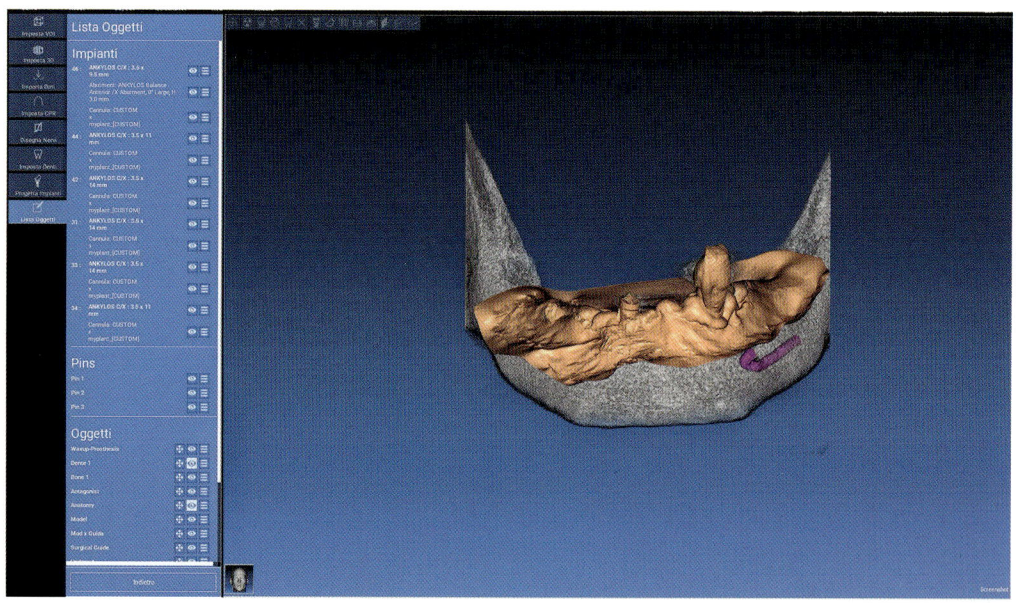

5.13 The STL files originating from the optical impression are matched to the DICOM files obtained from the CBCT examination, using the residual teeth – although they need to be extracted – as markers, enabling to plan the implant position.

WORKFLOW FOR PARTIAL EDENTULISM WITH PRESENCE OF METAL RESTORATIONS

In cases of partial edentulism with presence of metal restorations, the procedure is similar to that applied in cases of complete edentulism. In order to prevent any metal artefacts from affecting the possibilities of precise matching, an index with landmarks must also be fabricated in this case, as described above. A simple way to fabricate a radiographic template, in cases of partial edentulism with presence of metal restorations, is to insert landmarks in radiopaque material, which may be gutta-percha balls, into a clear guide (see 5.9).

WORKFLOW FOR PARTIAL EDENTULISM

In the case of a partially edentulous patient, who does not have many metal restorations, our technique does not require the presence of radiographic templates. Therefore, no landmarks are inserted in the mouth, according to the protocol used in cases of partially dentate patients. The removable prostheses are removed to perform both optical impressions and radiographic investigations. In cases where the patient still has some teeth, albeit in need of extraction, they are kept during this stage, so that they can be used as points of reference (markers).

Common workflow

From now on, the above pathways converge.

Matching will be carried out by using the residual teeth, if any, or the landmarks described above, to be able to match the 3D radiographic images which will be obtained with the CBCT technique. At least three markers or natural teeth are required, distributed along the entire arch (5.13 and 5.14).

Once the two scans are imported in the implant design software, the wax-up is matched, which will serve as prosthetic guide in identifying the proper implant positions. The virtual wax-up is produced in accordance with Skyn Concept principles (5.15).

The implant positions are identified, on one hand assessing the prosthesis, which will be fabricated through the mock-up and on the other, the bone anatomy (5.16).

The surgical index is then designed, starting from the number and position of the implants. Mucosa-supported indexes are generally used - unless there are areas to be regenerated, for which bone support is used to be able to open a flap.

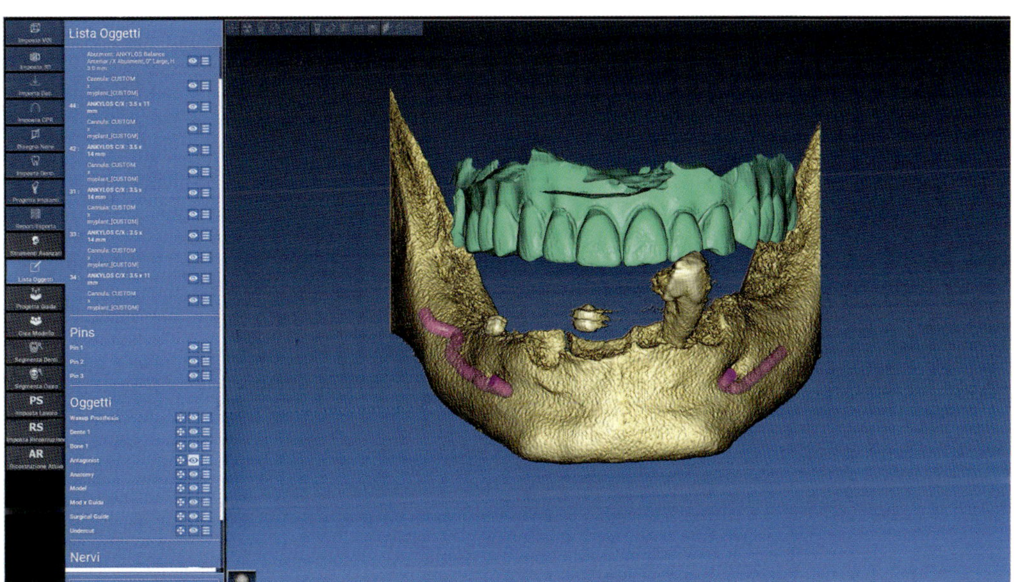

5.14 Should a minimum of three natural landmarks be unavailable, radiopaque markers are used.

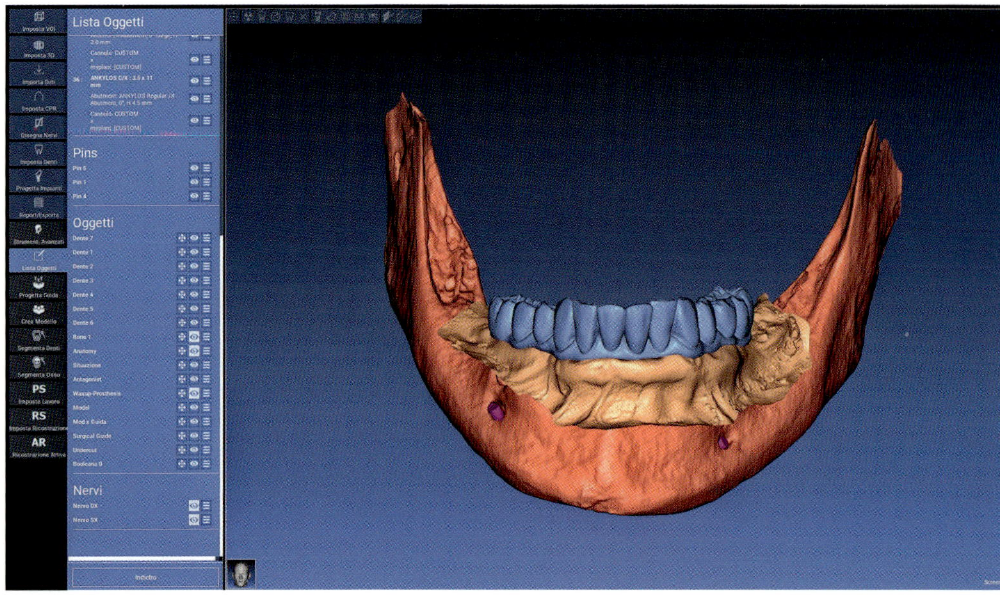

5.15 The mock-up is also imported.

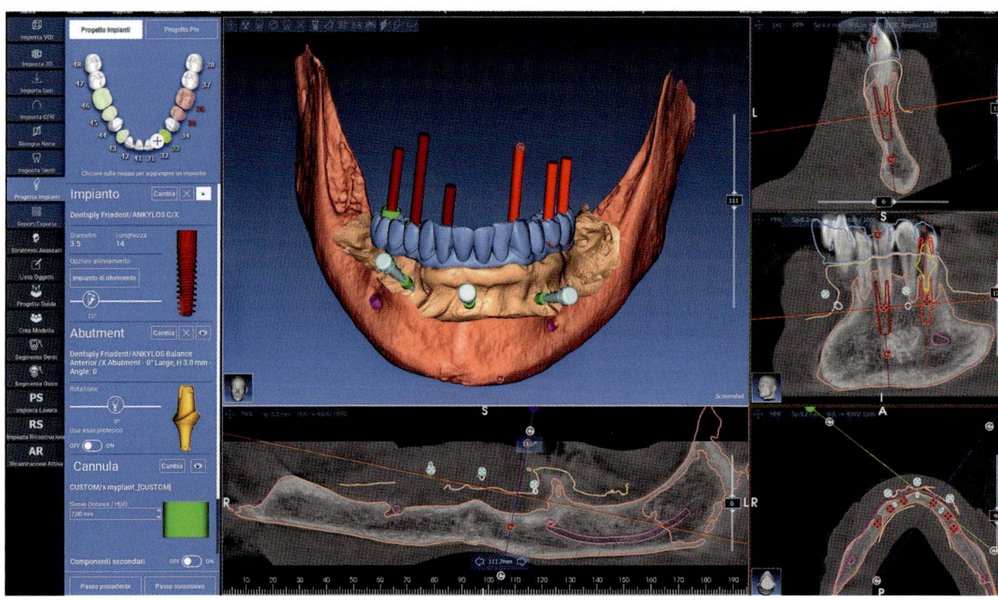

5.16 The implants are planned considering, on one hand, the mock-up, and on the other the available bone.

Prosthetic design also entails the selection of implant abutments. The Authors prefer using abutments for conometric prosthodontics, selecting them based on the abutment height and angle. The abutments must be parallel. In fixed conometric prosthodontics, it is important to check the spaces for proper placement of abutments and copings.

The components of the surgical index are designed with CAD software, specifically:

- the base of the index (Part B) (5.17), which will remain in position throughout the procedure.[9,10] It must include slots for the intra-osseous pins and retentive attachments for the interchangeable parts, which we shall refer to as type A secondary indexes. When designing the pin position, the clinician

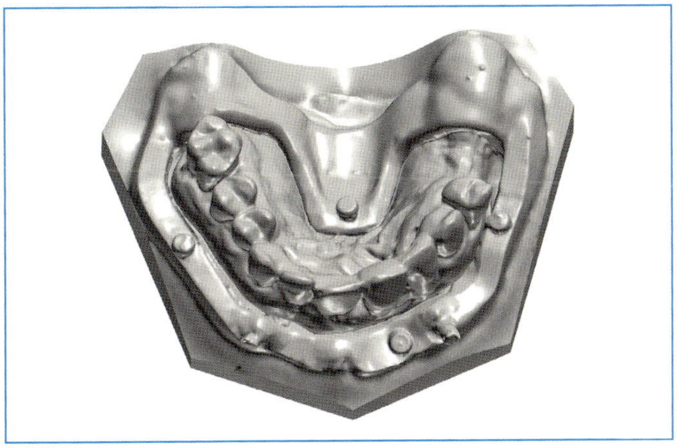

5.17 Part B of the index is designed.

ought to consider, on one hand, the position of the teeth to be extracted, and on the other, the position of the implant sites that are created so as not to generate interference;

- the interchangeable parts. These are the secondary tooth-supported – if any – indexes, that allow the pins to be fixated in the proper position. Therefore, Part A is supported by any teeth still present and is used to stabilize Part B, which will stay in place throughout the procedure (5.18). In the event of total edentulism, the mock-up is 3D-printed, set in occlusion and stabilized by the pressure of the antagonist, guaranteeing that thc desired position is obtained (5.19).

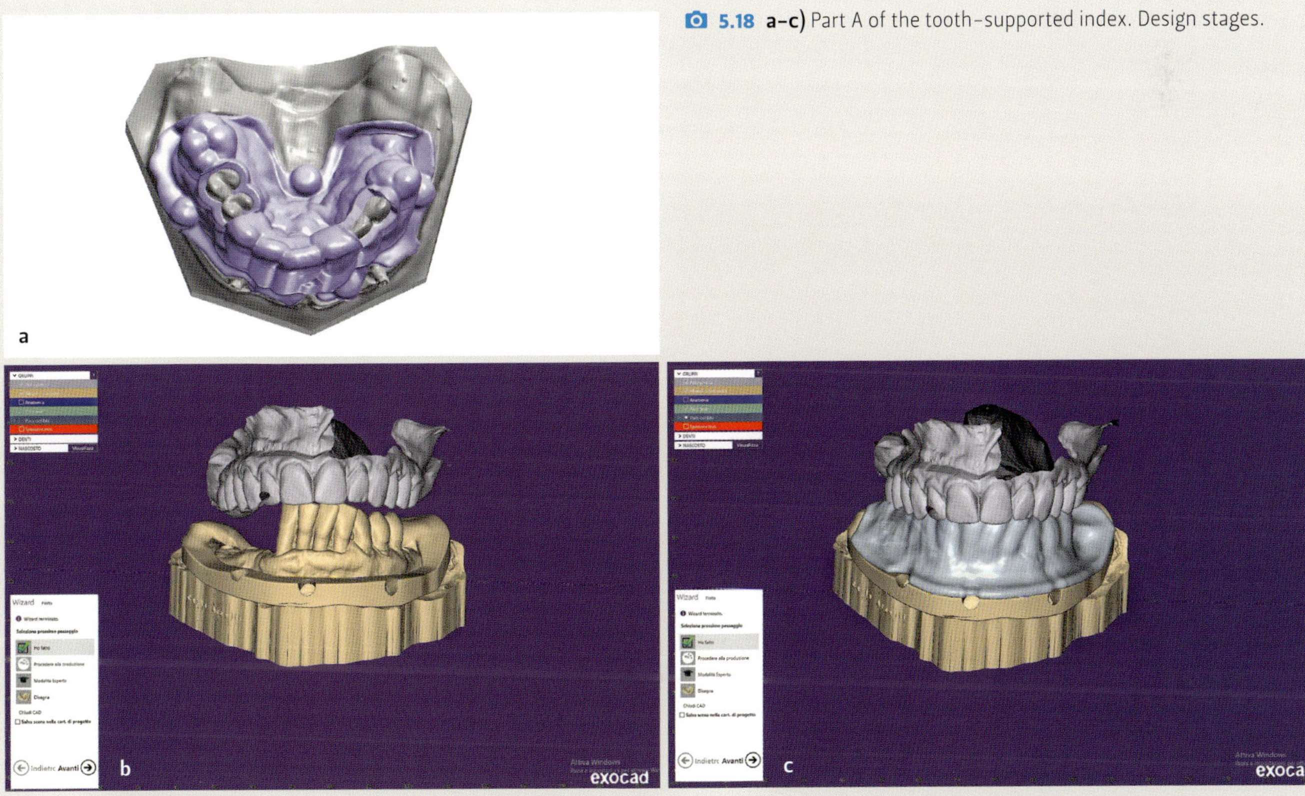

5.18 **a–c)** Part A of the tooth-supported index. Design stages.

The implant guide index (5.20) will be based on the designed prosthesis – preferably of conometric type – and must be fitted with connections for the retention attachments on the base of the index (5.21–5.23). Precision and maximum stabilization between the two components are essential.

All these components are physically manufactured once the design has been approved by the oral surgeon as well as by the prosthodontist, either machined by CAM milling machines or fabricated by 3D printing (5.24 and 5.25). In particular, the mesostructure of the prosthesis is fabricated in a glass fiber composite material, intertwined in a resin matrix, and the occlusal/esthetic component is fabricated in composite and lithium disilicate.

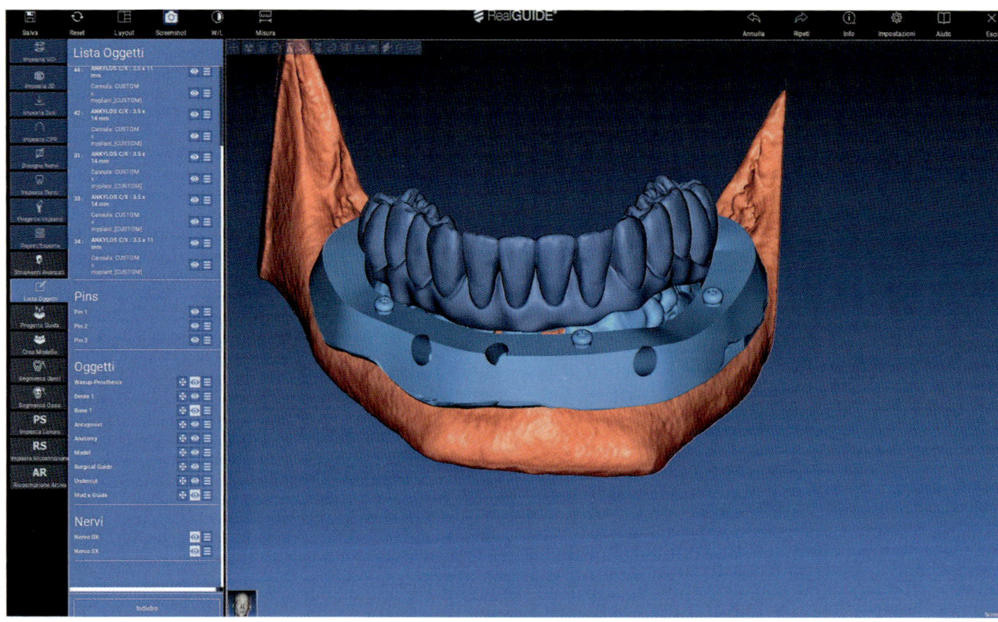

5.19 Mock-up as guide for stabilizing the prosthesis.

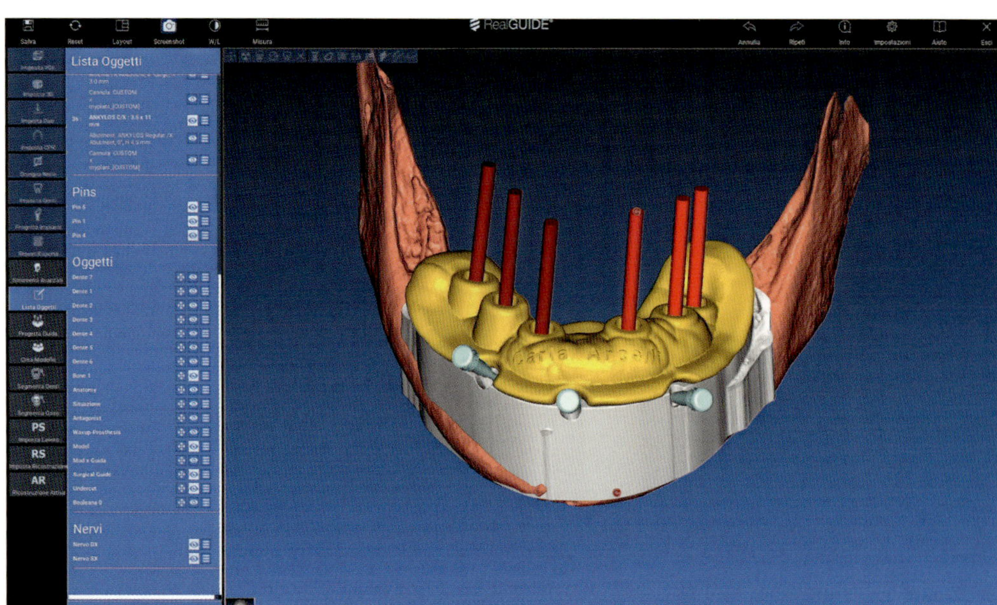

5.20 Design stage of the surgical guide in the CAD software. Index for implant insertion.

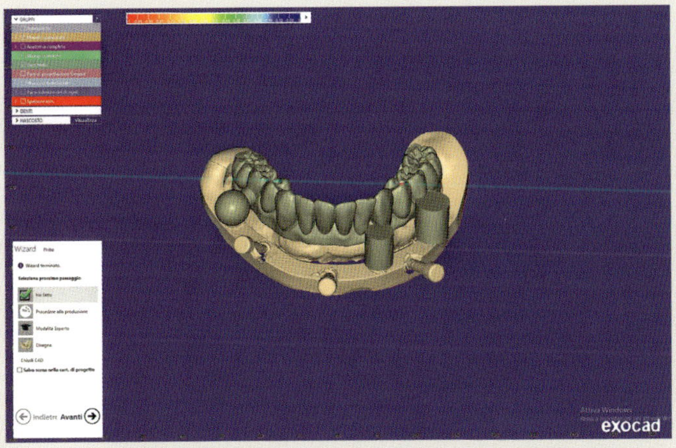

5.21 Prosthesis anchored to the retentive connections of Part B ready for rebasing, through which the conometric copings are encased.

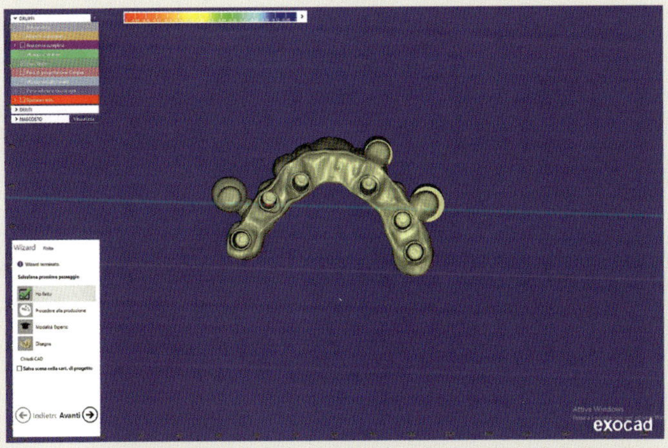

5.22 Detail of the housing that will hold the retention copings of the fixed conometric prosthesis.

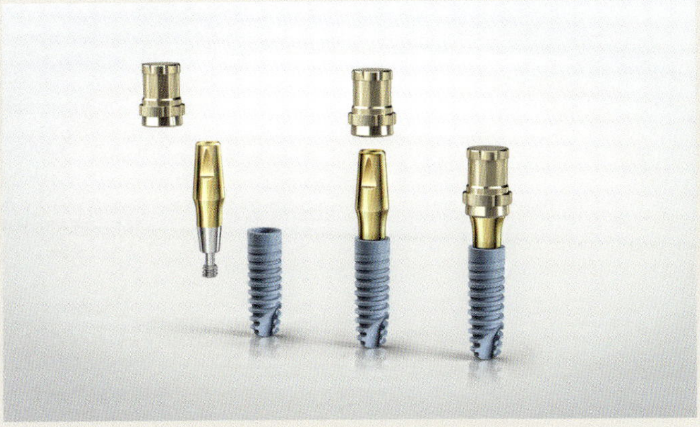

5.23 Conometric abutments and retention copings (Myplant two system).

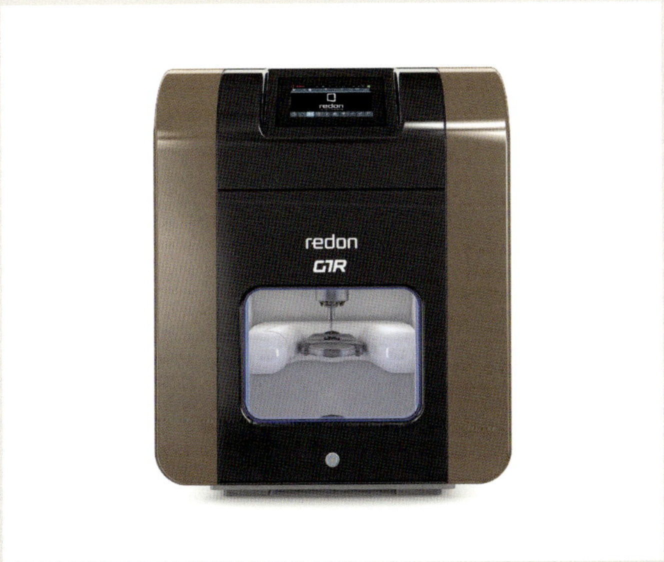

5.24 Example of a five-axis dry or wet milling machine that can be used to produce surgical guides, provisional prostheses, final prostheses and mesostructures in various materials.

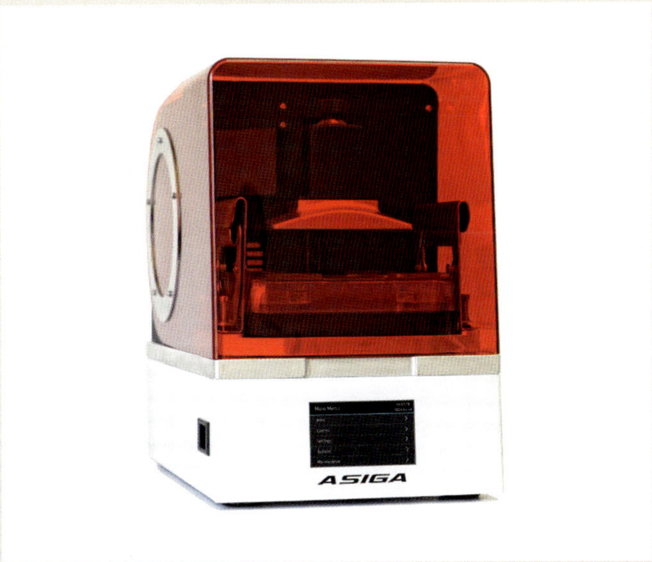

5.25 3D printer, which can be used to fabricate surgical guides.

The workflow described here, by making use of immediate loading fixed prostheses, makes it possible to avoid resorting to second stage healing screws, transfer abutments and, in case of using conometry, provisional abutments.

Let us go back to design and examine in detail the design steps in the case of a Toronto bridge.

The mock-up is designed, including the pink part (5.26), selecting the teeth from the natural teeth library (3 Shape, Skyn method) (5.27).

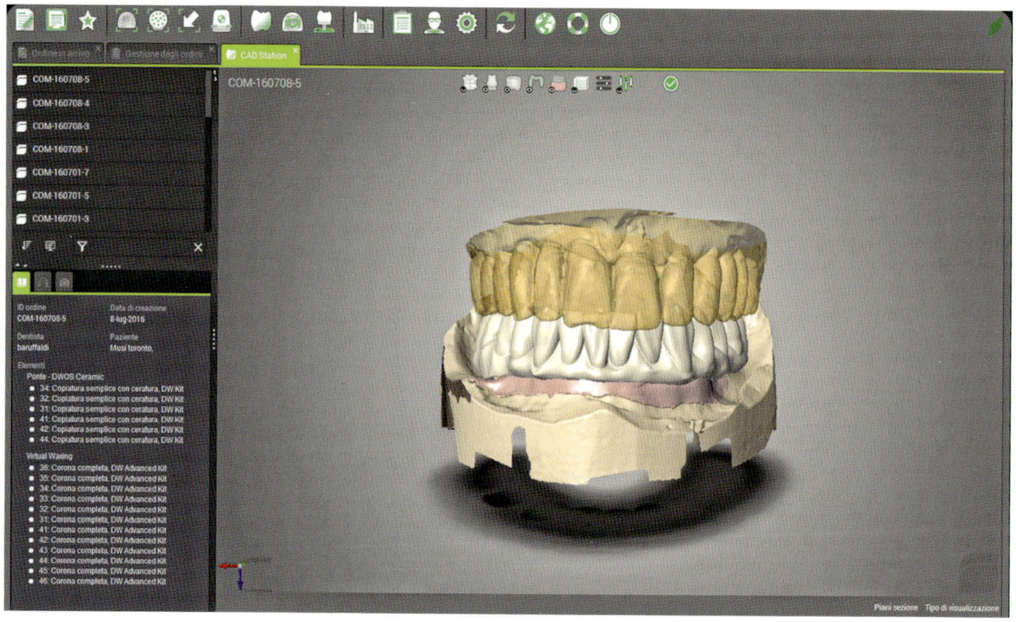

5.26 Mock-up modeled with CAD software (Co-Diagnostic, Dentalwings).

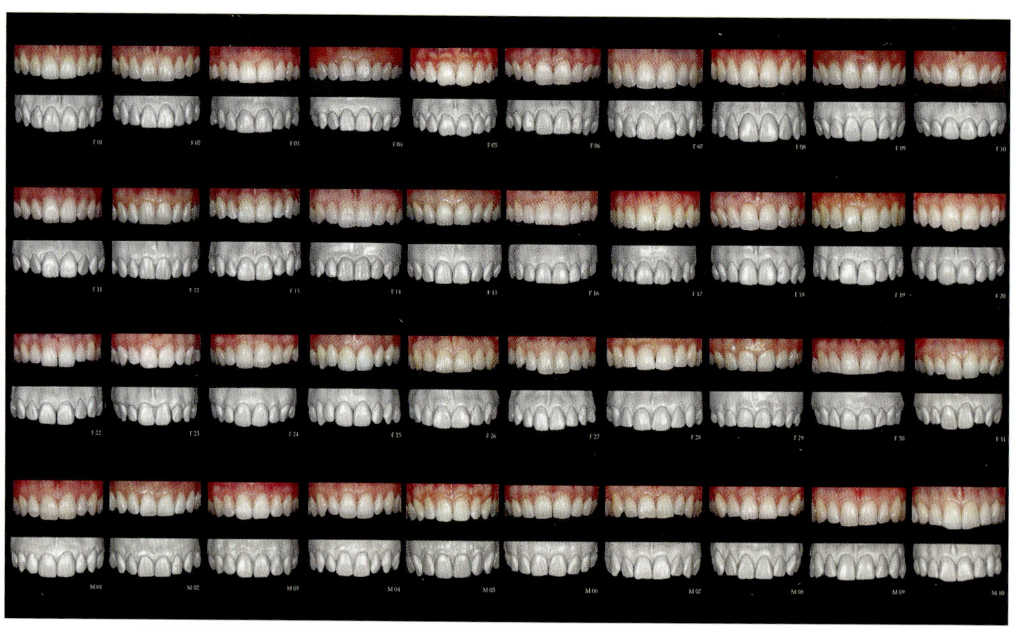

5.27 Example of library produced from impressions of natural teeth (Skyn Concept).

The implant position is planned on the basis of the designed mock-up.

For this to be possible, the software must include the selected implants, as well as the samples of prosthetic abutments for that specific type of implant. The overall dimensions of the prosthetic components are verified, in this case the retention copings, and the prosthesis is adapted, respecting the thicknesses and typical load resistance parameters of the selected material (5.28 and 5.29).

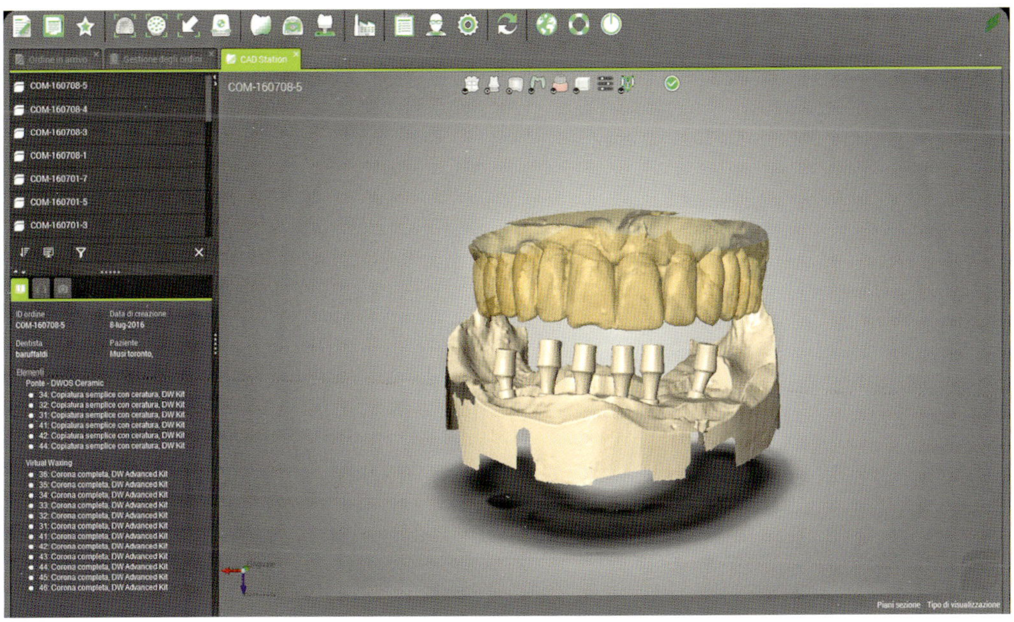

5.28 Abutments for conometric prosthesis, inclusive of copings.

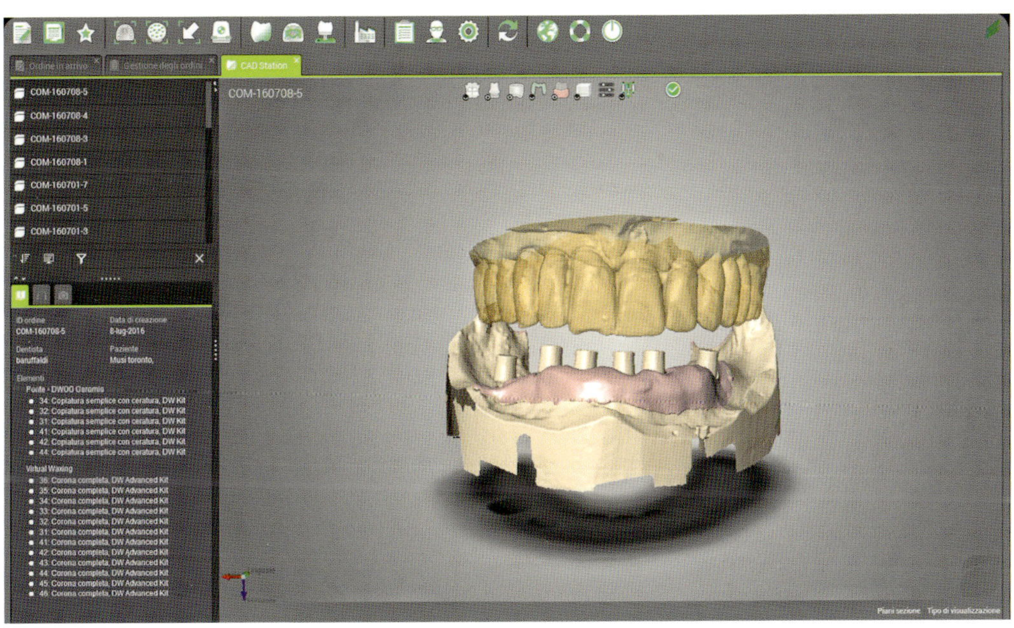

5.29 The same image but with visible soft tissues.

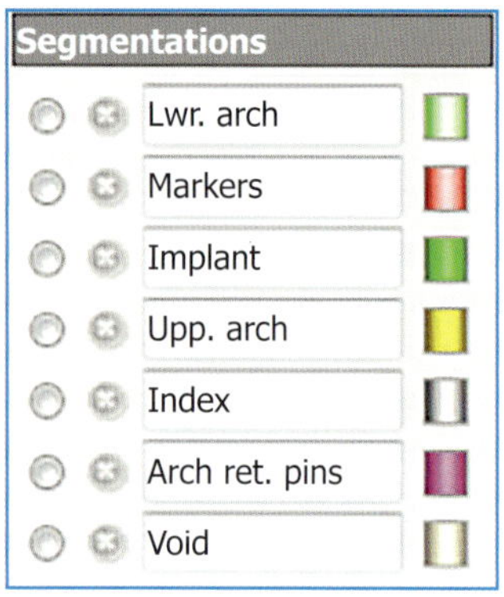

5.30 It is possible to visualize only the necessary information, using the various levels that can be displayed or hidden in the various stages of prosthesis modelling.

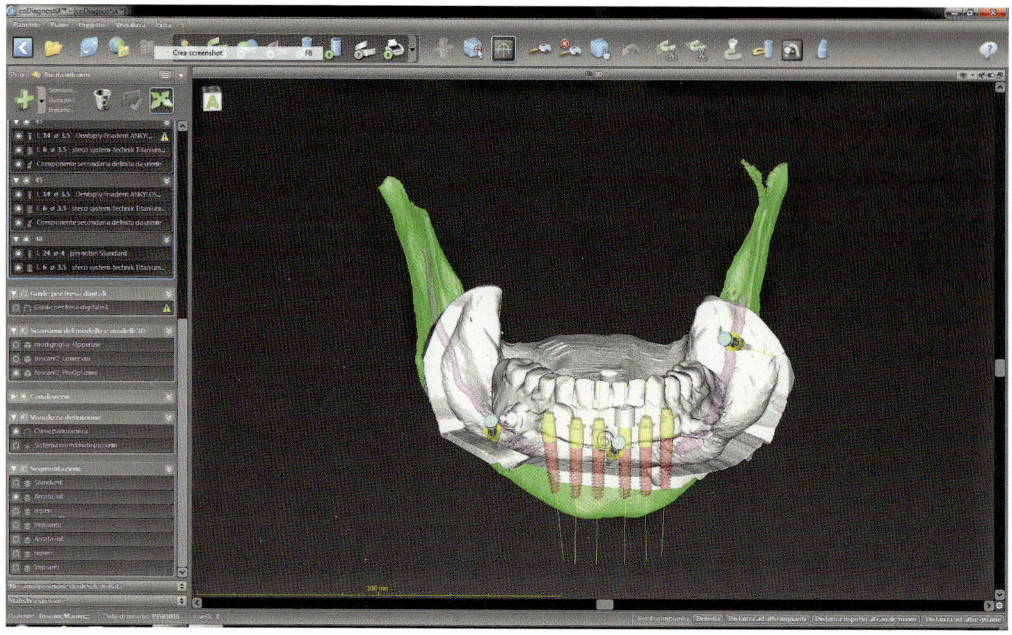

5.31 Denture used as radiographic template, including landmarks, implants – including prosthetic components – and intra-osseous stabilization pins.

CAD software allows different levels to be viewed or hidden, such as implants, soft tissues and hard tissues: in this way, it is possible to visualize only the information required at a given time (5.30 and 5.31).

After that, the pieces to be used are physically fabricated: Part B of the surgical guide can be produced with a resin DLP 3D printer, or in titanium, by means of a milling machine (5.32 and 5.33).

If opting for a milled part, a modified and open disc holder must be used, in order to allow the burs to work horizontally on the disc, to produce the guide holes for the intra-osseous pins. In both cases, the guide holes and precision attachments must be present, to stabilize the interchangeable Parts A of the index. The first top part, part A/1, used at the beginning of the surgical procedure, must be attached on one side to the precision attachments and on the other to the existing teeth. It is used to lock the intra-osseous pins in the desired and planned position; this step is indeed the only time when the situation in the mouth coincides with that of our initial data (5.34). As stated above, if no teeth are present, the copy of the prosthesis can be used as radiographic template, to secure the pins in the correct position, locked on Part B of the surgical index by means of the OT CAPs (5.35).

The next Part A to be made is the one used for bone leveling after the extractions, if required (Part A/2). Next up is Part A/3, which enables the insertion of preparation drills and implants in the desired position (5.36). It is recommended to use implant systems whose kit not only includes drills, but that guide all the way to implant insertion (5.37), in order to thoroughly follow the plan. This part of the guide must be completed by inserting the titanium sleeves – by press-fitting or gluing – of the implant system.

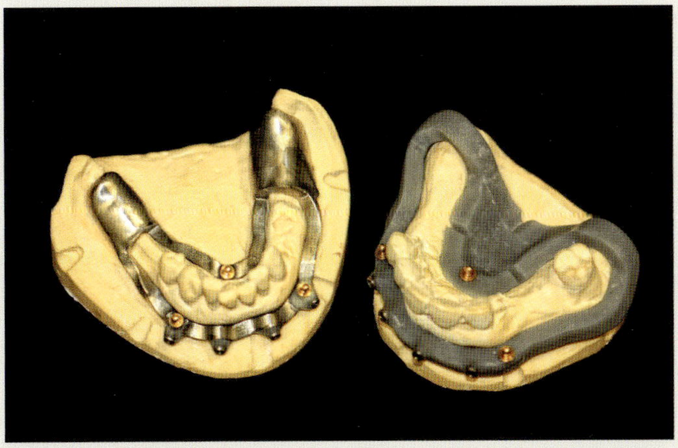

5.32 Part B of the surgical guide according to the DIGIT technique. Part B is fixed with intra-osseous pins at the beginning of surgery and is not removed until the end of surgery. The guide on the right was made in resin with 3D printer; the guide on the left was obtained from a solid titanium block, using a milling machine.

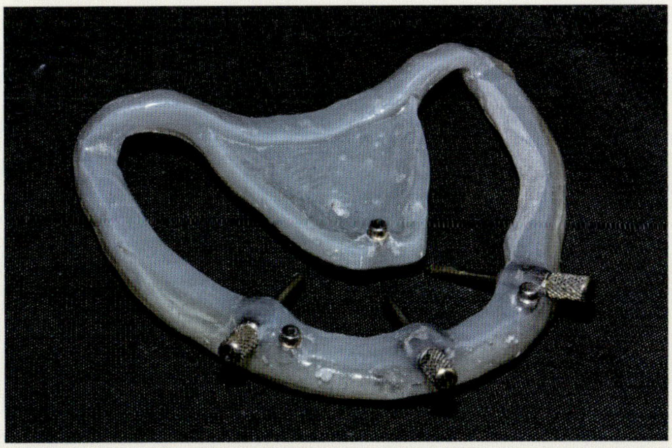

5.33 Resin 3D print of the first part of the guide.

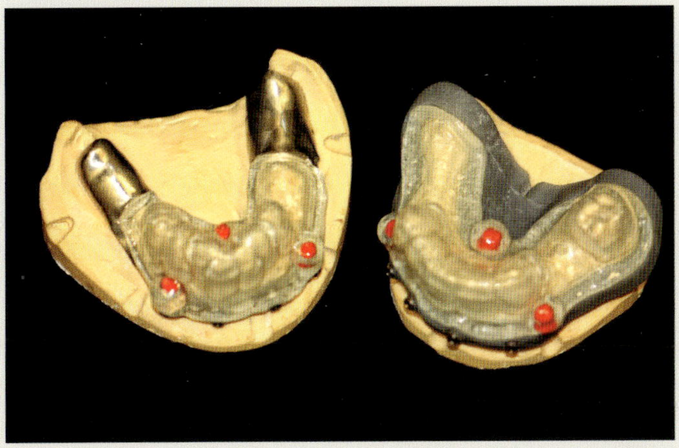

5.34 Part A/1 of the index.

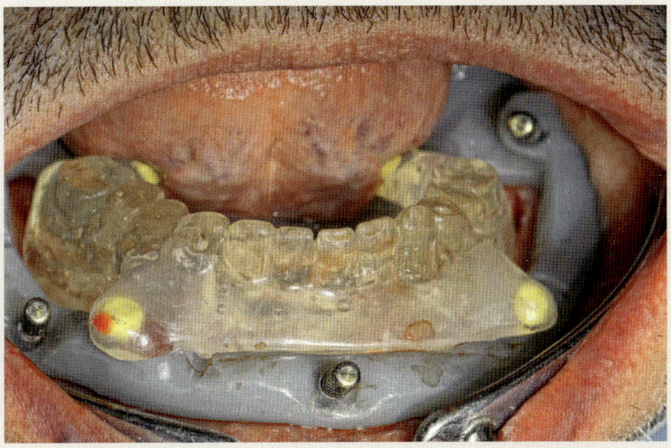

5.35 Copy of the mock-up, X-ray guide, used as A/1 guide in case of total edentulism.

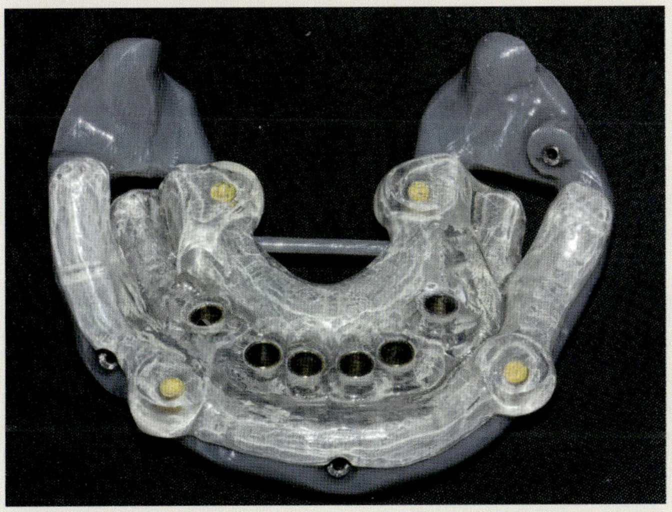

5.36 Part A/3 used for guided implant insertion.

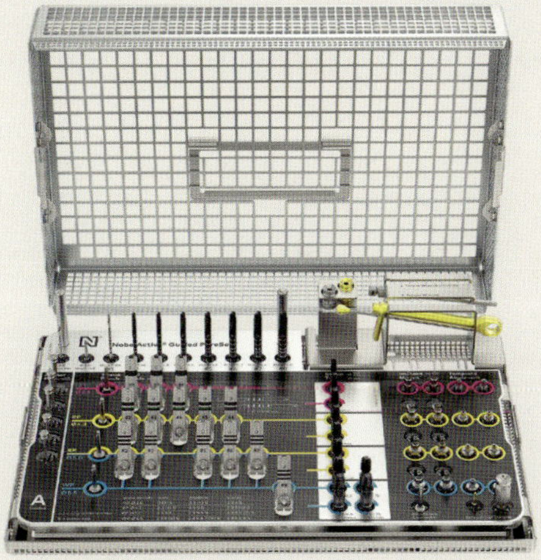

5.37 Implant kit for guided surgery.

It should be underlined that, if tilted implants and angled abutments are used, the final position of which must be certain, it is essential to mark the sleeves of the implant system used with a notch that identifies the final position of the anti-rotational system within the implant, in order to fix it in the desired position to properly match the abutment.

The part of the index used to insert the prosthetic abutments in the proper position is then fabricated. If angled abutments are to be used, it is necessary to use a part of the index guiding their insertion into the desired position (5.38). If non-indexed abutments are used, that is, without the anti-rotational system, or straight ones, no references are required, except the full insertion one. Conversely, where angled abutments need to be used, a guide must be prepared to help insert them in the proper position.

Finally, the fixed prosthesis may now be fabricated. With six implants as support, a Toronto-type prosthesis can be manufactured. As mentioned earlier, it is preferable to fabricate the prosthesis in composite on glass fiber mesostructure, using a conometric connection between prosthesis and abutment. With the DIGIT technique, which ensures extreme precision in the placement in the oral cavity, it is possible to move directly on to the use of the final prosthesis, skipping the provisional stage. Let us look at the steps.

If a CAD-CAM software is used, which contains a library of the selected implant abutments, the clinician may directly move on to the design stage, using as a guide the mock-up used in the first step of the work, to plan the position of the implants. Should this not be possible, an additional step must be carried out, consisting of a 3D printed model of the patient with leveled bone and holes in the planned implant insertion positions (5.39).

The digital implant analogs and the selected abutments are inserted in the model, then the model thus assembled is scanned (5.40 a,b). It is prefe-

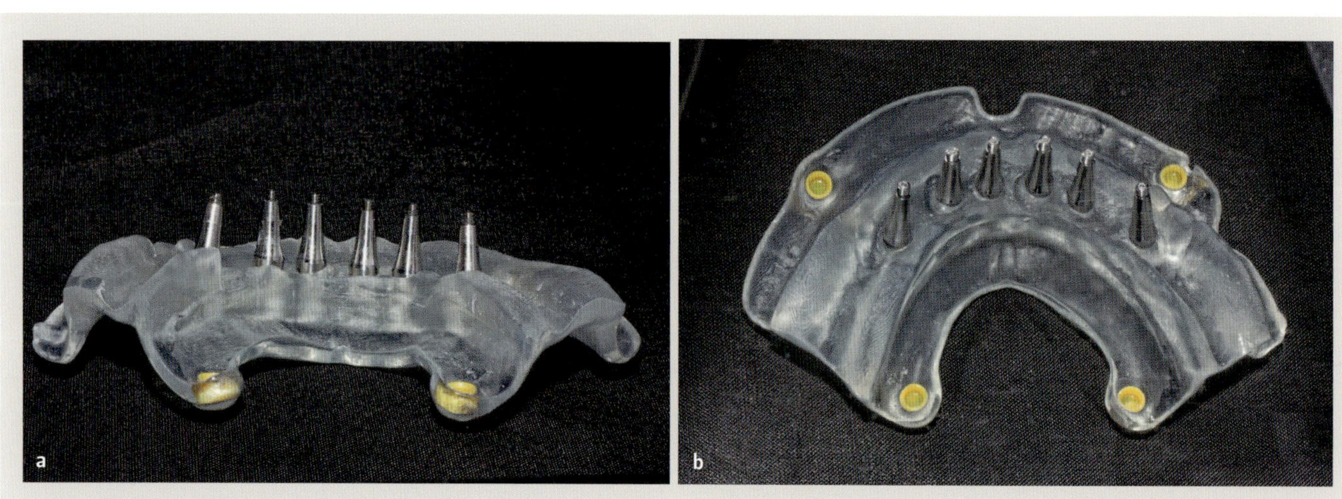

5.38 a,b) Guide for the insertion of non-indexed angled abutments.

rable to print the gingiva separately from the hard tissues, in order to carefully check the precision of the housings where the conometric copings are to be fixed. The final prosthesis is now modeled, thanks to the CAD program, using as a guide the virtual mock-up already used in the first stage of the technique (5.41 a-c).

The virtual model is exported into the CAM software, or sent to the 3D printer (5.42).

The prosthesis is printed in resin in a color - grey by preference - that best allows the result obtained to be evaluated. The printed piece is used to create a mold for the verticulator, i.e. the instrument used by the Authors to fabricate the prosthesis in composite with glass fibre mesostructure.

The next step is inserting the item in the verticulator and covering it with clear silicone (5.43). The silicone must be transparent to enable light curing of the composite that will be added (5.47) after the steps described below (5.41-5.46).

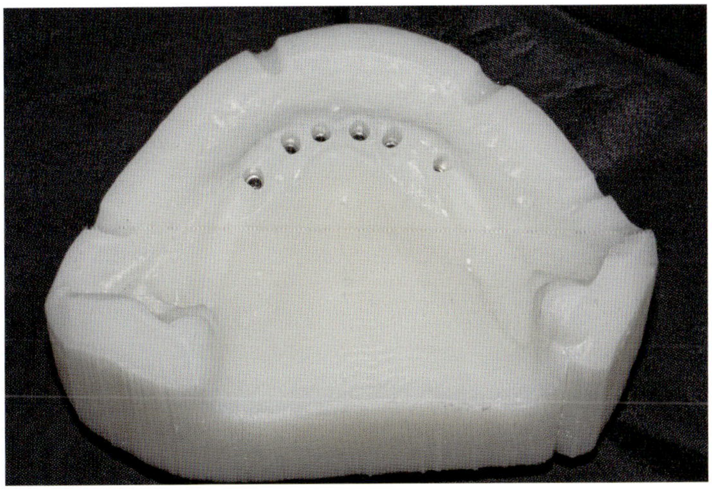

5.39 3D printed model with digital analogs of the inserted implants.

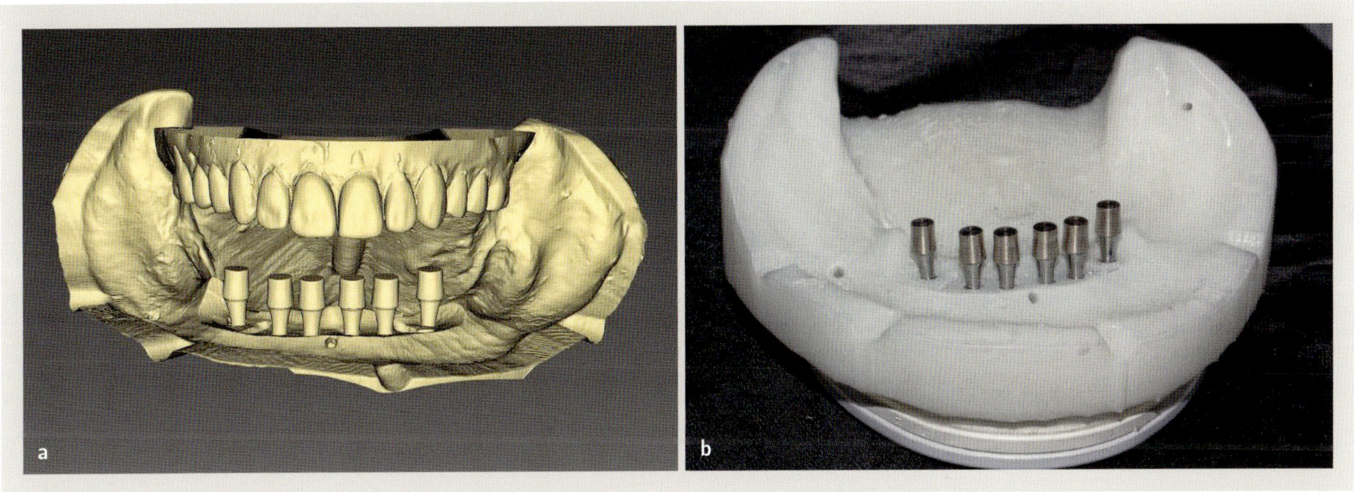

5.40 a, b) Abutments for conometric prosthodontics in position: in the CAD software (left) and in the model produced on the basis of this design (right), in which the digital analogs and the prefabricated abutments have been inserted and the corresponding copings fitted.

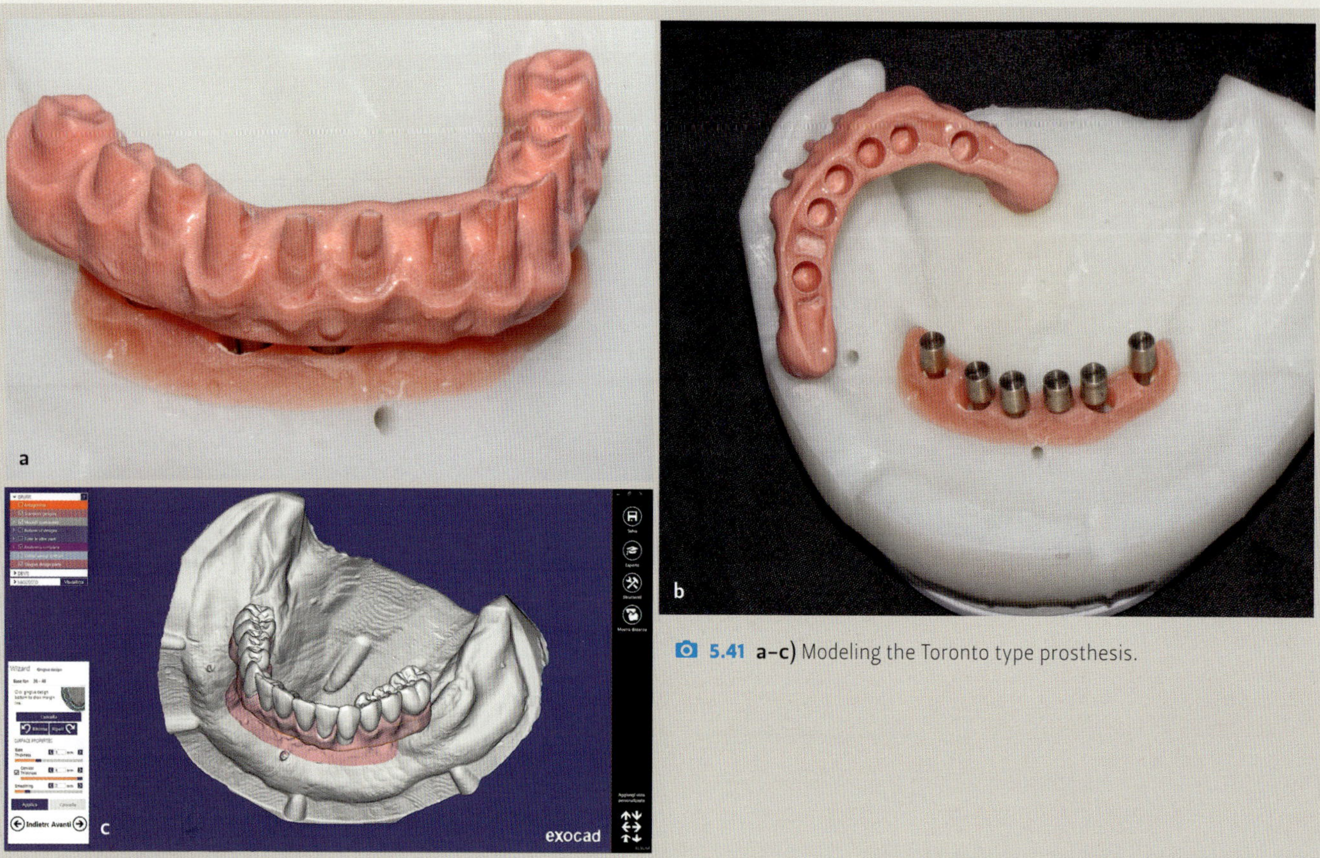

5.41 a–c) Modeling the Toronto type prosthesis.

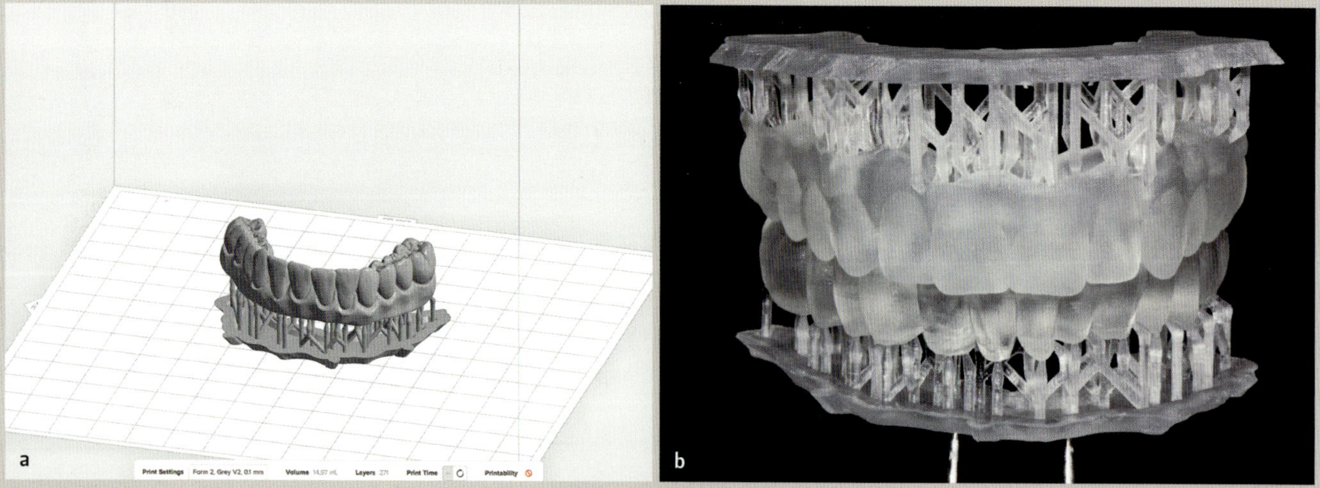

5.42 a,b) Final prosthesis printed in resin for models.

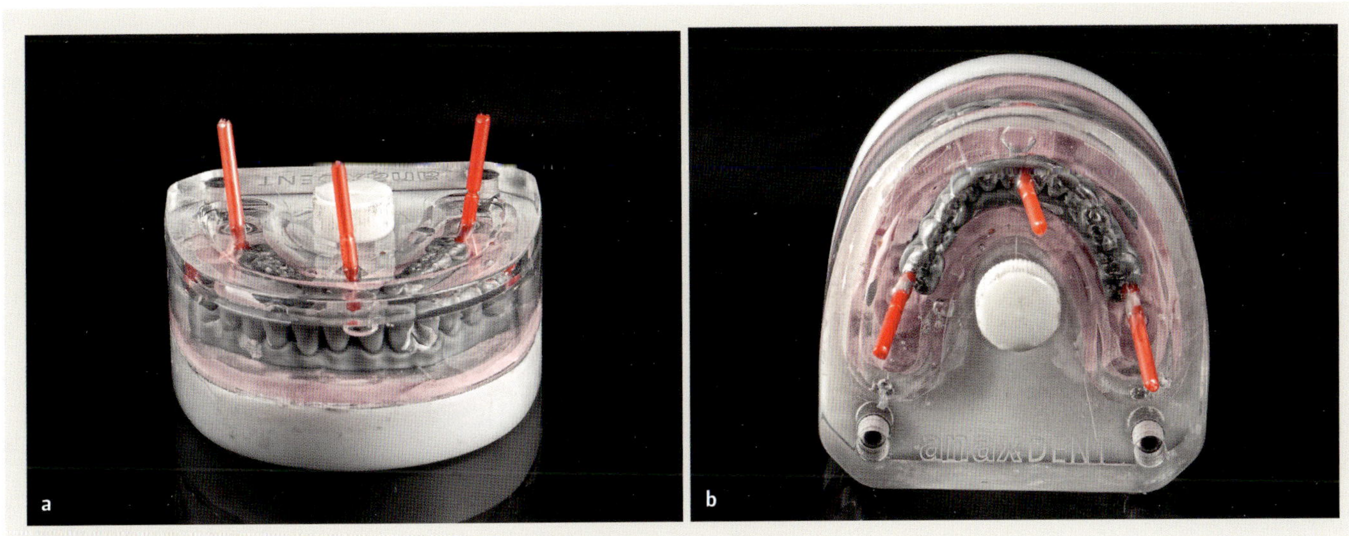

5.43 a,b) Final prosthesis inserted in the verticulator, in order to prepare the mold.

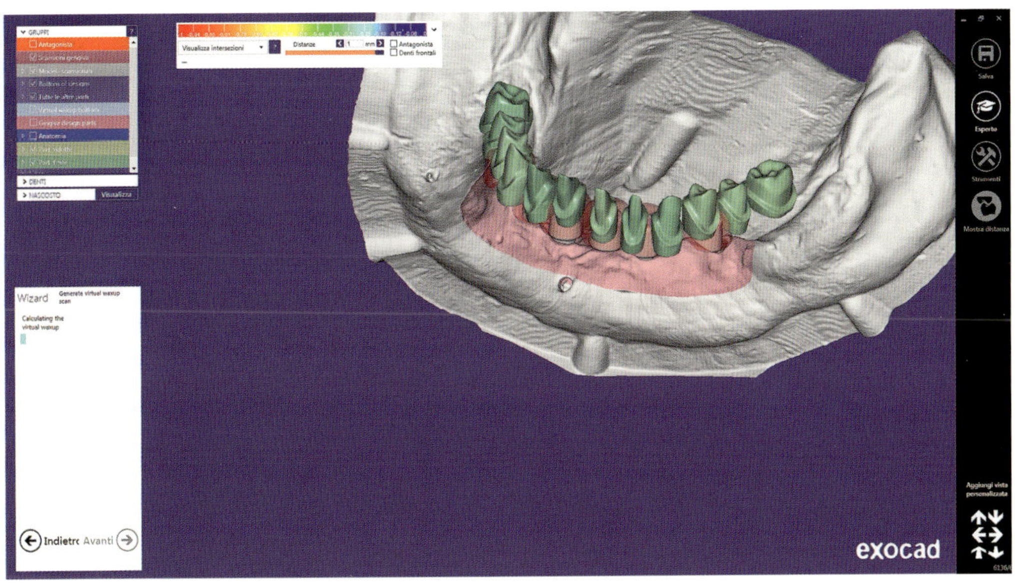

5.44 The prosthesis is reduced in the CAD program, in order to obtain the mesostructure design.

Back to the CAD program, starting from the prosthesis designed with the appropriate tools, the model is reduced and the mesostructure is created (see 5.44). The mesostructure is milled in PEEK (5.45) and placed inside the mold created in the verticulator, after removing the mock up (5.46 a,b). Before insertion, the clinician needs to check the conometric prosthesis copings for proper matching (see 5.47).

First, the dentin composite is injected in the space that is created around the mesostructure and light-cured. Then the item is removed from the shell and cut-back is performed, to leave space for the second injection of composite, i.e. enamel shade (5.48 a-d and 5.49 a,b).

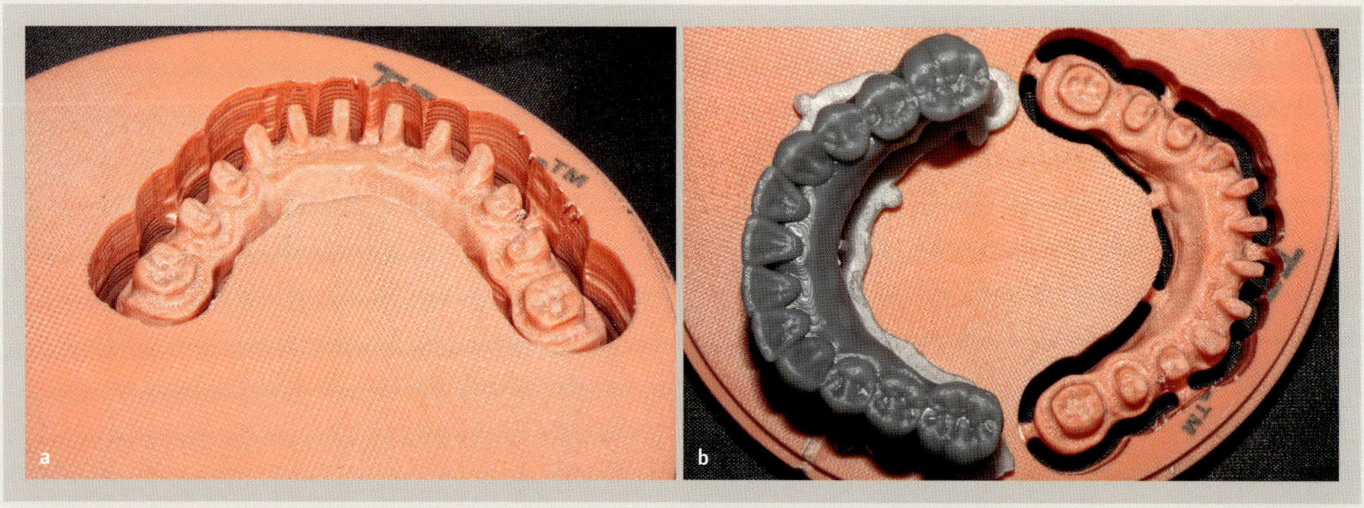

5.45 **a,b)** The mesostructure is milled in glass fiber (PEEK).

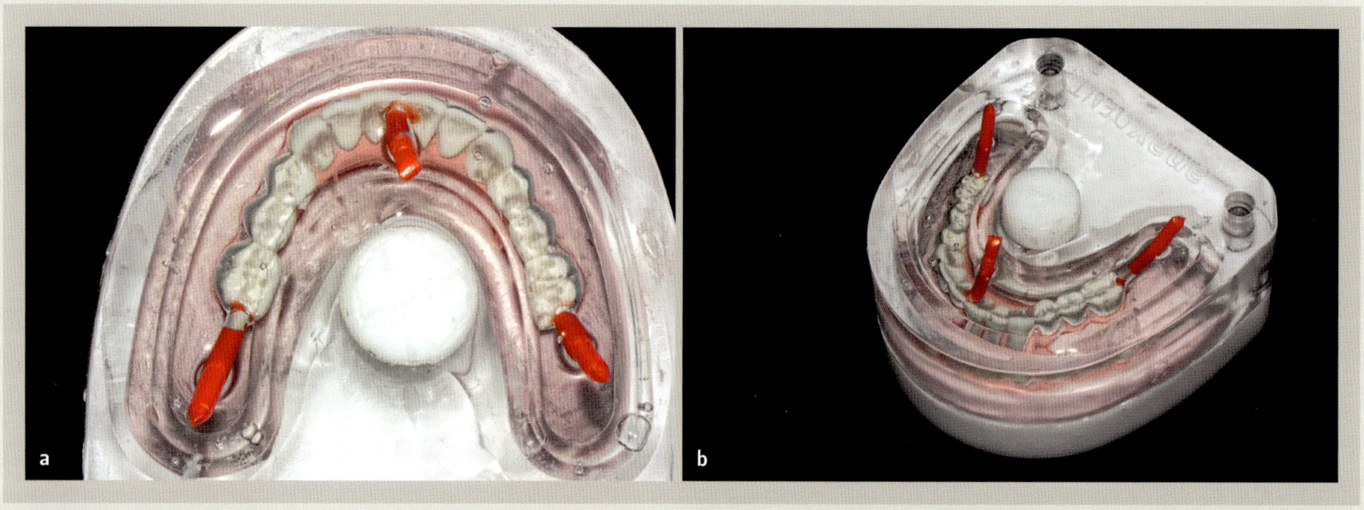

5.46 **a,b)** Mesostructure inserted in the verticulator.

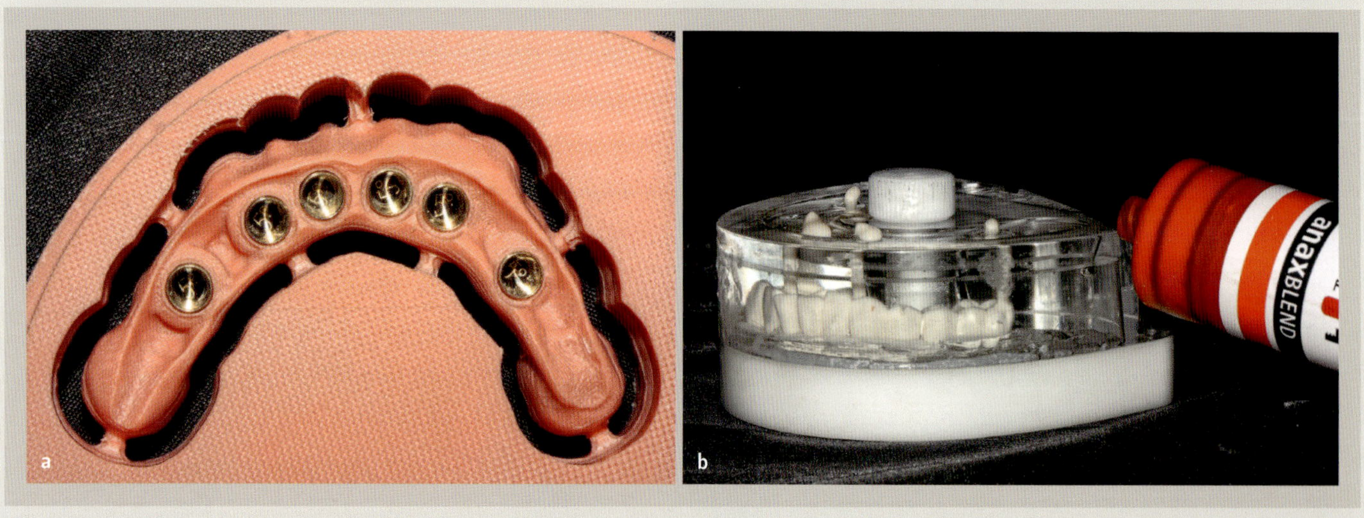

5.47 **a,b)** In this stage, the coupling with the retention copings is checked.

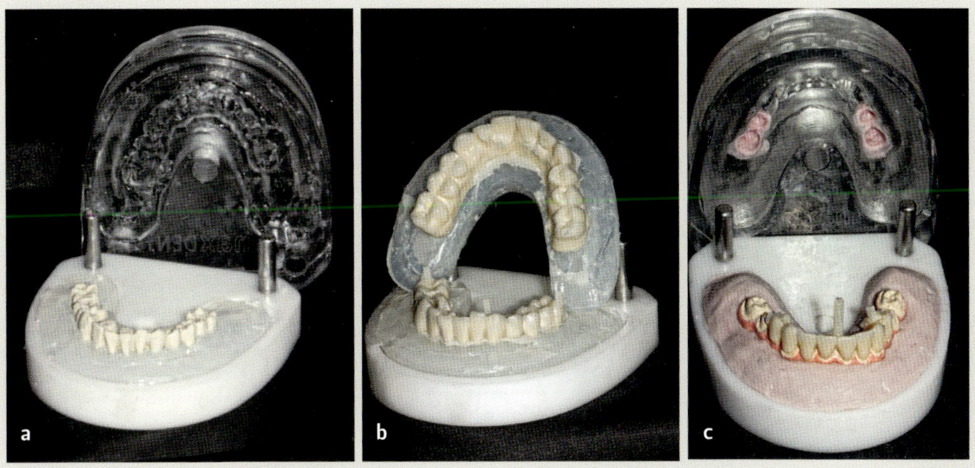

5.48 **a–c)** The dentin composite is injected first, then light-cured; the item is cut back to make room for the enamel composite, then inserted back into the shell and the enamel composite is injected. The procedure is repeated by applying the pink part.

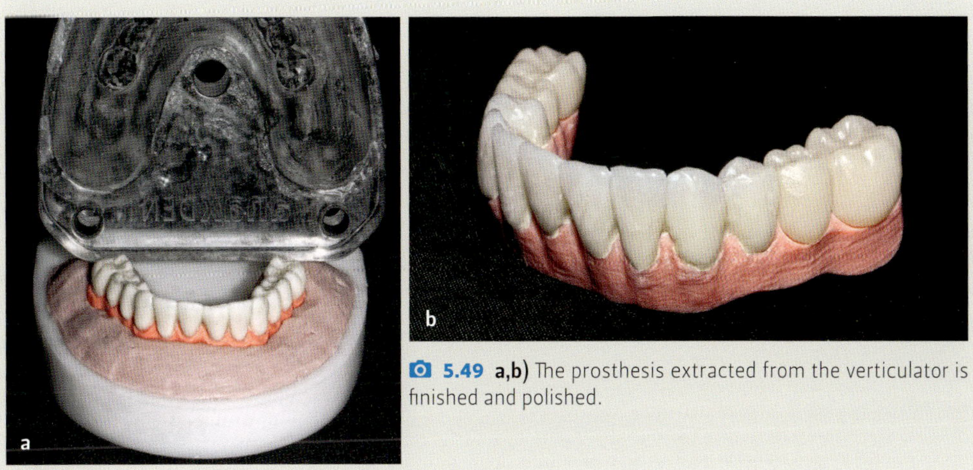

5.49 **a,b)** The prosthesis extracted from the verticulator is finished and polished.

The pink part may alternatively also be molded by hand, after removing the item from the mold; in which case, the previously printed repositioning model is used (5.50).

If the model into which the abutments were inserted has already been printed, after extracting the workpiece, it will be used as a repositioning model, to manually complete the veneering with the pink composite. Otherwise, the model inclusive of copings will be printed and used for the purpose. A variation introduced subsequently consists in inserting posterior teeth milled in lithium disilicate. This option enables greater control over time of the dimensional stability of the prosthesis, as well as maintenance of proper contacts (5.51). On the other hand, the fabrication of the main structure in glass fiber and of the functional and esthetic part in composite makes it possible to consider the prosthesis fabricated in this way as final. Indeed, it is possible to make any modification that might be required at any time by adding composite, once the tissues have healed completely.

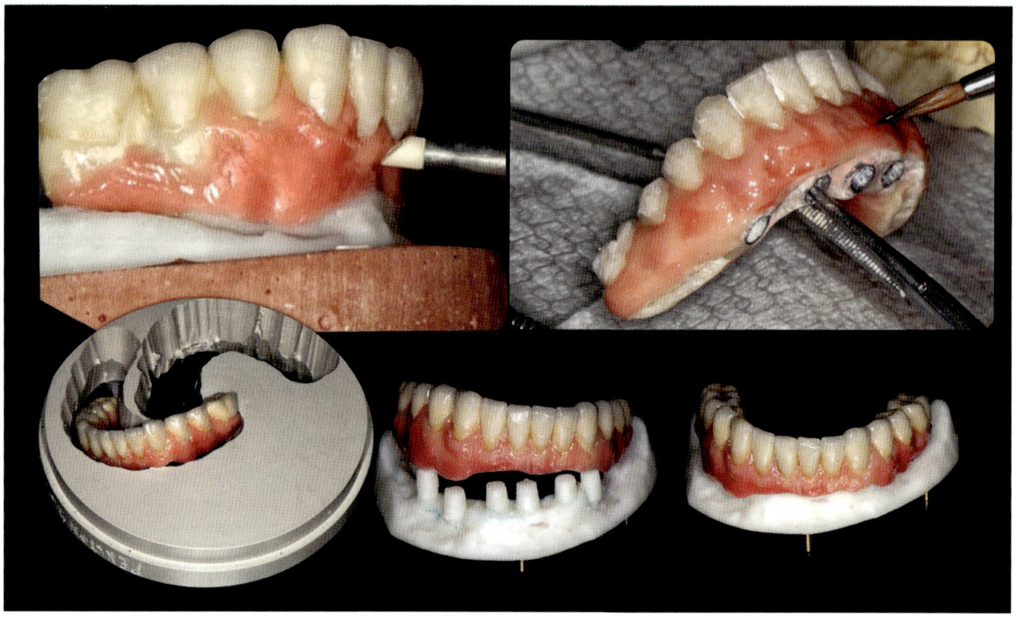

5.50 Manual production of the pink component. The model previously printed is used as support.

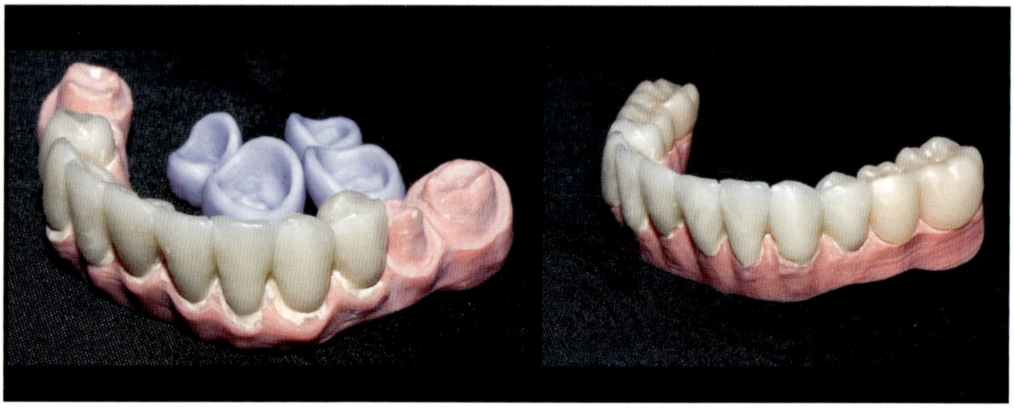

5.51 To ensure greater durability, milled lithium disilicate elements can be inserted on the posterior teeth.

The final step in the fabrication of the item, which is the special step in the Authors' procedure, consists in locking it to Part B of the surgical index, by means of light curing resin arms and Locator type attachments, or even individually milled attachments (5.52). This procedure makes it possible to reproduce in the mouth, in a reliable manner, the accurate position of the designed provisional prosthesis, allowing the position of the occlusion and of the VDO to be locked. Therefore, there is no longer the need to cement at least one coping before insertion in the mouth, because guidance is assured by the attachments on the index. The common attachments on the market may be used, or the pieces can be designed and milled individually (5.53). In the case of fabricating the final prosthesis, a further option is to design the mesostructure in zirconia, the occlusal part in lithium disilicate and the pink part in porcelain.

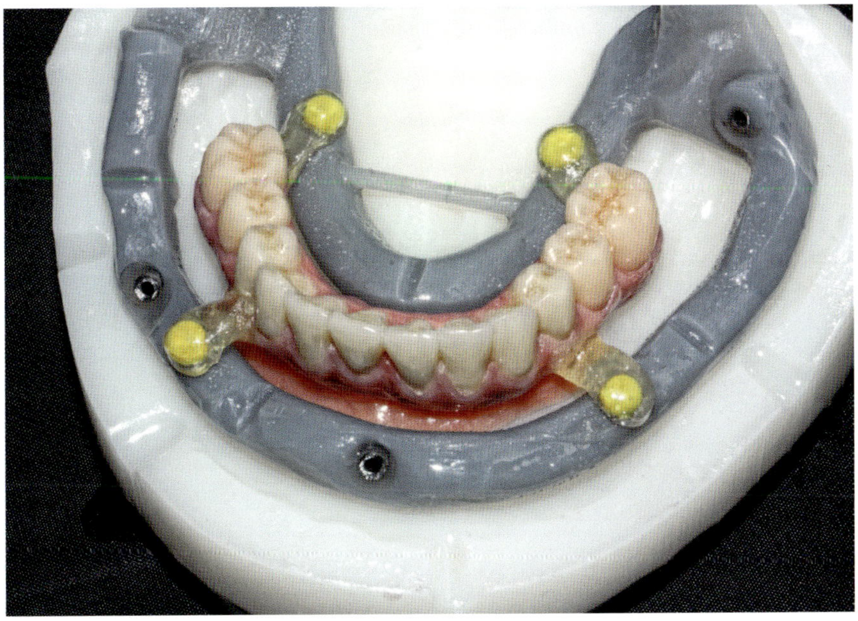

5.52 Prosthesis fixed to Part B of the surgical guide. In this way, it is possible to lock the conometric copings in the definite position in the mouth, immediately following the surgical stage, with no risk of misplacement. The patient might not actually be fully cooperative, as they might be sedated or still under anesthesia.

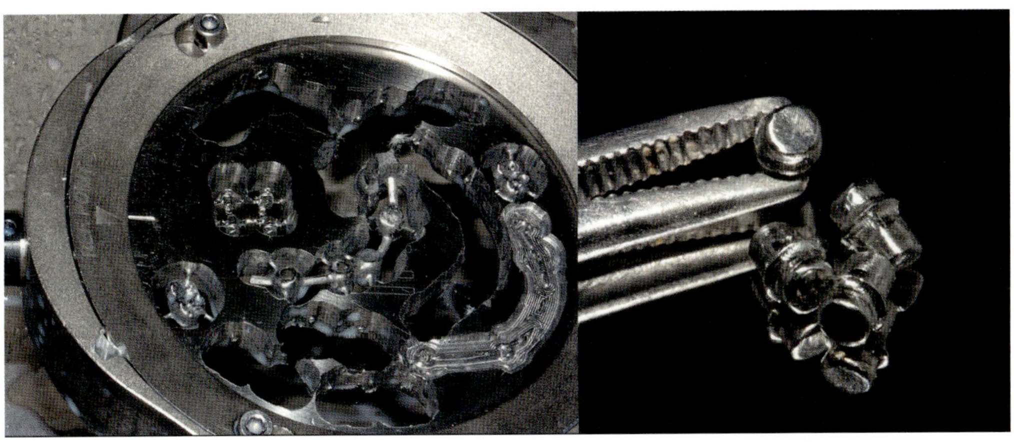

5.53 Retentive titanium attachments, produced in house.

Clinical stage

To describe the clinical stage, a double full arch rehabilitation case will be illustrated. Both upper and lower arches were restored by means of a Toronto type prosthesis on six implants per arch.

The patient's teeth in both arches were affected by grade 3 mobility, and needed to be extracted. Two removable partial dentures with severe signs of wear were present, with loss of VDO (5.54-5.57).

SURGICAL PROTOCOL

All surgical procedures were carried out under local anesthesia. The upper surgical index and all A parts, printed in resin, were sterilized with an ethylene oxide solution. Part B, prepared for the mandible and milled in titanium, was sterilized in autoclave.

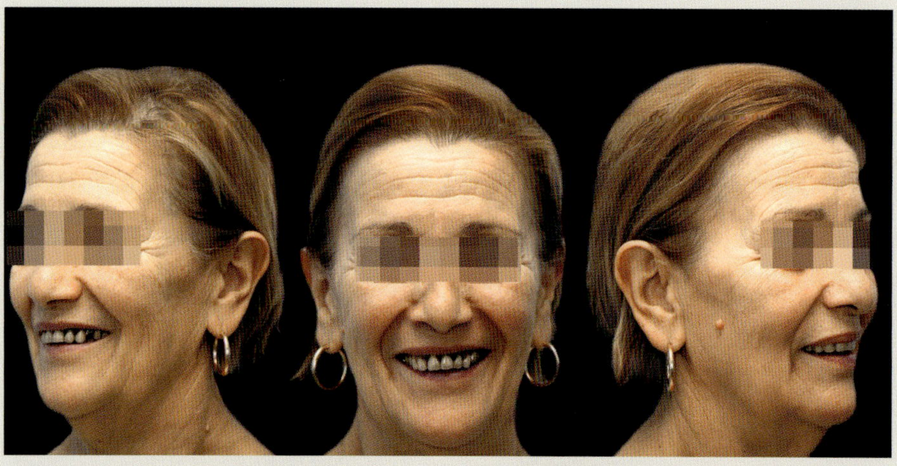

5.54 Initial photographs of the patient.

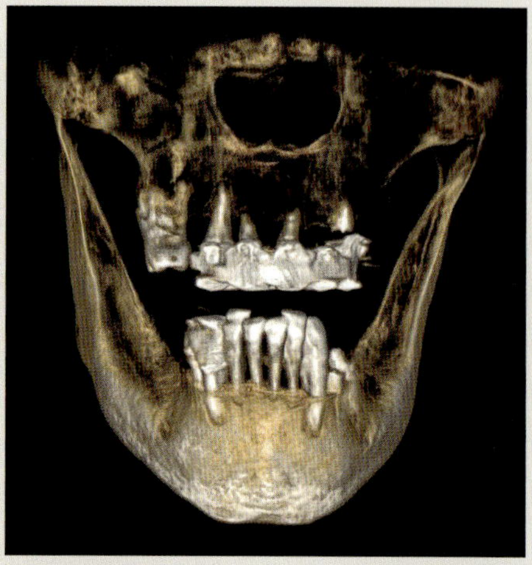

5.55 Panoramic radiograph and optical impression.

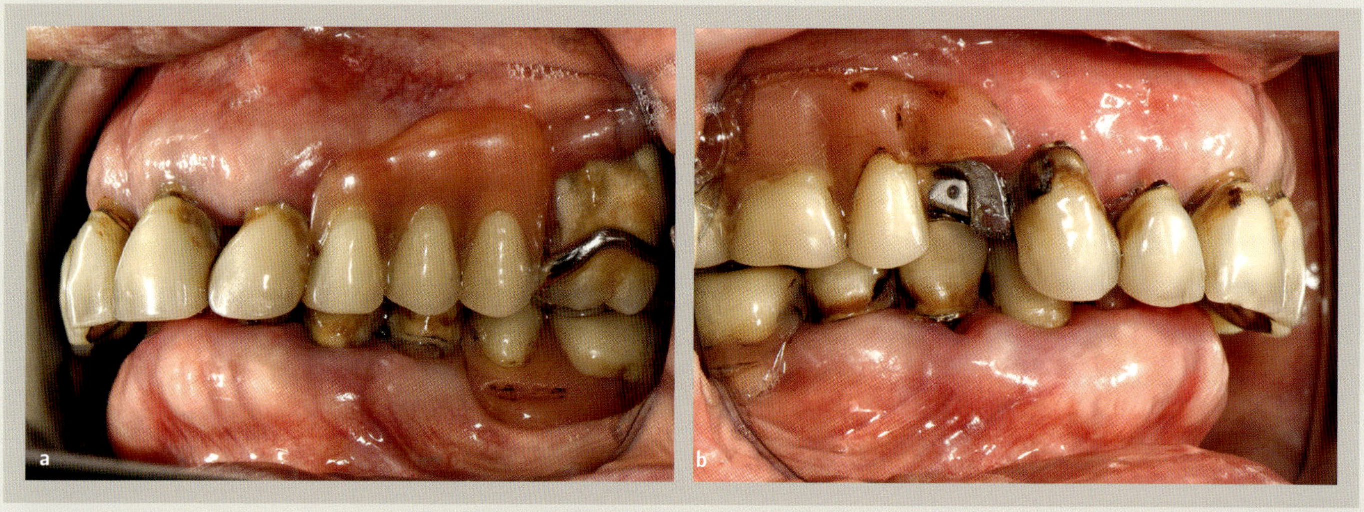

5.56 Initial situation of the patient, with poor oral hygiene due to low motivation, teeth with grade 3 mobility and worn removable partial dentures, at the level of the mandible as well as of the upper jaw, with collapsed VDO.

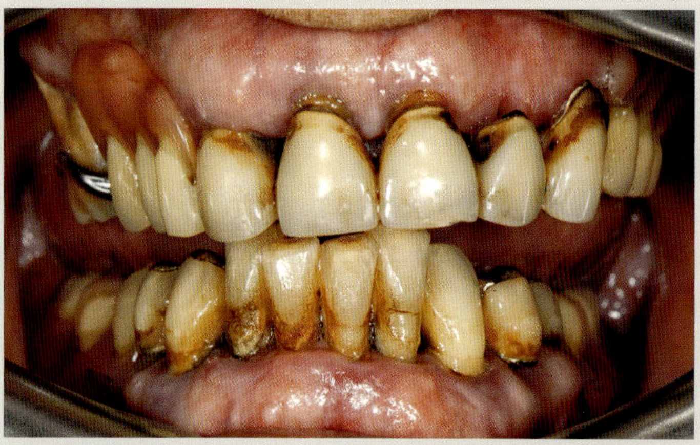

5.57 Note the presence of removable prostheses with clasps and the poor oral hygiene of the patient.

One hour before the procedure, antibiotic prophylaxis of 2 grams of amoxicillin and clavulanic acid was administered. The patient was asked to rinse for one minute with 10 ml of 0.2% chlorhexidine-based mouthwash, used for its immediate antibacterial effect and for its prolonged permanence in the oral cavity.

Local anesthesia was administered through local infiltration of 4% articaine, with adrenaline 1:100.000. To reduce the post-operative oedema, it is possible to administer dexamethasone sodium phosphate, by intramuscular injections.

In the first stage the required information was collected through CBCT examination and intraoral scan. The acquired data were imported and matched in the CAD software (5.58). The teeth were removed and the bone was leveled virtually. Then the prosthesis was designed, starting from the mock-up, according to the Skyn method, making use of libraries of natural teeth.

The implants of the desired type were inserted; the position was identified by using the mock-up as guide (5.59 and 5.60 a,b).

The surgical guides were designed on the virtual renderings, divided into two parts, as described.

The pins were inserted on the buccal side of the alveolar process, through Part B of the guide, avoiding any interference with critical anatomical structures, teeth to be extracted or implants to be inserted (5.61 a,b). Part B for the mandible was milled in titanium, while Part B used in the maxilla was 3D printed in resin. OT-Cap attachments were inserted on both indexes (5.62).

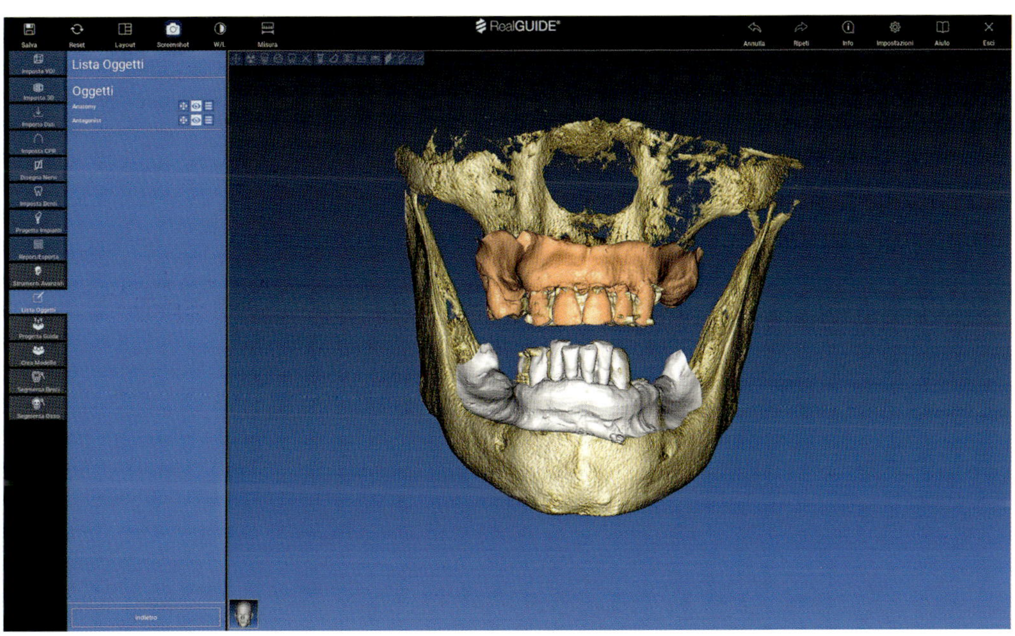

5.58 The models in STL format have been imported and matched to the CBCT in the design software.

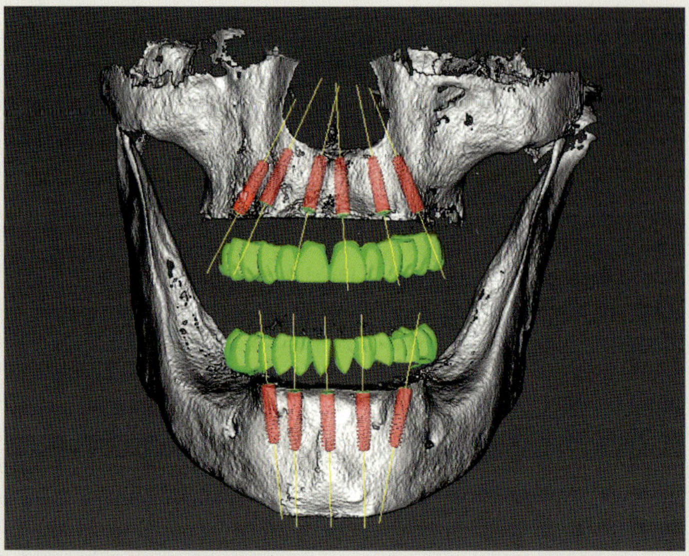

5.59 The implants are inserted using the mock-up as guide; the alveolar bone is also leveled.

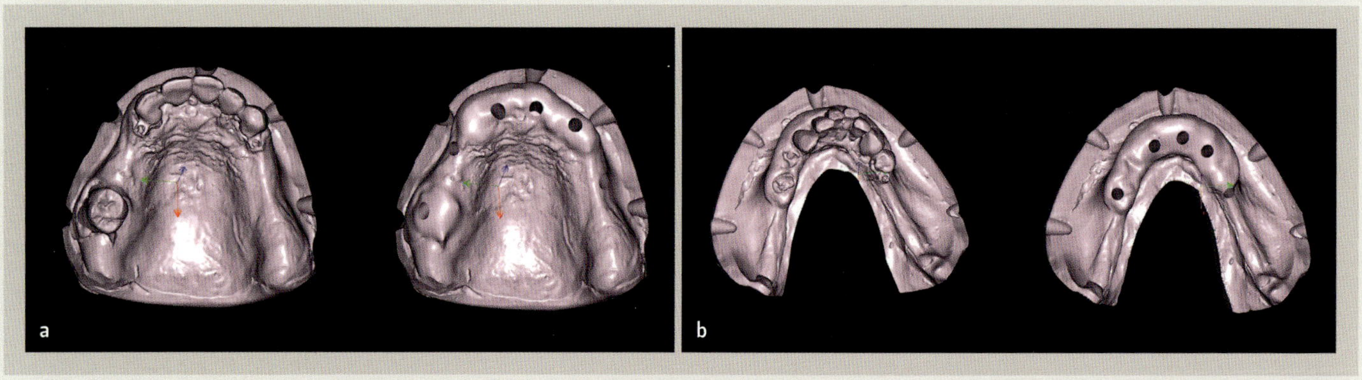

5.60 a,b) The upper and lower jaws before and after treatment. After removing the teeth and leveling the bone, the implant positions are identified. Maxilla and mandible are modified with computer software.

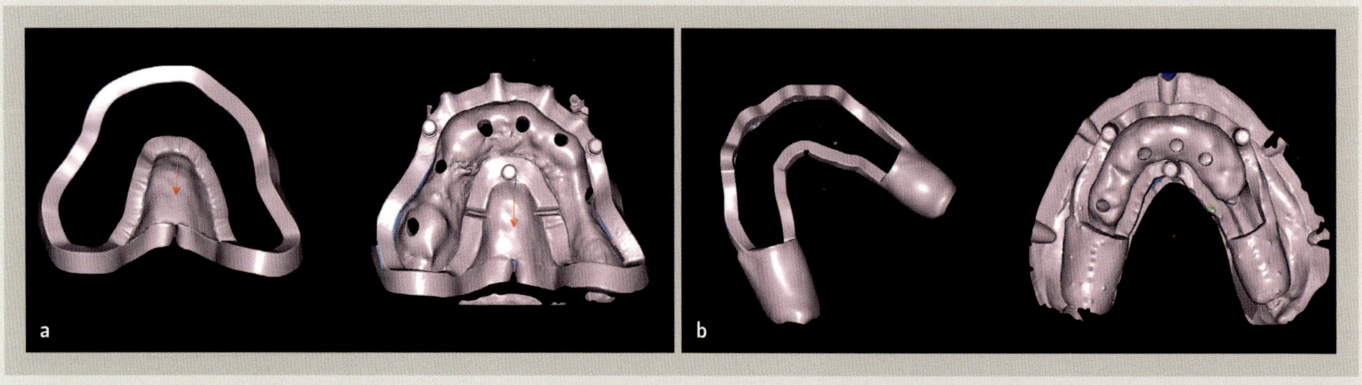

5.61 a,b) Part B designed in the upper and lower jaw.

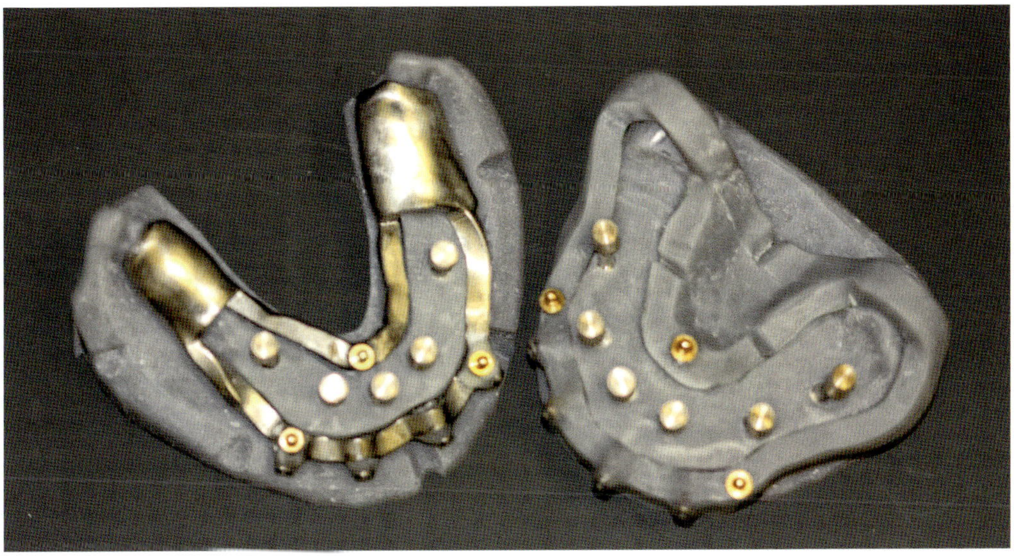

5.62 Part B for the mandible, milled in titanium; Part B for the maxilla, printed with 3D printer in biocompatible resin.

Parts A were then printed: A1 for placement; A2 for alveolar bone leveling; A3 for implant insertion (5.63).

At this stage, having prepared all the hardware required for the procedure, the surgical stage began, starting from the mandible. Before extracting the teeth, the surgical stent was inserted in the mouth, with the two assembled Parts: B and A1. The proper position was established using the dental support, and Part B was secured with intra-osseous pins (5.64). The residual teeth were used to ensure the proper housing of the base index (Part B) and its fixation with the pins, thanks to the first dental support index (Part A1), connected via retentive attachments.

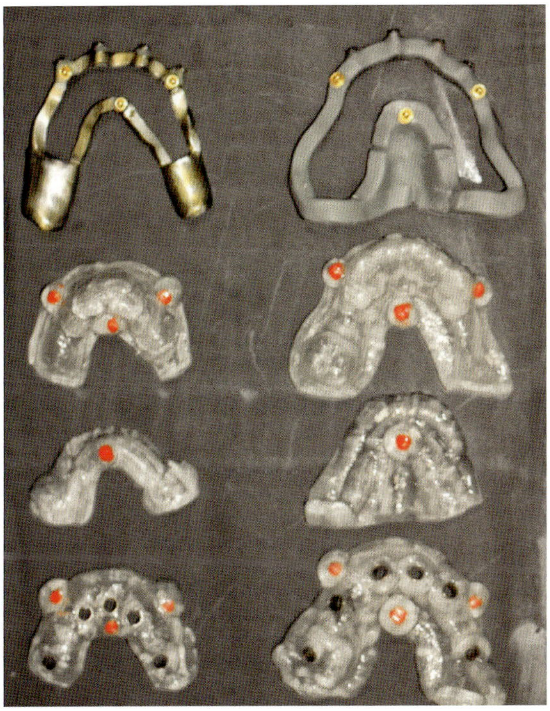

5.63 From top to bottom, on the left the sequence for the mandible and on the right, for the maxilla. Above, Part B of the guides; followed by Part A1 used to correctly position Part B in the mouth; Part A2 to level the bone and finally, Part A3 used to insert the implants.

Having fixed points of reference allowed the position of the base index from the virtual design to be transferred to the patient's mouth. *After removing the first secondary index, the compromised teeth and/or implants are extracted with the utmost care*, to preserve the integrity of hard and soft tissues (5.65).

We should point out that in the event of wholly edentulous arch, the base index is fixated using a silicone bite.

After fixating Part A2, designed for bone leveling - if required -, the intended set of drills are used in sequence to prepare the implant sites, until the diameter and depth planned in the design stage are achieved, using Part A3 (5.66 a,b).

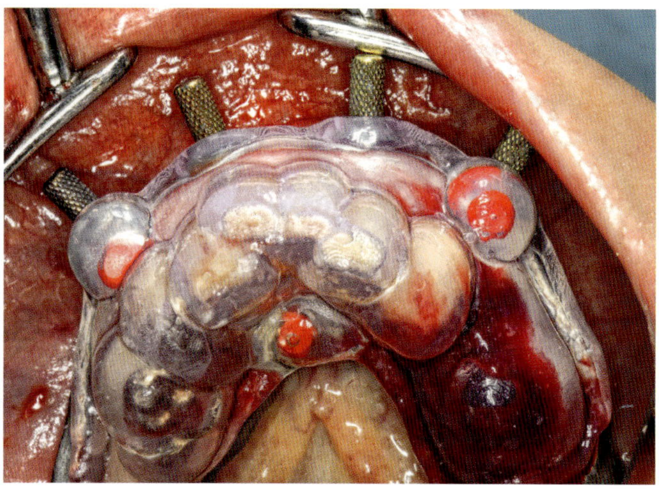

5.64 Surgical guide assembled in the mandible. Part B coupled to Part A1, with ball attachments and pins inserted in place.

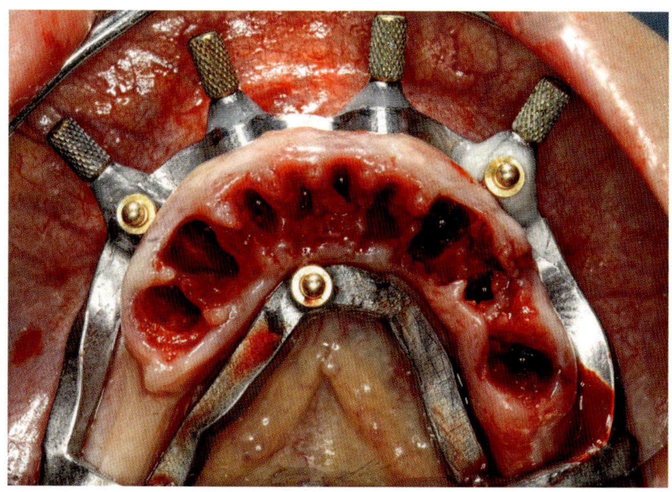

5.65 After removing Part A1, keeping Part B in place, the teeth are extracted.

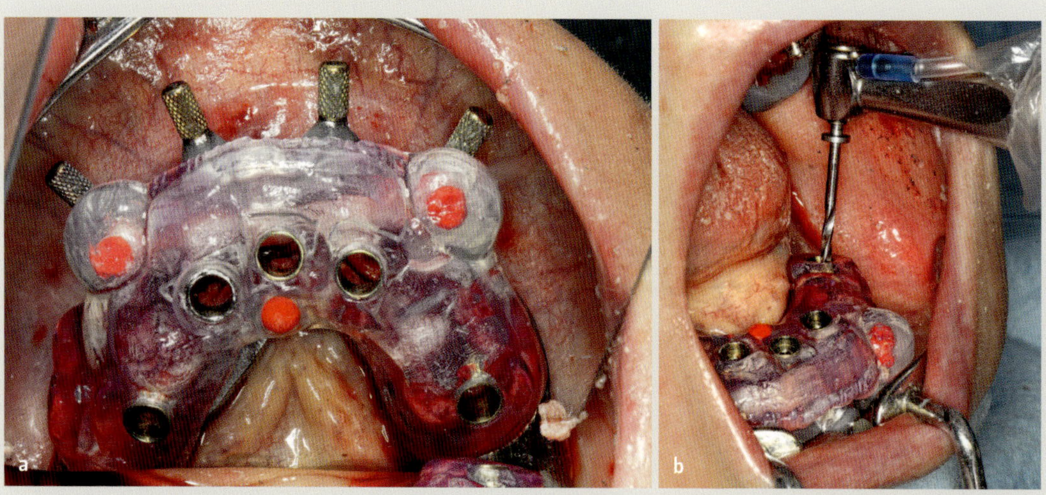

5.66 a,b) Sequence of burs of the specific kit, using Part A3.

We should point out that in the event of wholly edentulous arch, the base index is fixated using a silicone bite.

After fixating Part A2, designed for bone leveling – if required –, the intended set of drills are used in sequence to prepare the implant sites, until the diameter and depth planned in the design stage are achieved, using Part A3 (5.67).

Once all the implants had been placed, the final abutments were screwed onto them. The abutments should then be tightened, according to the specifications provided by the manufacturer, only after the proper position of the implants has been confirmed. In this case, it was not necessary to use the guide index for abutment placement, because straight, non-indexed abutments were used (5.68–5.74).

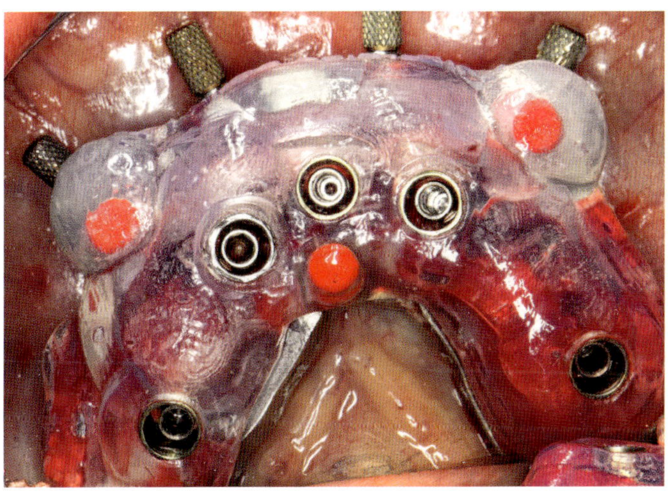

5.67 Guided implant insertion.

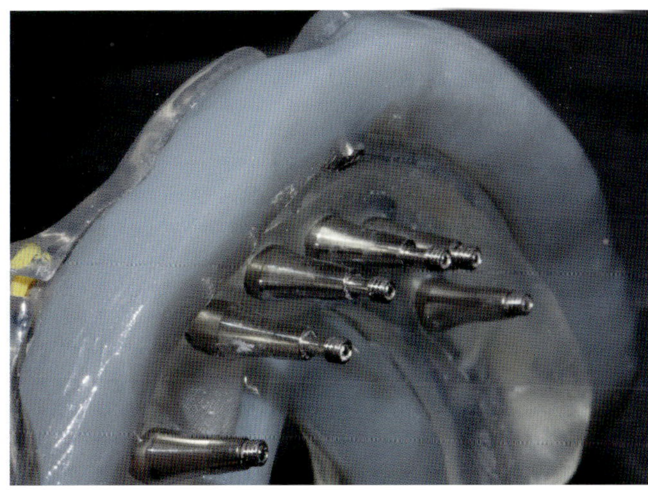

5.68 Part A3 for proper placement of implant abutments.

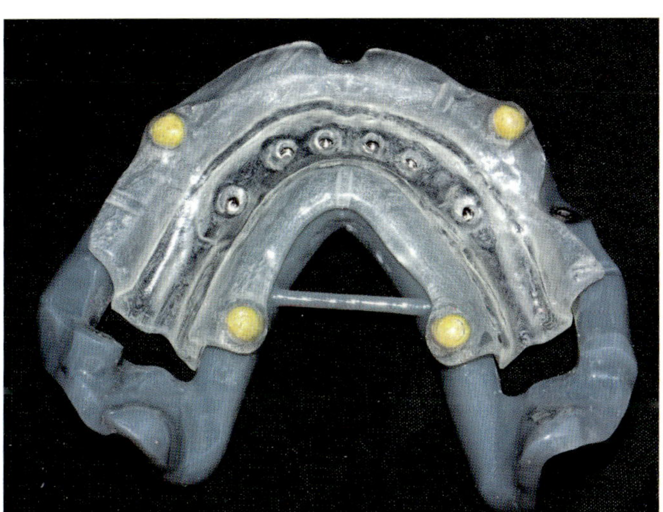

5.69 Occlusal view of the same part A3.

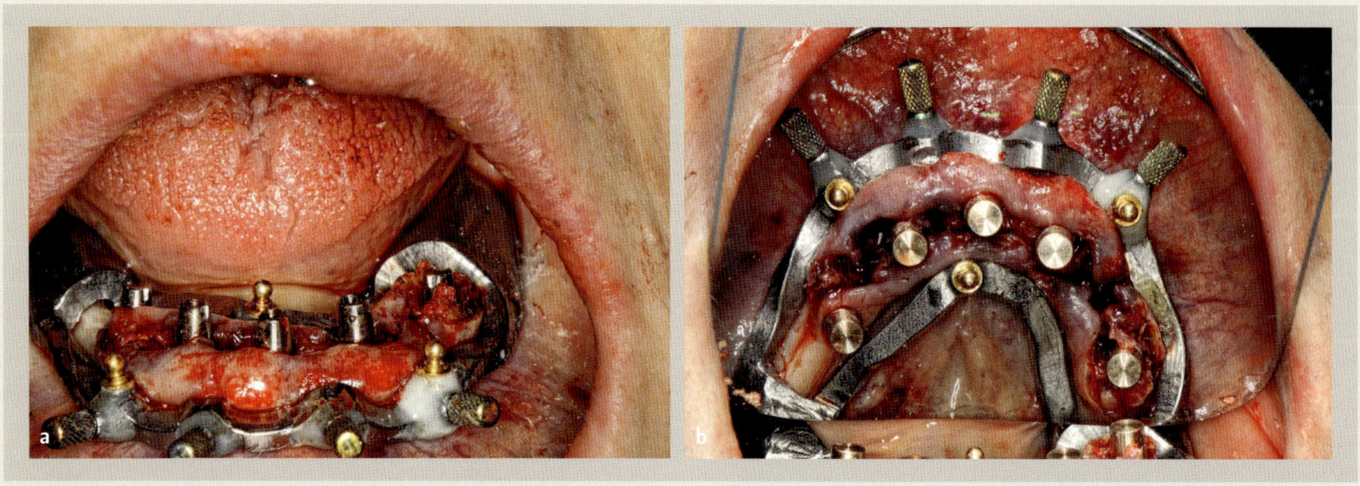

5.70 **a)** Inserted implant abutments. **b)** The retention conometric copings are placed on the abutments and activated.

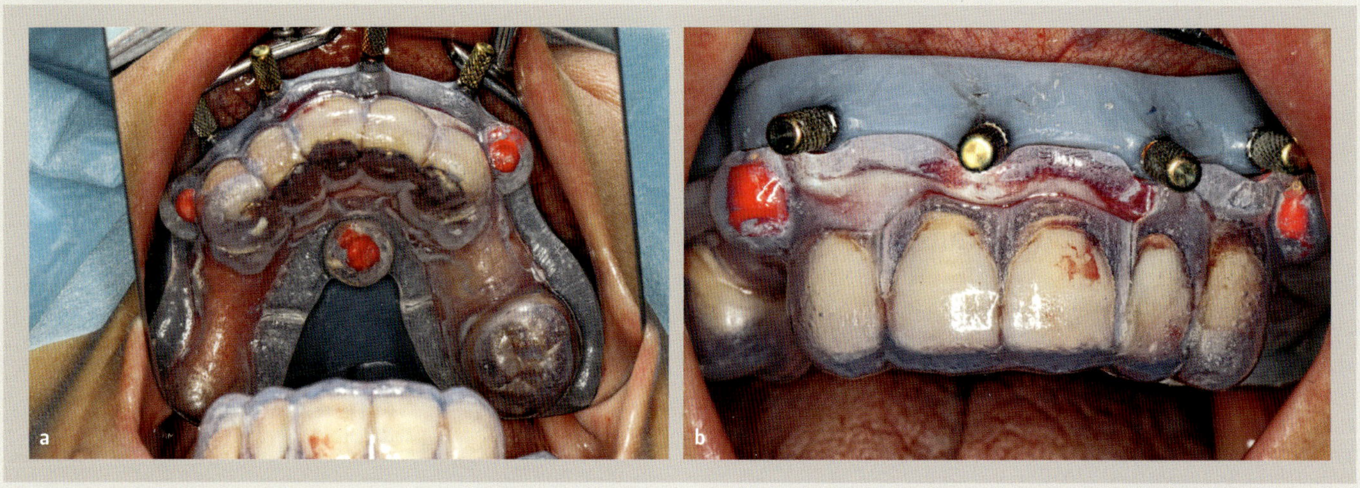

5.71 **a,b)** The procedure is repeated in the same session in the maxilla. Here, part A1 and B of the index are inserted in the desired position and part B is stabilized with the intra-osseous pins.

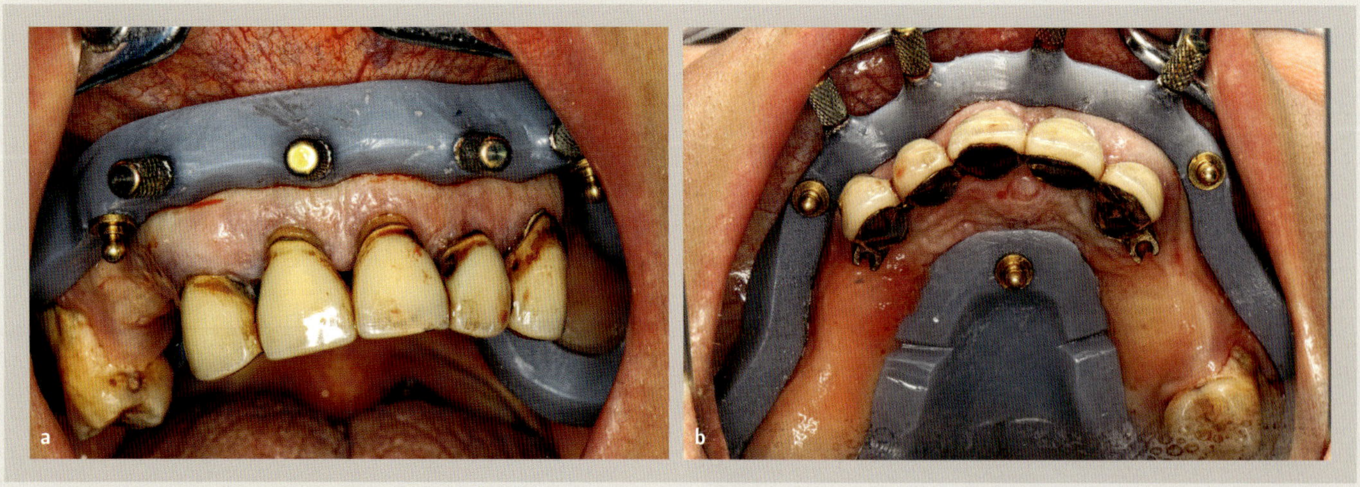

5.72 Part A1 is removed and part B is left in place.

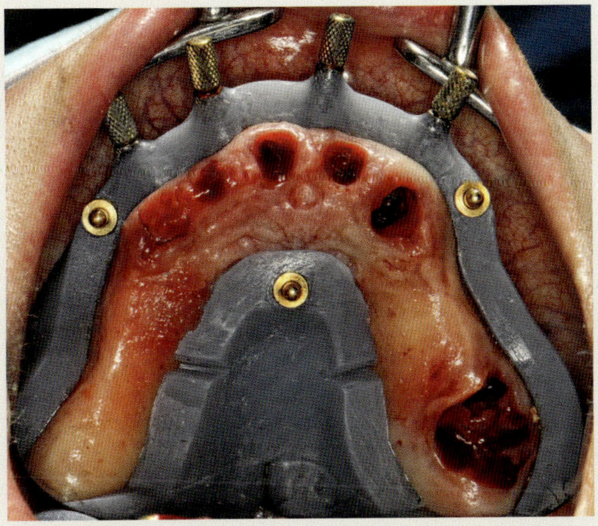

5.73 The compromised teeth are extracted.

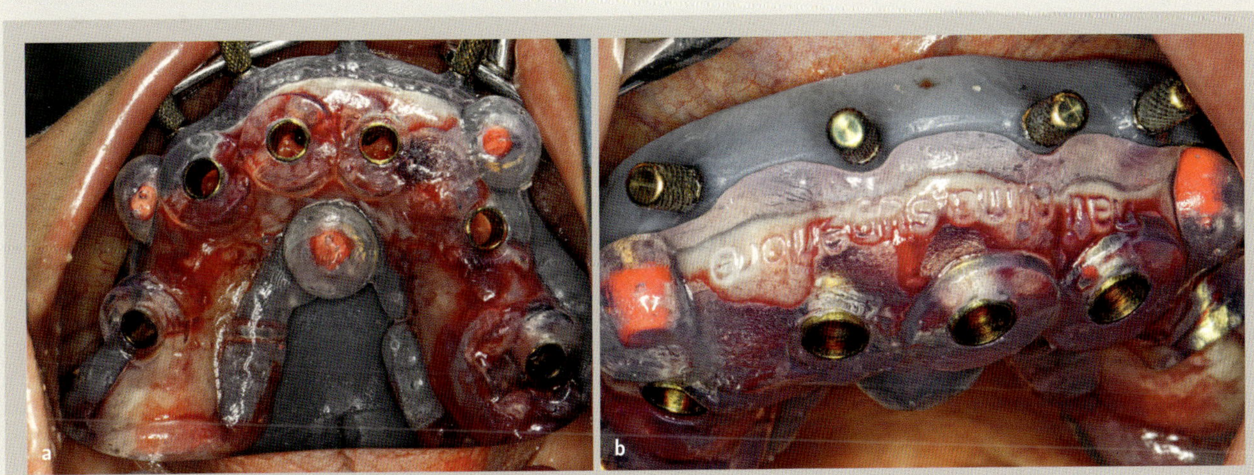

5.74 Part A3 is fixed in position and the implant sites are prepared.

It is essential for the abutments to be parallel to avoid failed prosthesis insertion. The activated retention copings are placed on the abutments (5.75).

The same procedure was performed for the maxilla (5.76 and 5.77). Should it be required, it is possible to place a suture with resorbable thread. According to the proposed technique, the provisional prosthesis was also placed by means of the guide of the same intra-osseous pins used to lock the implant guide.

Once the rubber dam was applied to prevent infiltrations, the prosthesis was rebased on the abutments, through the corresponding holes (5.78 and 5.79). After rebasing, the required occlusal corrections were carried out, followed by accurate polishing. At this stage, the attachments to the surgical guide were also removed (5.80). The prostheses were secured in the mouth by conometry and a post-operative control X-ray was taken (5.81 and 5.82).

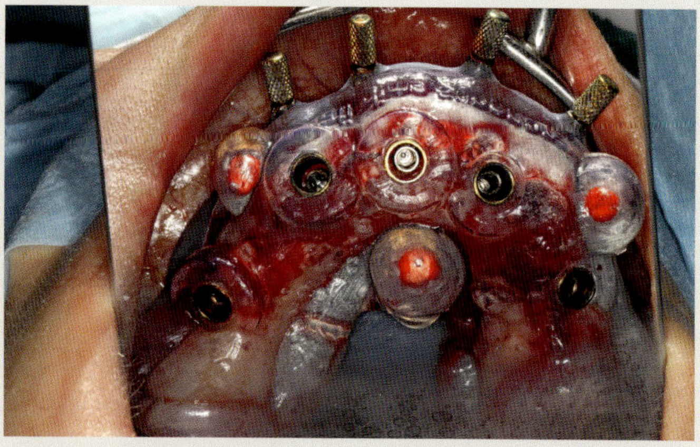

5.75 Implants in position.

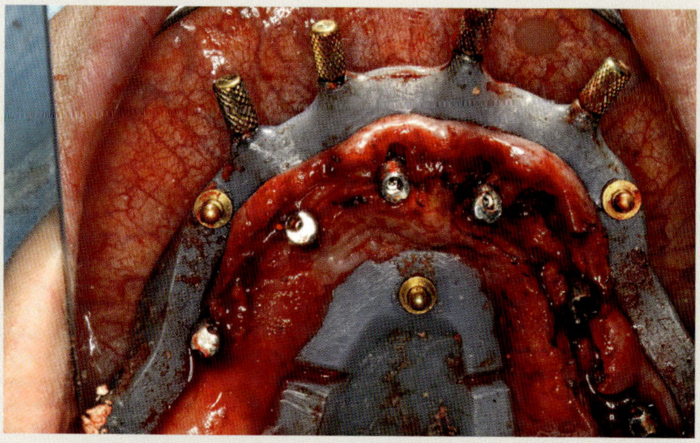

5.76 Abutments inserted in the proper position.

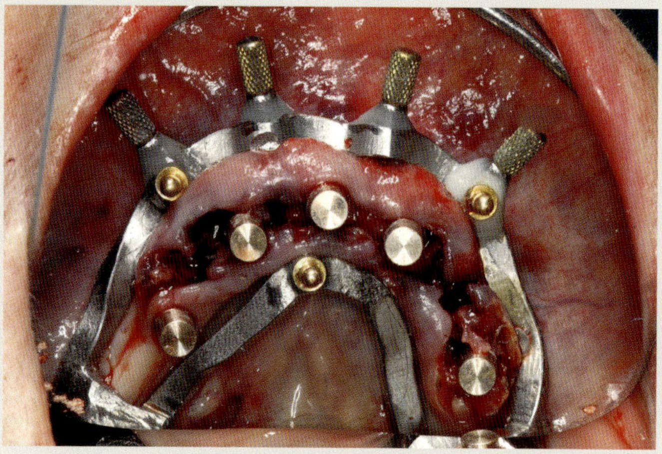

5.77 Conometric copings inserted on the abutments and activated, ready to be fixed by rebasing on the prostheses prepared prior to the procedure.

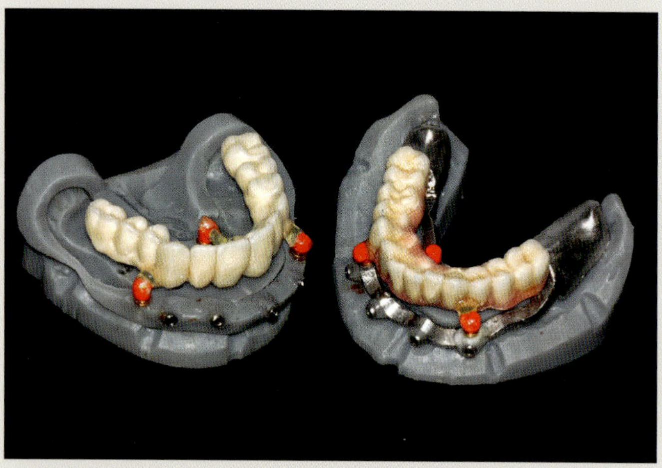

5.78 The upper and lower prostheses inserted on the 3D printed resin models printed, including the attachments for placement in the desired position.

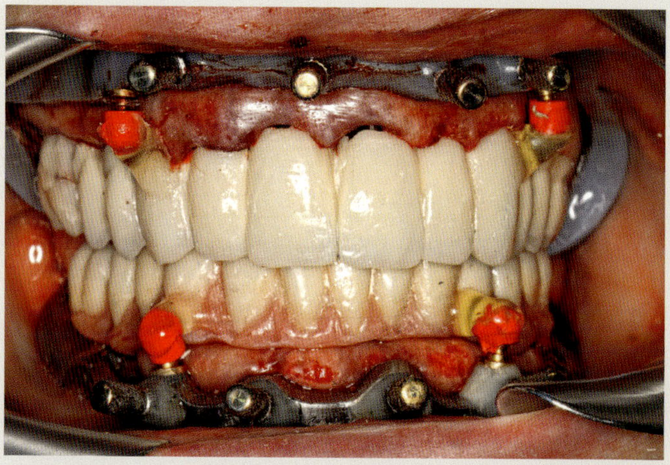

5.79 The two prostheses are tested in the mouth prior to direct rebasing, which will serve the purpose of locking the retentive conometric copings in the framework.

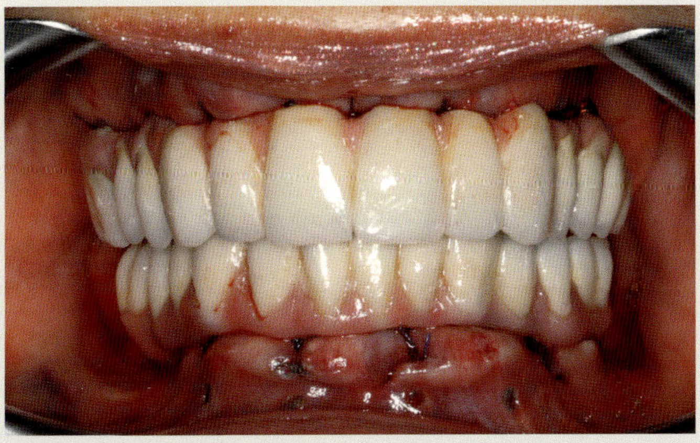

5.80 After rebasing, the prostheses are finished and the arms containing the attachments are removed.

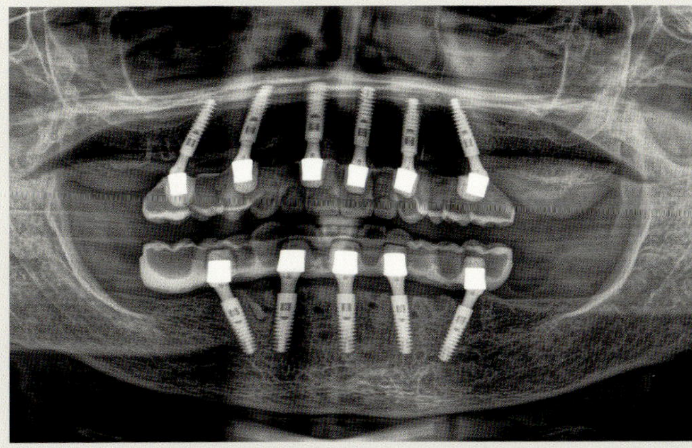

5.81 Post-operative X-ray.

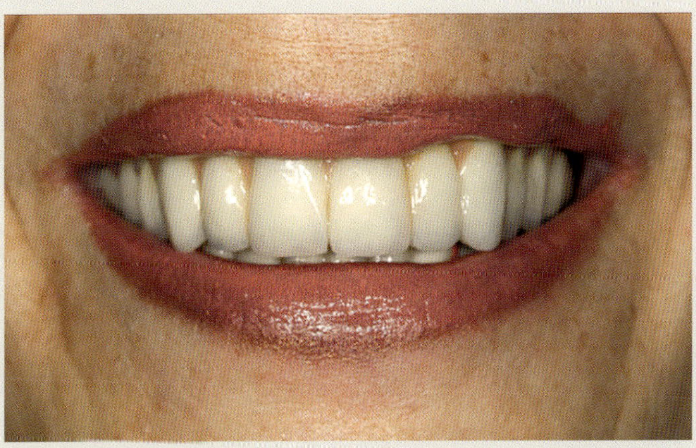

5.82 Patient's smile.

The patient was discharged a few hours after entering the office, with the fixed prostheses in place (5.83). A follow-up visit was scheduled seven days after the procedure (5.84 a-d), followed by more follow-ups after two weeks, one month and, finally, two months after the surgery.

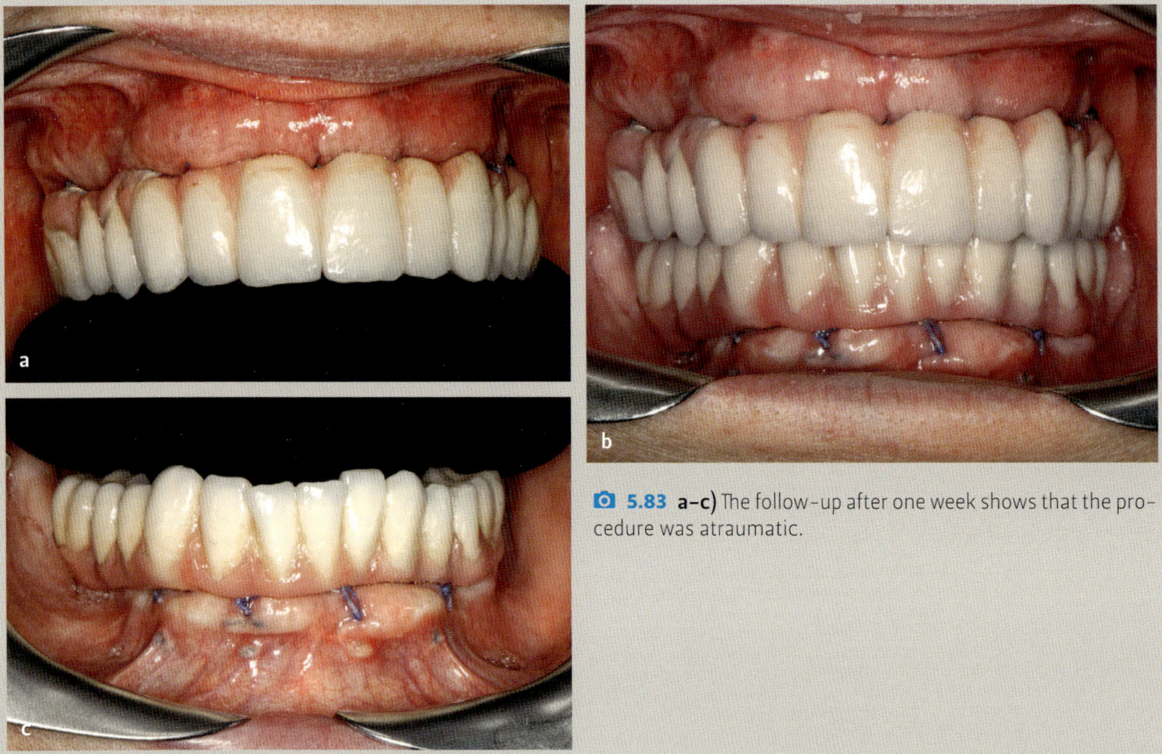

5.83 **a–c)** The follow-up after one week shows that the procedure was atraumatic.

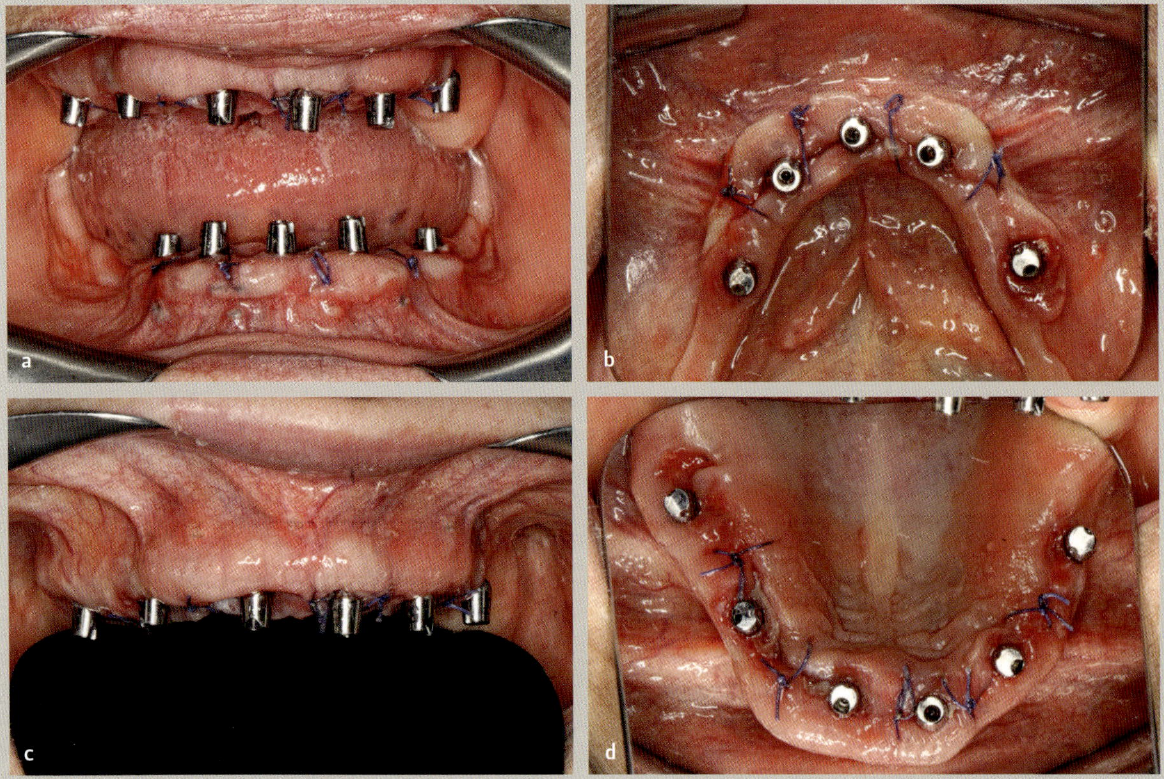

5.84 **a–d)** Ten days after the procedure, the prostheses are removed and hard and soft tissues are checked.

POST-SURGICAL PROCEDURES

The patient was prescribed drug therapy with painkillers for post-operative pain control, until the symptoms resolved. In addition, two one-minute rinses per day were prescribed with a 0.2% chlorhexidine-based mouthwash, for two weeks. For the first month after surgery, it was recommended to follow a soft diet, in order to limit the occlusal load and to reduce micro-movements, which might affect the osseointegration process.

Patients must be instructed on oral hygiene procedures and be included in a maintenance program, which consists in carrying out quarterly professional hygiene sessions. Clinical and radiographic examinations must be repeated every six months after prosthetic loading, to assess the success and survival rate of the implants placed.

Appendix

An alternative to the use of the verticulator is made possible by the introduction to the market of composite blanks, which means that the prostheses already prepared to accommodate the PEEK mesostructure can be milled.

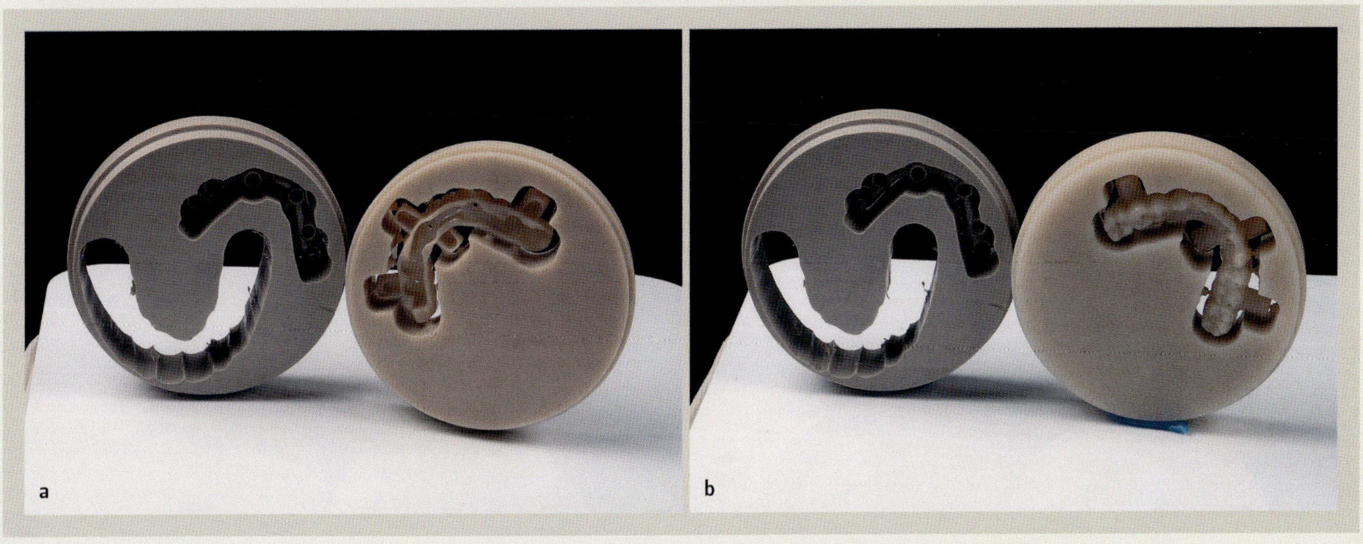

5.85 a,b) The PEEK disc in which the mesostructure was milled (left) and the composite resin prosthesis (right).

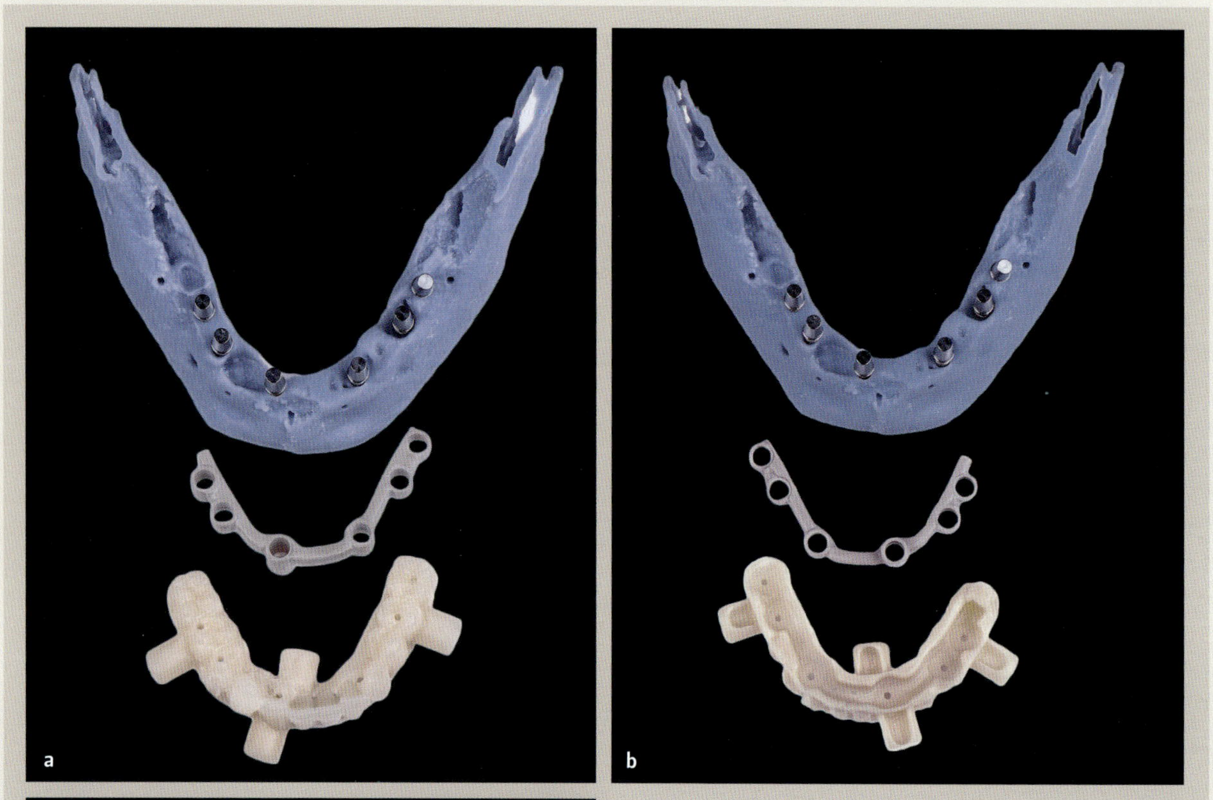

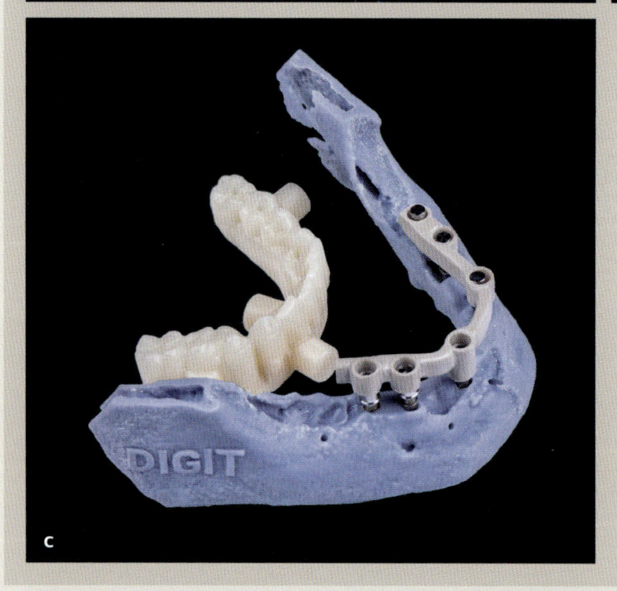

5.86 a–c) In this case the superstructure, including the spaces for the attachments – in compliance with the DIGIT method – was milled in composite. The PEEK reinforcement on the conometric copings can be observed.

REFERENCES

1. **Orentlicher G, Horowitz A, Kobren L.** Computer-Guided Dental Implant Treatment of Complete Arch Restoration of Edentulous and Terminal Dentition Patients. *Oral Maxillofac Surg Clin North Am* 2019;31(3):399-426.
2. **ten Bruggenkate CM, van der Kwast WA, Oosterbeek HS.** Success criteria in oral implantology. A review of the literature. *Int J Oral Implantol* 1990;7(1):45-51.
3. **Baruffaldi A, Poli PP, Baruffaldi A, et al.** Computer-aided flapless implant surgery and immediate loading. A technical note. *Oral Maxillofac Surg* 2016;20(3):313-319.
4. **Beretta M, Poli PP, Tansella S, et al.** Virtually guided alveolar ridge reduction combined with computer-aided implant placement for a bimaxillary implant-supported rehabilitation: A clinical report. *J Prosthet Dent* 2018;120(2):168-172.
5. **Beretta M, Poli PP, Maiorana C.** Accuracy of computer-aided template-guided oral implant placement: a prospective clinical study. *J Periodontal Implant Sci* 2014;44(4):184-193.
6. **Schneider D, Marquardt P, Zwahlen M, et al.** A systematic review on the accuracy and the clinical outcome of computer-guided template-based implant dentistry. *Clin Oral Implants Res* 2009;20 Suppl 4:73-86.
7. **Tahmaseb A, Wismeijer D, Coucke W, et al.** Computer technology applications in surgical implant dentistry: a systematic review. *Int J Oral Maxillofac Implants* 2014;29 Suppl:25-42.
8. **Meloni SM, De Riu G, Pisano M, et al. et al.** Full arch restoration with computer-assisted implant surgery and immediate loading in edentulous ridges with dental fresh extraction sockets. One year results of 10 consecutively treated patients: guided implant surgery and extraction sockets. *J Maxillofac Oral Surg* 2013;12:321-325.
9. **Baruffaldi A, Poli PP, Baruffaldi A, et al.** Computer-aided flapless implant surgery and immediate loading. A technical note. Oral Maxillofac Surg 2016;20:313-319.
10. **Baruffaldi A, Baruffaldi A, Baruffaldi M, et al.** A suggested protocol to increase the accuracy of prosthetic phases in case of full-arch model-free fully guided computer-aided implant placement and immediate loading. Oral Maxillofac Surg 2020;24(3):343-351.

The SKYN concept

Livio Yoshinaga, Alfonso Baruffaldi

SKYN is a new concept in the dental sector, pointing to an innovative method for communication, diagnosis and planning in dentistry, with a focus on digital tools. The technique is also integrated with the design of a laboratory workflow, based on digital instruments, using CAD-CAM/CAE. Although it is able to "talk" to all CAD-CAM systems on the market, the SKYN Concept design process uses the 3Shape Dental System platform exclusively with the specific digital UHD (Ultra High Definition) library and the proprietary MillBox milling strategy (CIMsystem) for Roland®, Imes-Icore®, VHF® and Redon®.

SKYN Concept uses clinical protocols fully integrated with the laboratory workflow. The key feature of SKYN is replicating the natural morphology, using CAD-CAM technology, with no need to design each individual tooth. Guided by a simple 2D design, the SKYN Concept uses just a picture and a video as complete digital documentation, in addition to information derived from the intraoral scan, to execute 3D designs. At the same time, psychology and architecture of work environments are applied, since SKYN recommends a new communication protocol and a special "smile design" room, with a "designer" architecture, to maximise patients' satisfaction and positive feedback.

Copying nature is not enough. It is necessary to start from natural morphology and combine shapes and the best morphology, to enhance nature and create what we call "super-natural smiles". This improved morphology is then turned into a digital library, using the 3Shape Dental System software platform with UHD resolution (6.1).

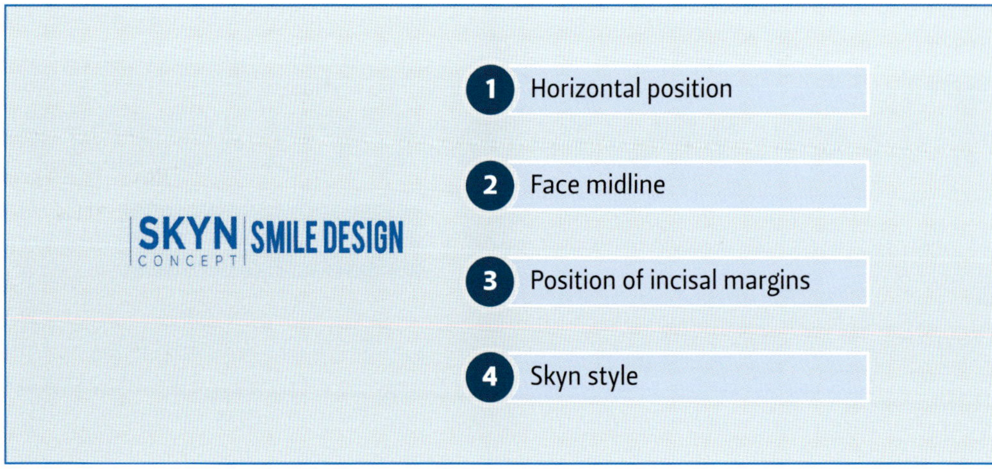

6.1 Skyn concept technique workflow.

Computer-aided smile design was introduced around 1986, when teeth were drawn on a picture of the patient's face, using the DOS system and a Targa card on Intel 286 machines. The output device was a thermal printer, which could immediately produce photo prints with the desired modifications. The purpose was to help dentists communicate with patients, to visualize the changes in their aesthetics. A decisive advance in the technique took place around 2016, when together with Christian Coachman, we developed what nowadays is called DSD (Digital Smile Design). Since then Smile Design supports not just the patient, but the dental technician as well. DSD has finally turned a possibility into an actual visible design, just as in architecture. In this way, the dental technician can have a plan to follow, with measurements and references that originate from the patient's face. The next step was to transfer the design into 3D: CEREC was the first platform used.

A direct mock-up, replicating natural teeth, was executed intraorally or on a model. CEREC then used Biocopy to "copy" in 3D the real morphology, with a technique based on AST (Anatomic Shell Technique). This process was developed jointly with Dr Paulo Kano (dentist, Brazil). The next step was achieved thanks to the 3Shape software, with Dental System able to use digital libraries and techniques to improve natural morphology, as well as a complete workflow, with digital control of the preparation, which led to what we now know as SKYN Concept. This clinical and CAD-CAM workflow was then implemented and improved by other specialists, such as Florin Cofar, Lorant Stumpf and Alejandro Pineda, who significantly contributed to the technique. The crucial point in its evolution was the foundation of the SKYN Concept headquarters in Sao Paulo where Dr Kano opened a training centre and a digital laboratory. Many questions were finally answered through mentoring by Dr Fabricio Guarnieri, digital expert dentist, technician and smile designer.

Picture 6.2 shows the superior simplification level achieved with DSD: SKYN Smile Design uses just one picture, one video and a complete intraoral scan. Using the picture, analysis and decision making are based on four elements:

1. the orientation of the face on the horizontal plane;
2. the face midline position, in order to compare it with the teeth midline and decide whether to move it or not, when designing the new central teeth position;
3. incisal margin position, to control its exposure;
4. which smile style would be best.

At this stage, patient involvement is recommended, as they help make the choice, defining the esthetics they identify with.

The four criteria are identified in a single picture. As, the whole gingival tissues will be perfectly replicated through the intraoral scans no further pictures are necessary.

A video complements the documentation with which we can acquire much essential information and get to know the patient better. The upper, lower and occlusal scans complete the data acquisition; in case of occlusion problems, a second scan in centric relation (CR) is added. The scans are matched to the photo using markers. In this way, it is possible to perfectly position our digital model, in order to apply our 2D designs and superimpose the library of 3D Supernatural teeth (6.3 and 6.4).

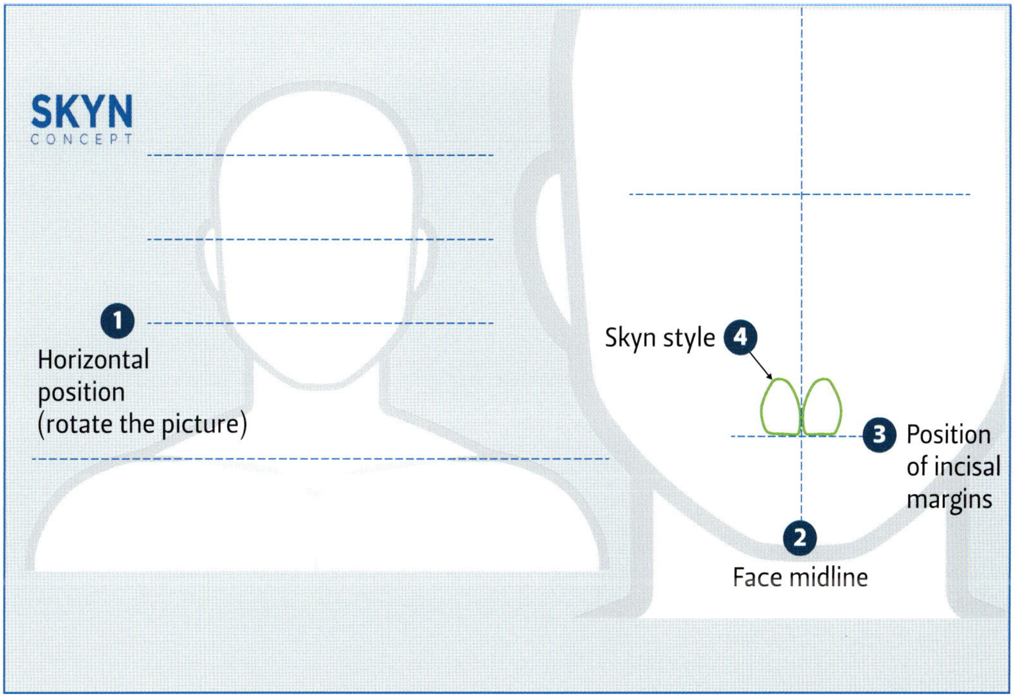

6.2 Skyn Smile Design diagram obtained from a single picture.

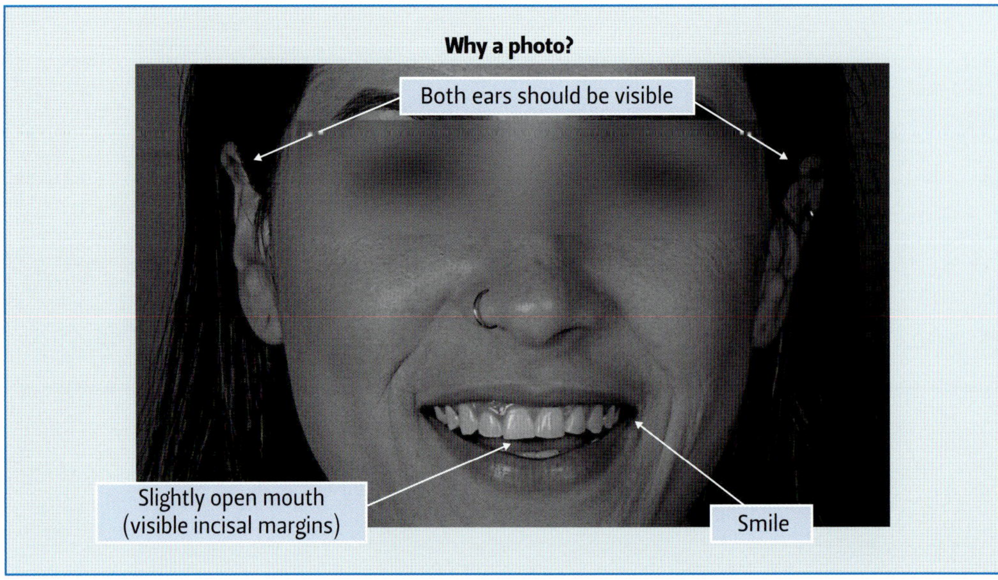

6.3 References in the patient's picture.

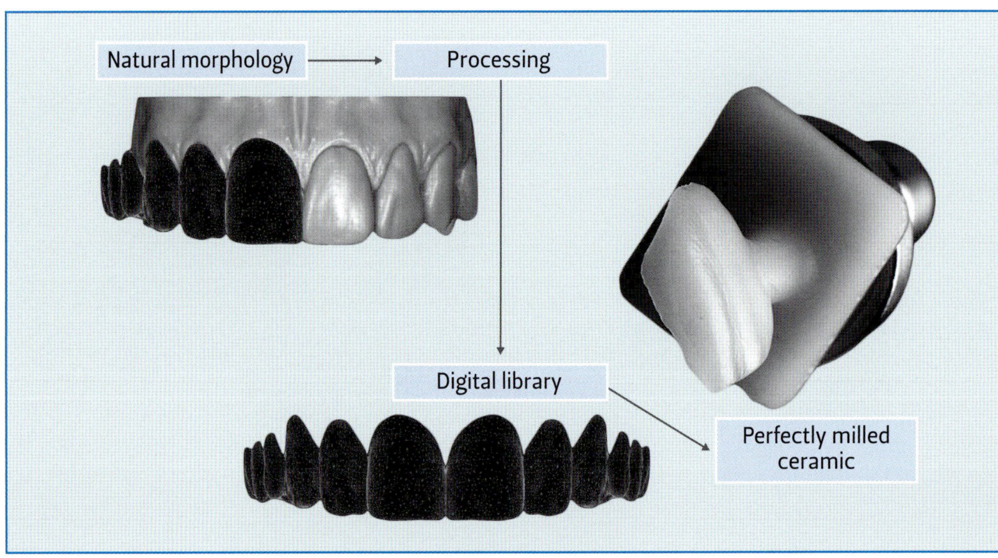

6.4 Overlay of the supernatural library on the patient's picture.

The workflow is distinguished and shown in blue (dentistry) and in green (dental technician) (6.5)) and each step leads to the next, so dentists as well as technicians know exactly what to do and when to do it, with perfectly synchronised steps and actions.

During the first appointment, a complete case documentation is acquired (one picture, one video and intraoral scans); this will be complemented with a 2D smile design, resulting in a mock-up. Then, on the second appointment, the mock-up is applied and a "before and after" video presentation is shown to the patient. Once accepted, the preparations and the digital control of the preparation ensure all spaces are respected, as well as rounded edges to make the milling process easier.

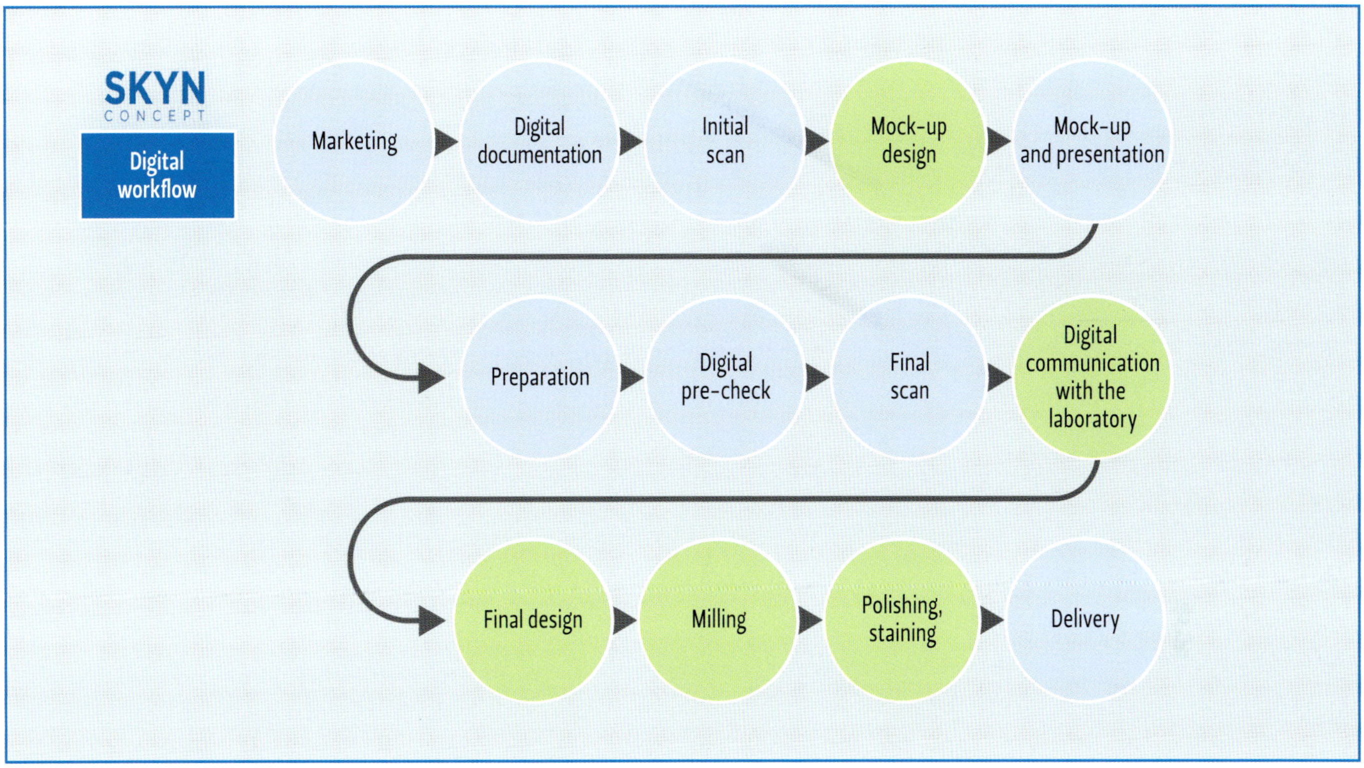

6.5 Workflow for the dentist (in blue) and for the dental technician (in green).

The laboratory then receives and designs the final STL files (crowns, veneers, inlays and onlays), and carries out the milling process, using the proprietary milling strategies.

Finally, a ceramic restoration is obtained, which needs only to be polished, stained and glazed, if required. Cementation is carried out with no need for touch-ups and with contact points that are already perfect, defined in the design stage.

If the gingival architecture is less than ideal, an optional workflow is required (6.6). The mock-up will act as the guide: gingival surgery is performed, and a digital surgical check is carried out, to ensure the design has been complied with. The osteotomy is then performed and the new gingival shape is scanned and sent to the dental technician, who adapts the initial design to the new gingiva, then prints another 3D model and produces a new mock-up, to guide the final preparation.

If orthodontic treatment is required, it might not be possible to execute a mock-up, therefore a 2D simulation will be used.

Orthodontic appliances and aligners are entirely designed using digital systems and define the final reference position of the prepared teeth, in the event that a veneer or crown needs to be placed on the aligned teeth. A final scan is taken and sent to the dental technician after orthodontic treatment; the design is adapted to the new situation, then a new 3D model is produced and the final mock-up is used to continue the preparation stage, as described above (6.7).

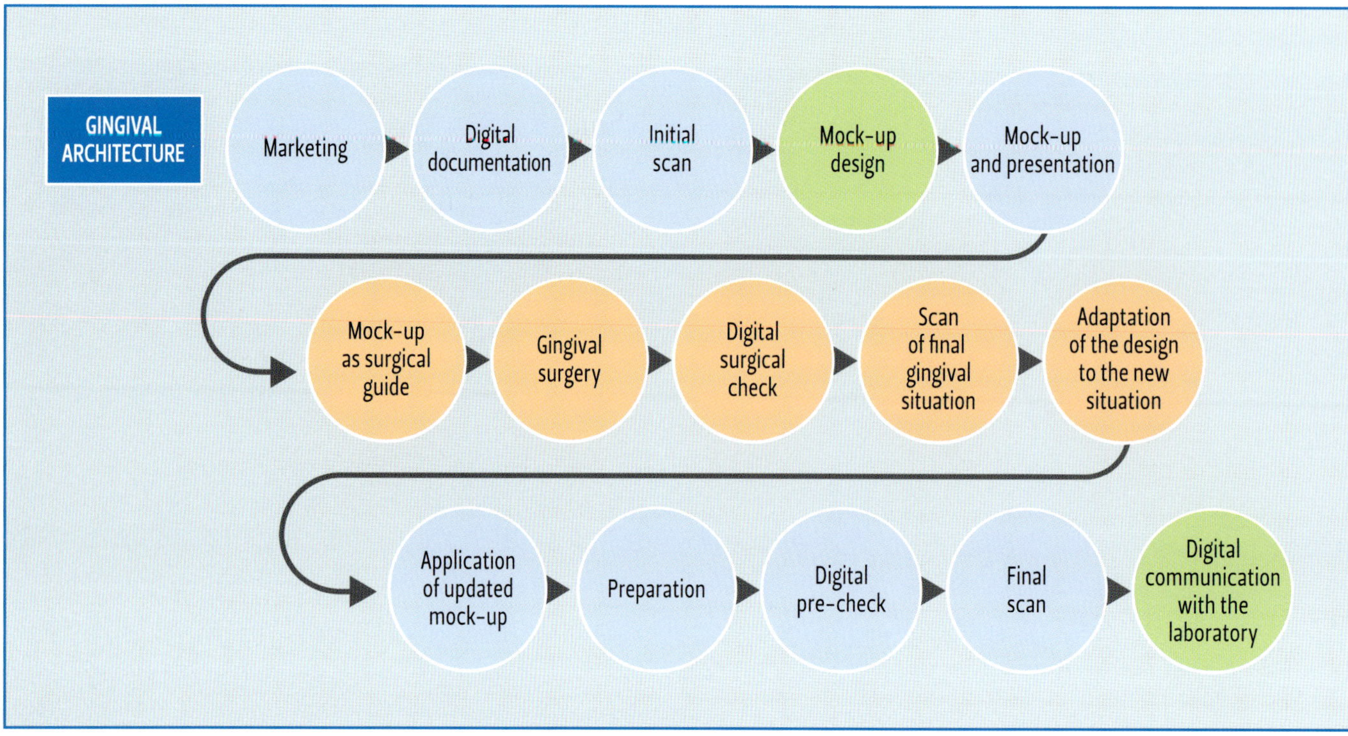

6.6 Optional workflow to be used in case of non-ideal gingival architecture.

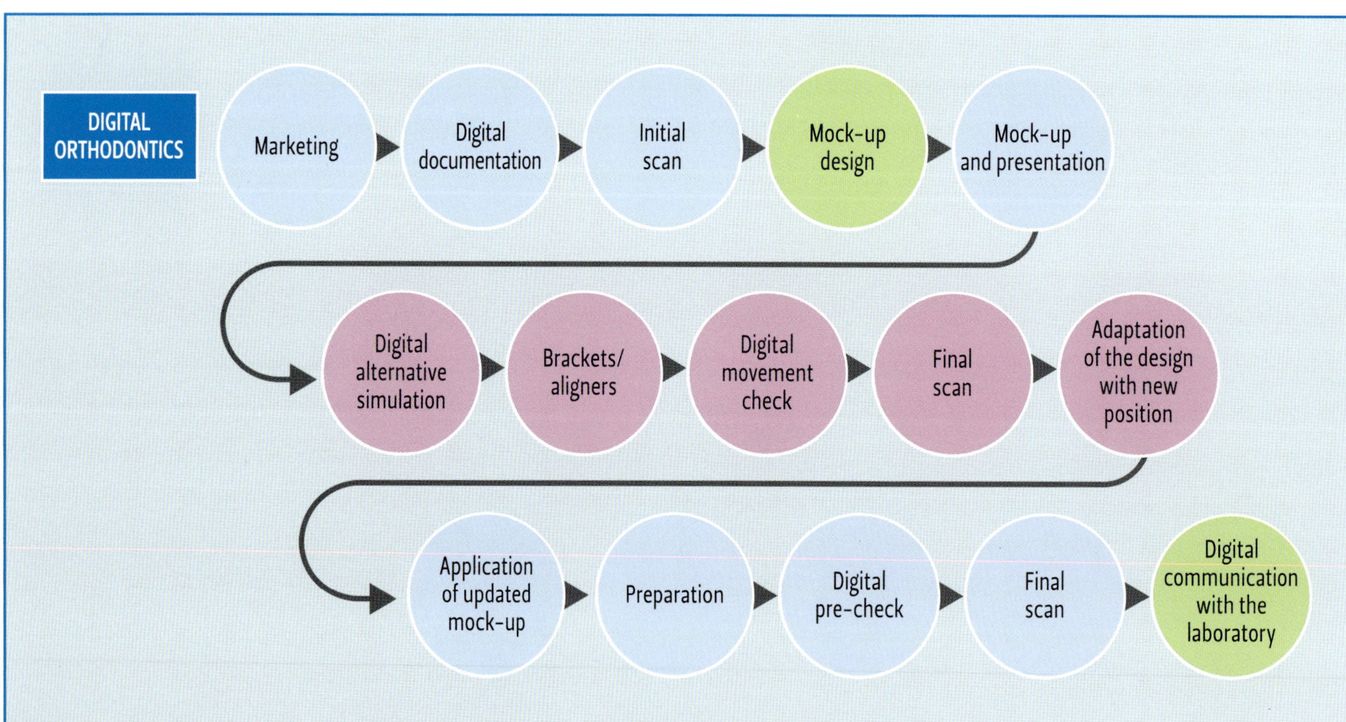

6.7 Optional workflow to be used in case of orthodontics.

Although types of workflow may vary, implants may be planned based on the initial situation or placed taking into account the final crown position. This ensures that both esthetics and function are complied with when the crown is designed according to the SKYN Concept technique. The position of the implant is always planned according to the DIGIT method, developed by Baruffaldi A. et al,[1,2] which is integrated into the SKYN Concept Implant Workflow. In general, implants may be planned at various stages of treatment plan, according to the situation. The DIGIT technique adds to the method the value of predictability and precision required by SKYN Concept, so that all cases may be treated in the most suitable manner (6.8).

The final result is natural looking ceramic restorations of extreme beauty and functionality. No touch-up is required after milling and no models need to be used for adaptation and contact points. Indeed, both have been defined and designed during CAD.

Thanks to the use of the proprietary SKYN Concept strategies, developed at CIM Systems - Italia, perfect milling can be obtained.

An important factor to focus on is marginal precision, which is also critical for healthy gingival tissues, which determine approximately 40-50% of tooth morphology.

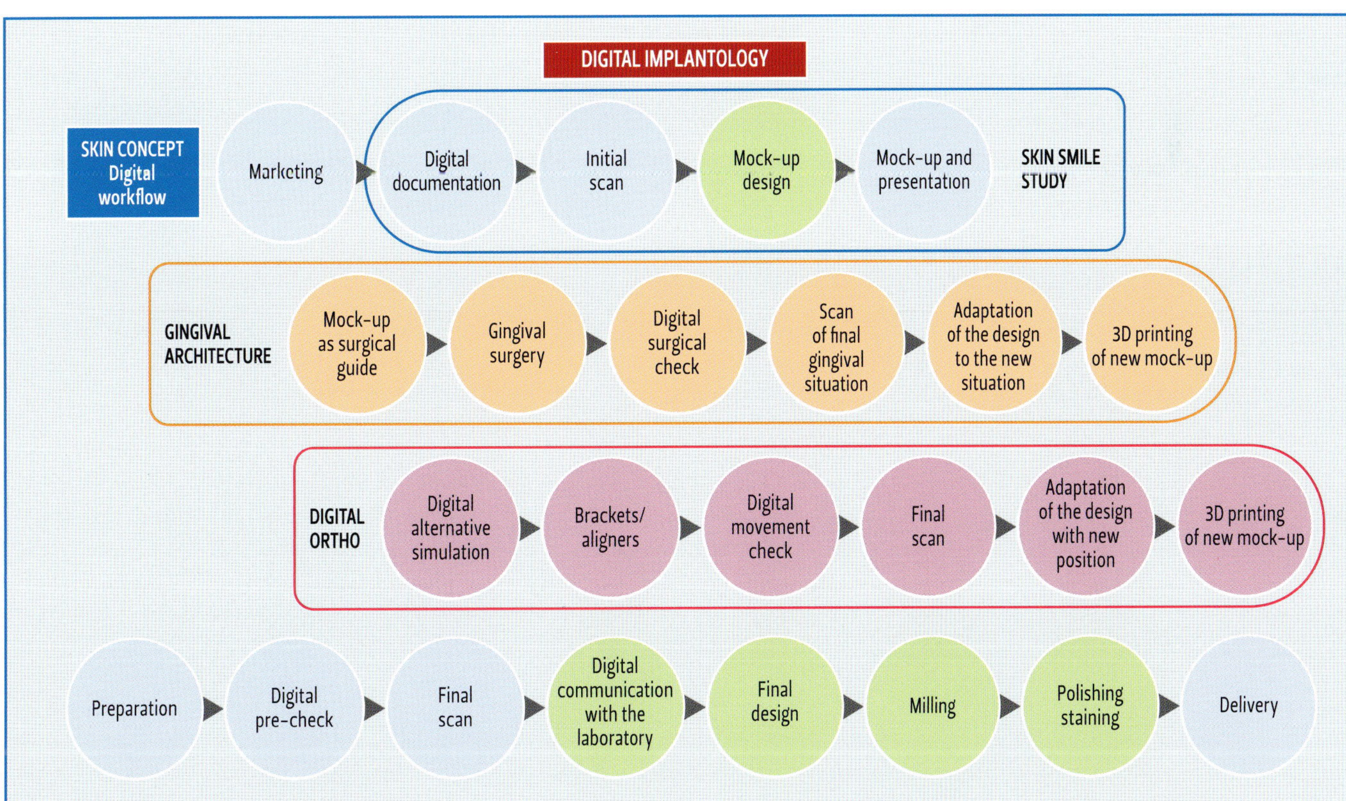

6.8 Workflow in case of implant insertion.

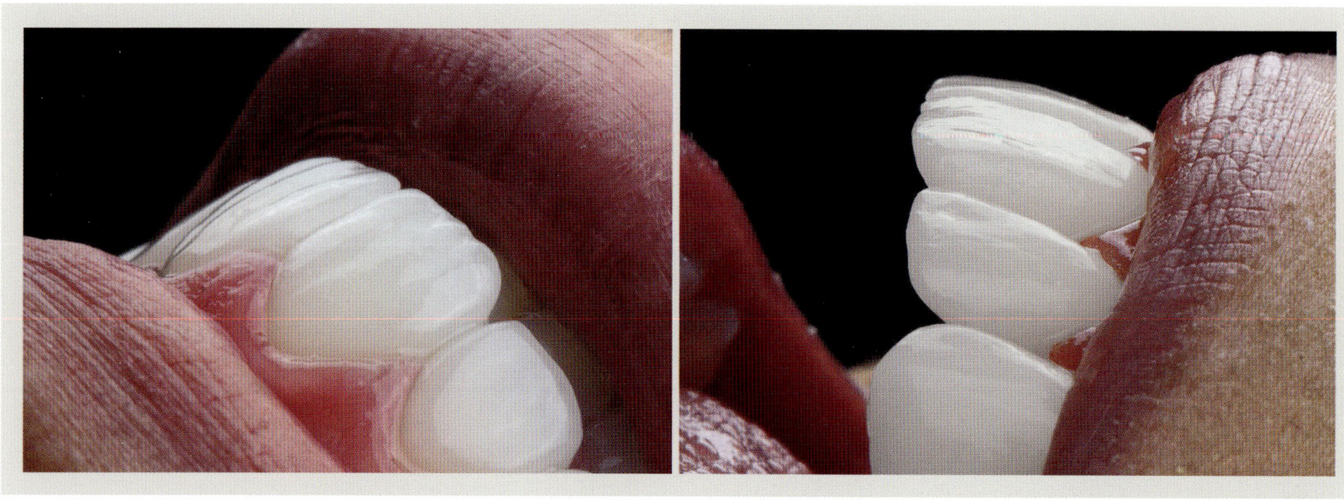

6.9 Examples of veneers and crowns produced with Empress CAD.

IPS Empress CAD Multi (Ivoclar, Schaan, Liechtenstein) is our choice for ceramic restorations in the anterior regions. It is a leucite-based material, which has excellent biomimetic features and represents the gold standard among the ceramic materials currently on the market. This product stands out for the shaded tone and transparency, which are essential for a natural smile (6.9).

An example case for SKYN Concept which required the preparation of veneers, crowns on natural teeth and implants is presented below.

Clinical case

A multidisciplinary case designed and executed with SKYN technique is illustrated below. The workflow involved Prof. Paolo Generali from the University of Modena and Reggio Emilia (Italy), for the clinical part, and the Odontodigitale dental laboratory (Piacenza, Italy) for the dental-technical part

The patient requested the replacement of a PFM bridge in the upper arch, supported by teeth 1.3 and 1.1, and with teeth 1.2 and 2.1 as pontics (6.10).

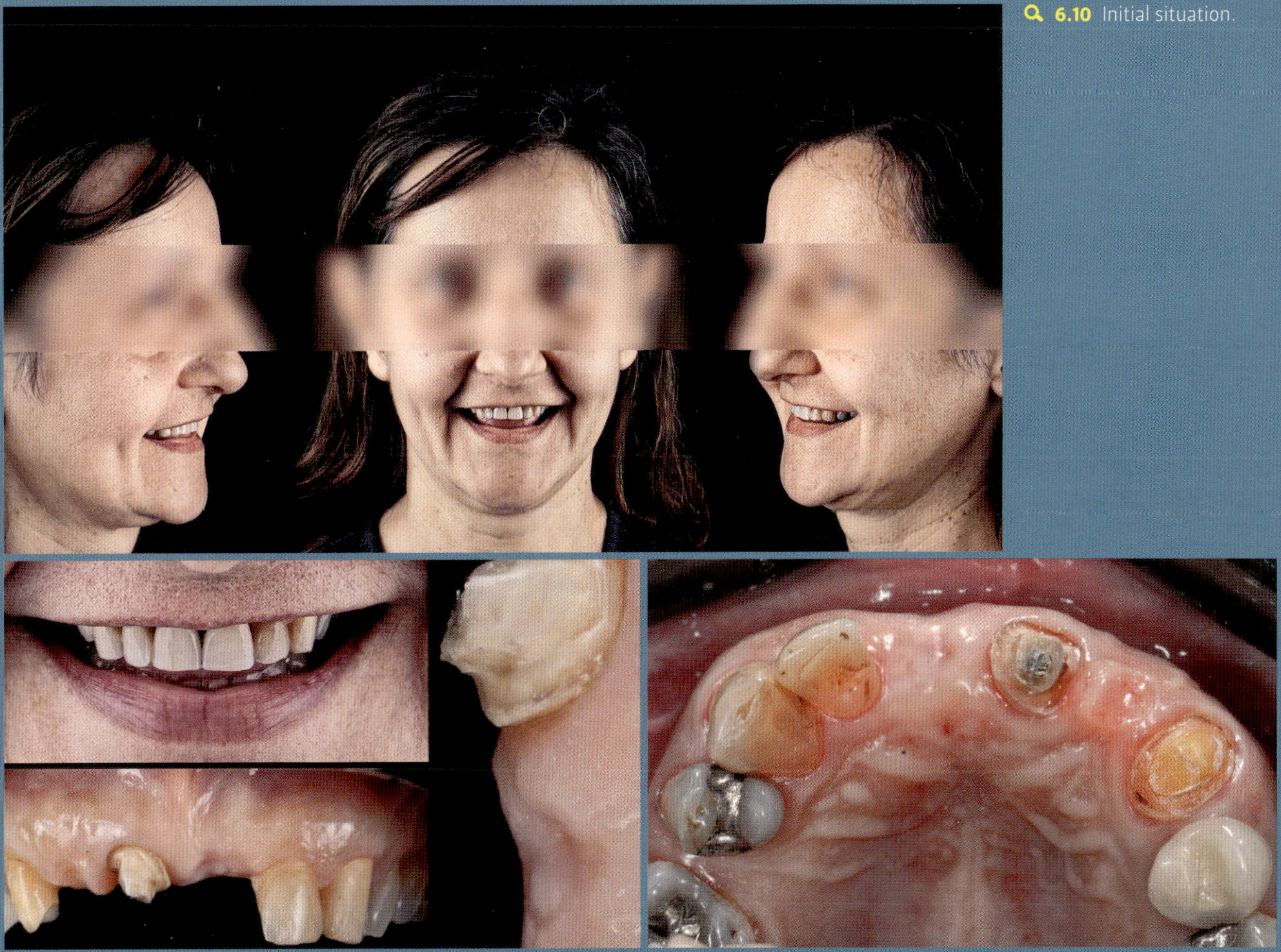

6.10 Initial situation.

A rehabilitation was planned with the insertion of two implant-supported crowns replacing the pontics, and restoring the remaining teeth with ceramic crowns and two veneers on teeth 2.2 and 2.3 (6.11).

After taking an impression with an intraoral scanner (6.12), a virtual wax-up was designed, using anatomies contained in the digital SKYN libraries (6.13). The wax-up was used to produce a model with a 3D printer, and a silicone index was created for intraoral transfer of the design, by means of composite resin (6.14).

Once the design was approved by the patient, the next step consisted in using the wax-up for implant planning. A CBCT scan and guided implantology software were used (6.15).

Implant planning made it possible to 3D print a surgical guide (6.16), which was used to guide the insertion of the implants in the intended position.

After the osseointegration period, the impression of implants and natural teeth was taken (6.17).

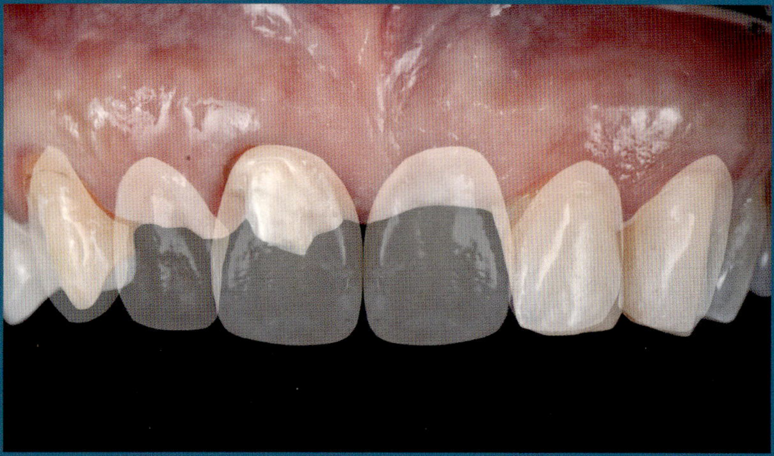

6.11 To replace the existing prosthetic work, a rehabilitation was planned with implant- and tooth-supported crowns and veneers.

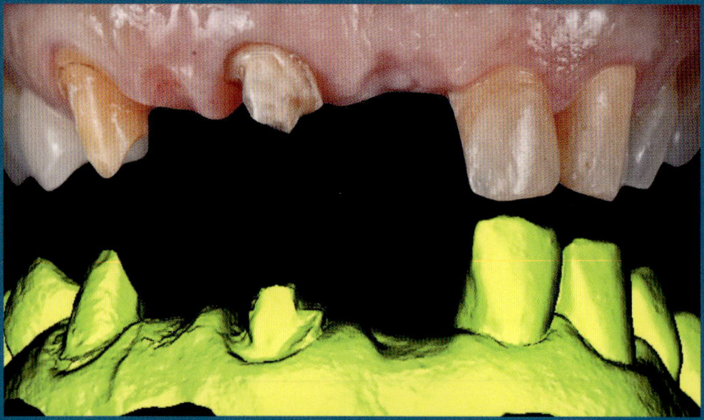

6.12 Digital impression.

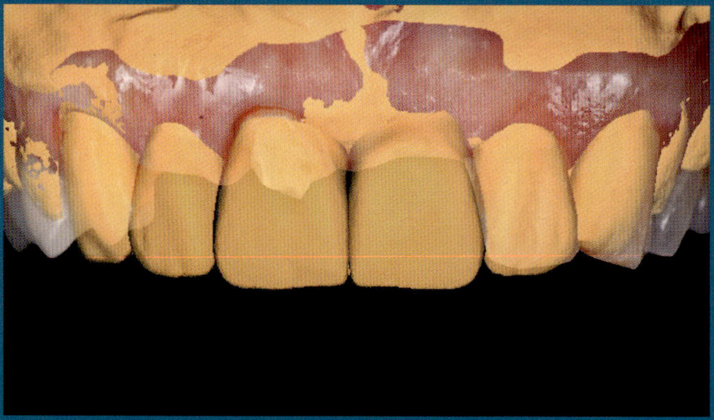

6.13 Digital wax-up with dental SKYN libraries.

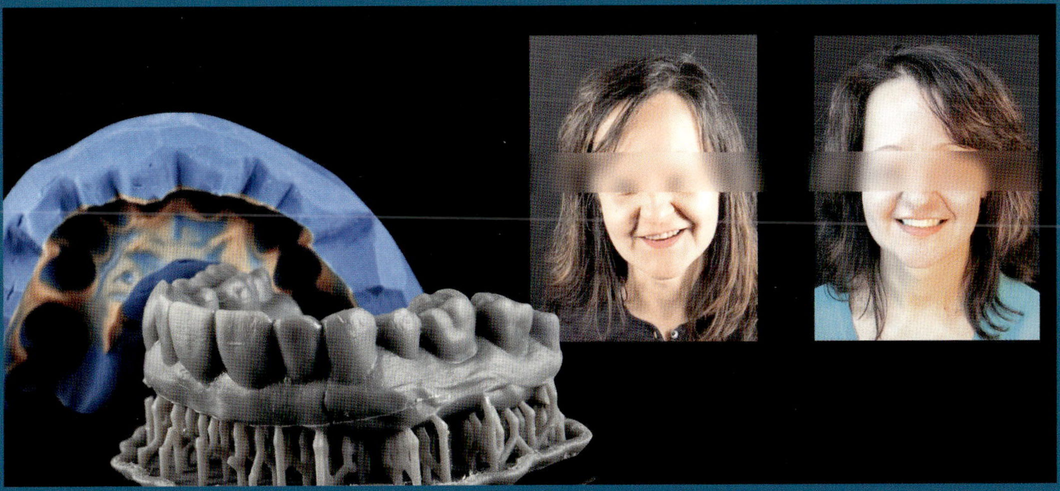

6.14 The wax-up is replicated with a 3D printer and transferred intraorally.

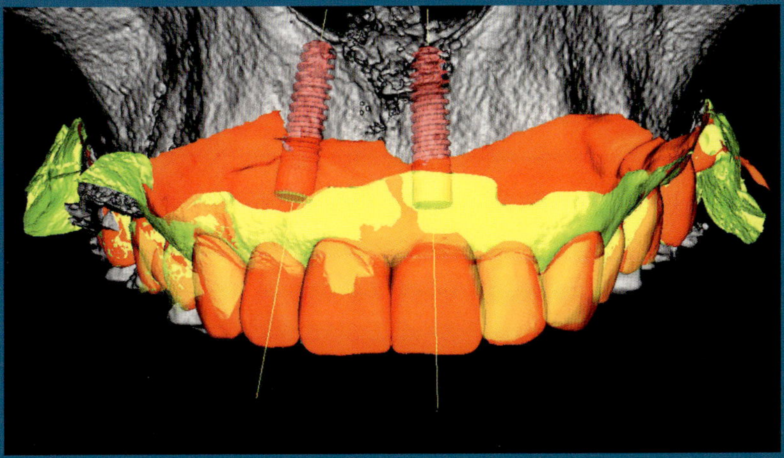

6.15 Digital wax-up enables prosthetically guided implant planning.

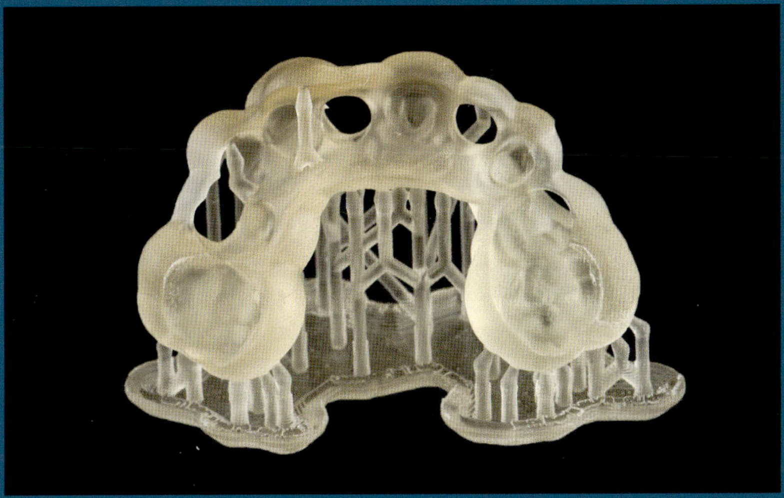

6.16 The surgical guide is fabricated with a 3D printer.

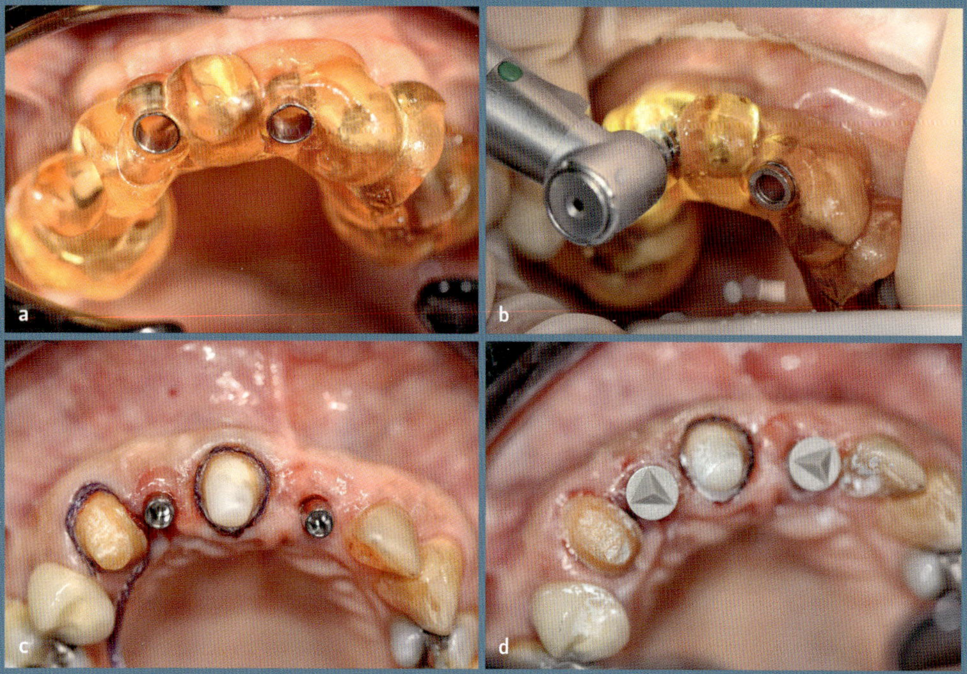

6.17 **a)** Placement of the surgical guide; **b)** guided implant insertion; **c)** implant abutments insertion; **d)** placement of scan bodies for digital impression.

By means of the CAD-CAM software, the design initially proposed was copied, and replicated in the final restorations (6.18a-c). Restorations were made in ceramics, with a milling machine able to replicate the details of the anatomies selected in the design stage, at the very beginning of the treatment. After the milling stage, the items required only polishing and staining, so as not to modify the digitally created texture (6.18d-6.24). Each step of the rehabilitation was guided by the design that had been initially approved. The techniques and instruments used ensured the exact transfer of digital information at each step to increase the predictability of both the clinical and dental technical parts.

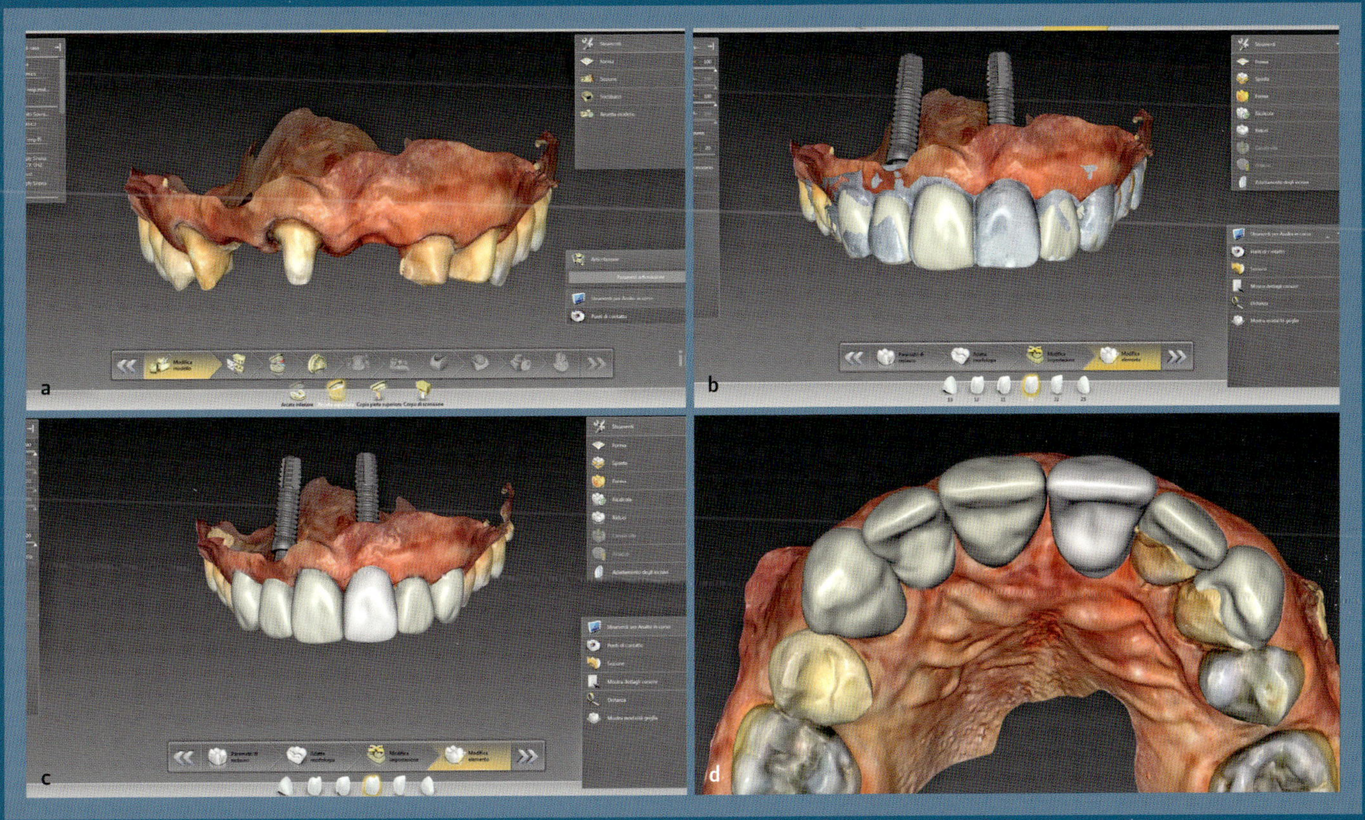

6.18 **a)** Importing the impression into the CAD-CAM software. **b,c,d)** Designing the final crowns and veneers that replicate the initially proposed design.

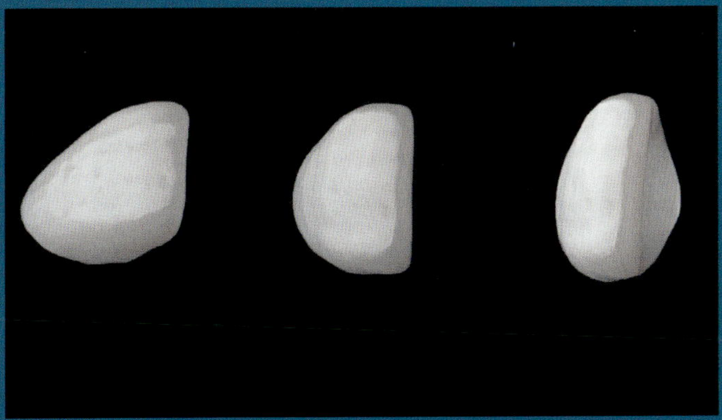

6.19 Detail of one of the items after the milling stage.

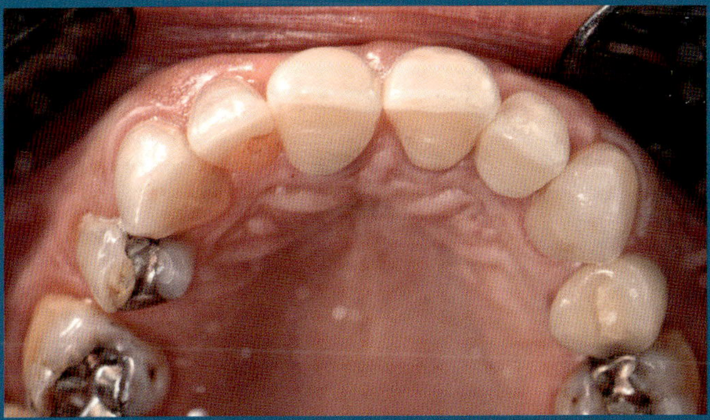

6.20 Occlusal view of the rehabilitation.

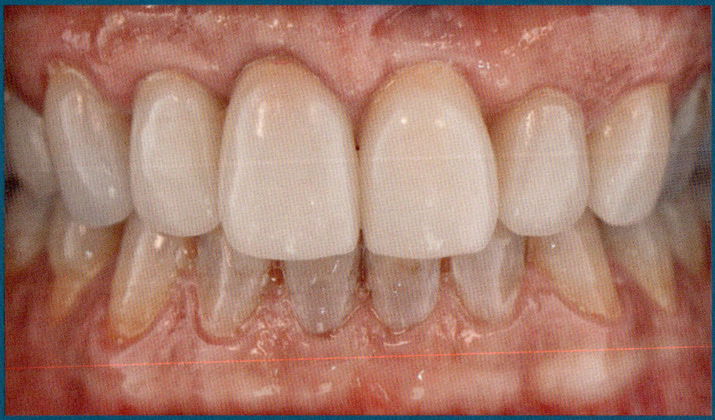

6.21 Frontal view of the rehabilitation.

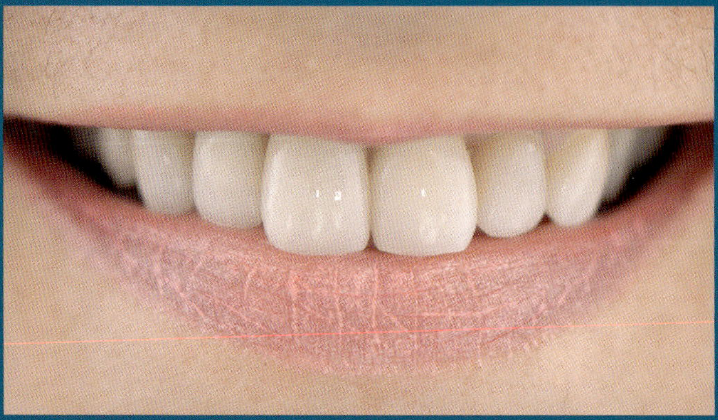

6.22 Integration of the restorations.

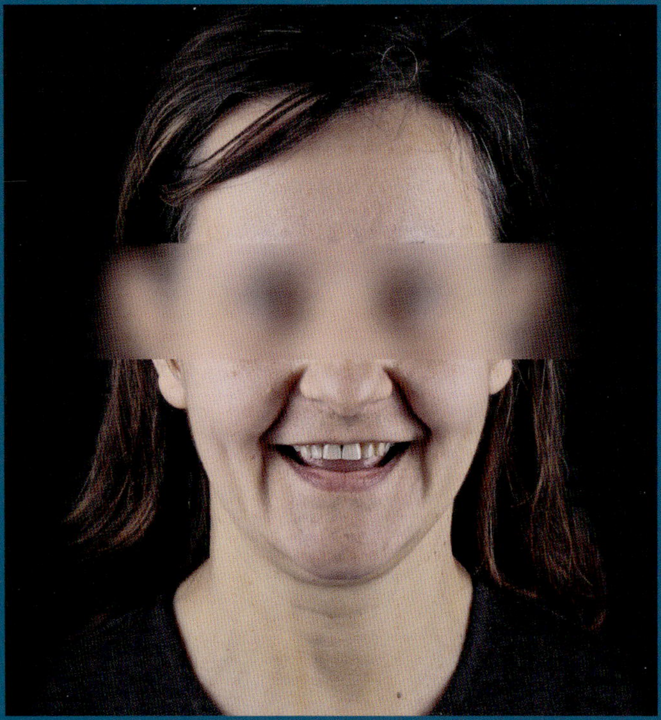

6.23 The patient before the rehabilitation.

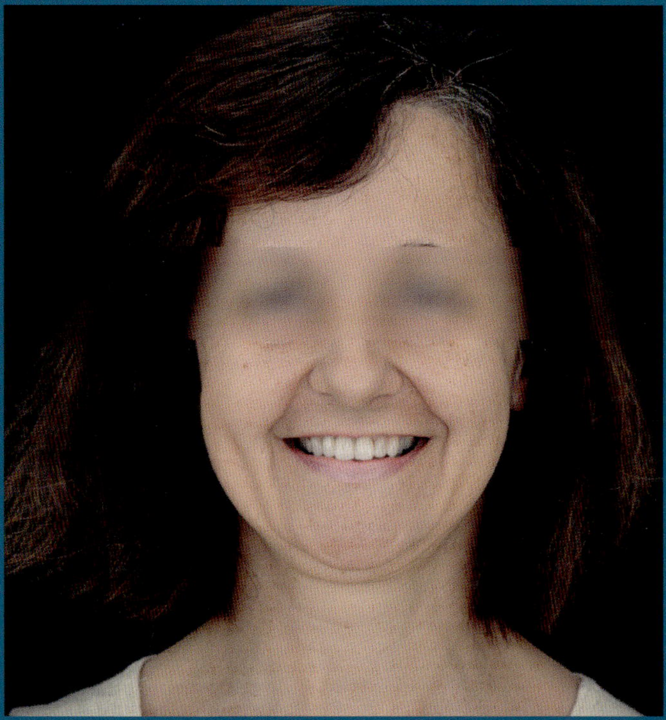

6.24 The patient at the end of the rehabilitation.

Clinical cases

Alfonso Baruffaldi

In this chapter, some cases exemplifying the DIGIT technique, taken from our clinical practice, will be illustrated.

In some of them we show how some frequently occurring variables in oral surgery are addressed, such as the need for bone tissue regeneration or the inability to immediately load certain implants. Our guided surgery technique makes it possible to load these implants even at a later stage, upon final prosthesis delivery. The position, inclination, depth of the implants and consequently the type, position and dimensions of the implant abutments do not change compared to that in the initial design, which allowed all the items required for the temporary prosthetic rehabilitation to be fabricated. However, the possibility remains to take a digital impression after healing, using specific ScanPosts (scan bodies that enable, by matching with implant libraries included in the system, the identification of the exact position of the implant: type, inclination, insertion depth, diameter, position of the anti-rotation system) for conometric abutments. The initial design will be superimposed on it, to get to the fabrication of the final prosthesis - even in different materials from the composite resin that the temporary prosthesis is fabricated with - without the need for intermediate try-in. Should a try-in be required, this will be made very straightforward by the easy removal and installation of the conometric retention prosthesis itself, with obvious time saving for the dentist.

Clinical Case 1

Female patient, 70 years old

The patient presents with the need to restore proper mastication in the lower arch, complaining of tooth mobility and widespread gingival inflammation. The patient is under therapy with levothyroxine for hypothyroidism. No other significant systemic conditions are present.

The objective examination of the lower arch highlights the presence of teeth 38 (residual root), 35, 34, 33, 32, 31, 41 and 42. The periodontal support is extremely reduced, with grade 3 mobility of all teeth, except 33 and 35 with grade 1 mobility. No mucosal lesions were found.

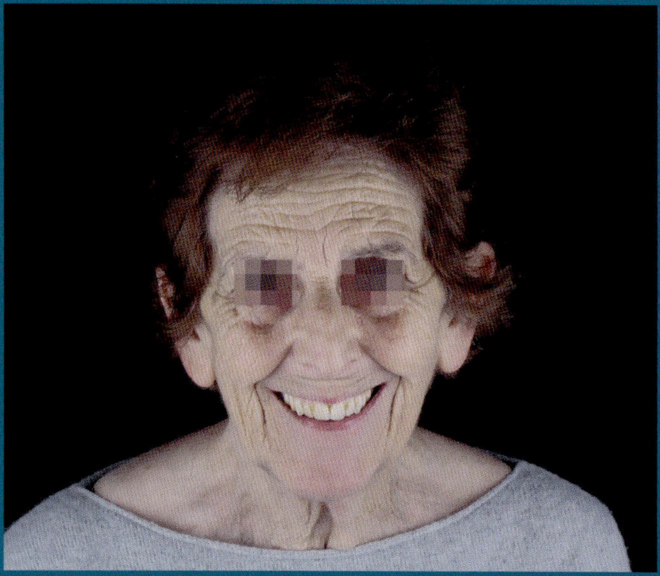

7.1 The patient has no specific esthetic demand for the lower arch but requests the hygiene procedures of the future prosthesis to be made as easy as possible.

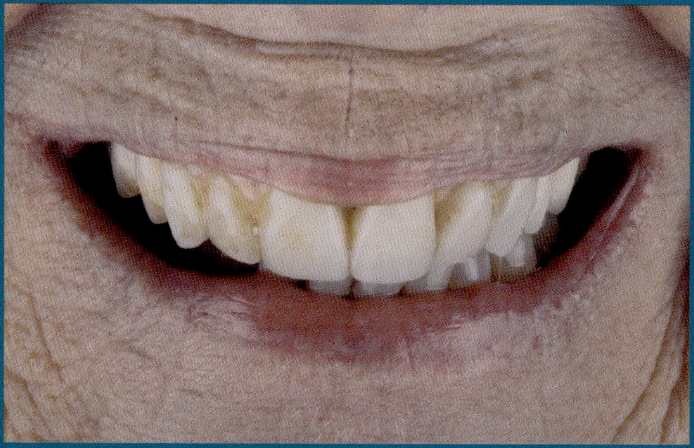

7.2 The patient's smile. The partial edentulism of the teeth in the fourth quadrant can be seen.

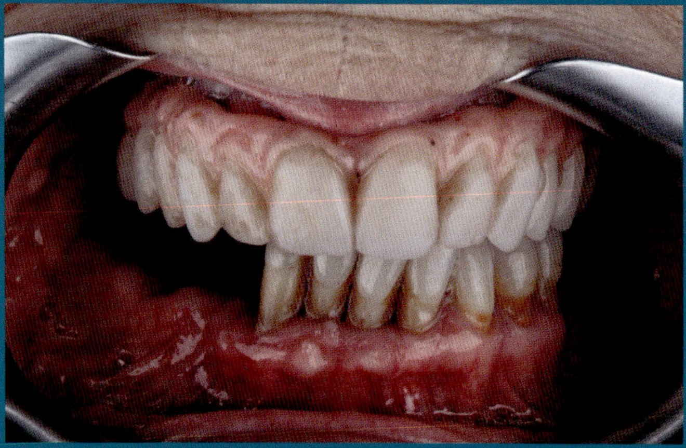

7.3 Occlusal relationship between the upper Toronto type prosthesis and the lower arch.

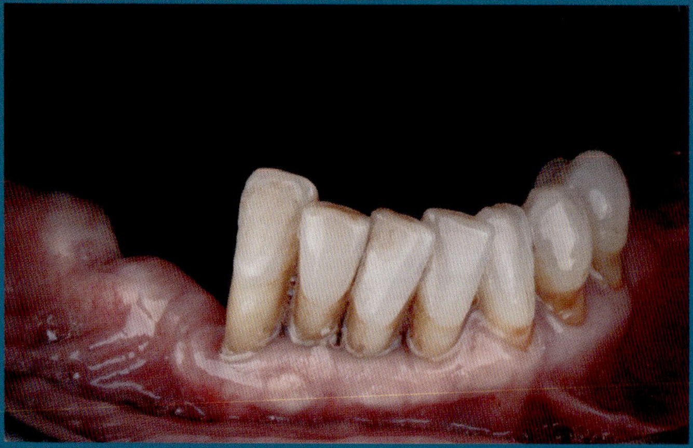

7.4 Bone resorption due to teeth loss can be observed in the fourth quadrant.

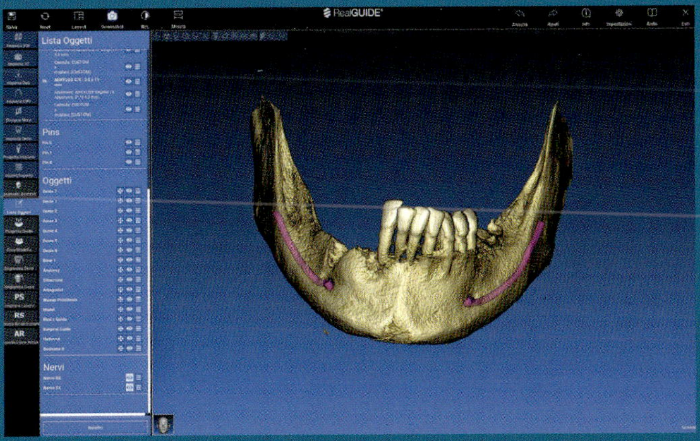

7.5 CBCT view in the design software.

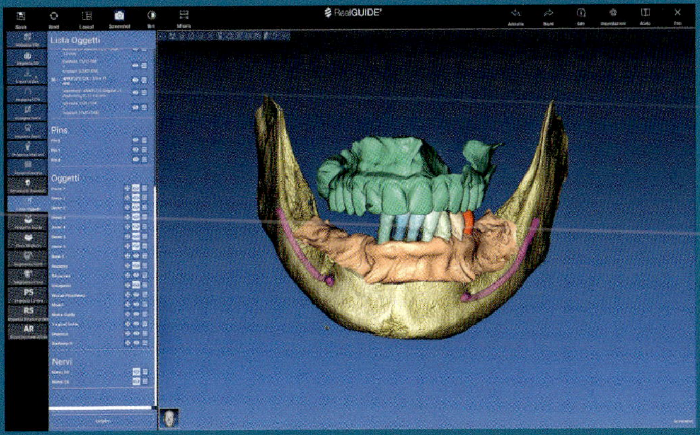

7.6 Matching the CBCT and the optical impression.

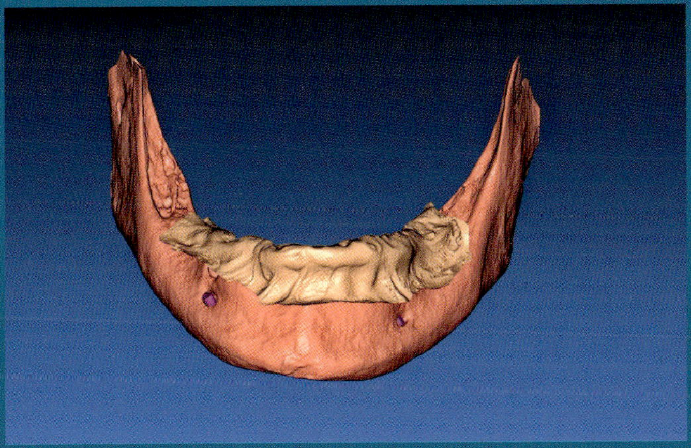

7.7 The teeth in the lower arch are virtually extracted.

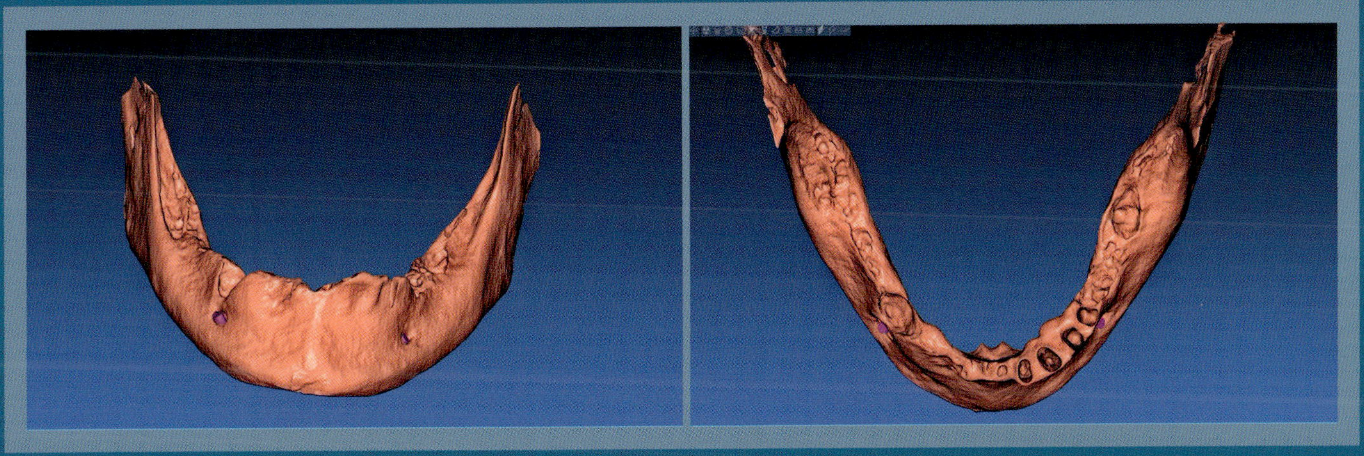

7.8 Virtual images of the widespread bone resorption of the lower arch.

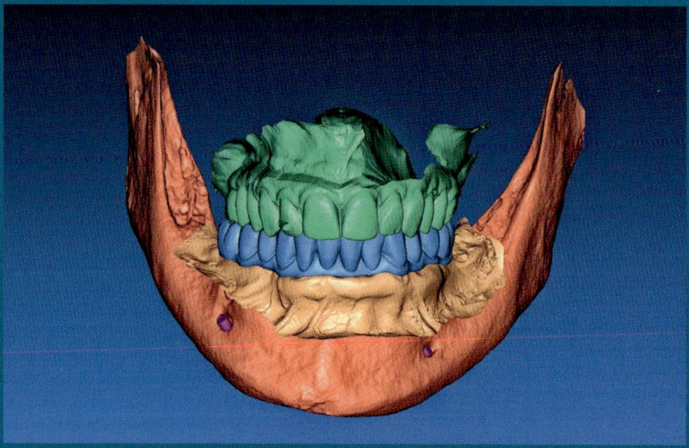

7.9 Design of the lower prosthesis, which will feature conometric connections with the implants.

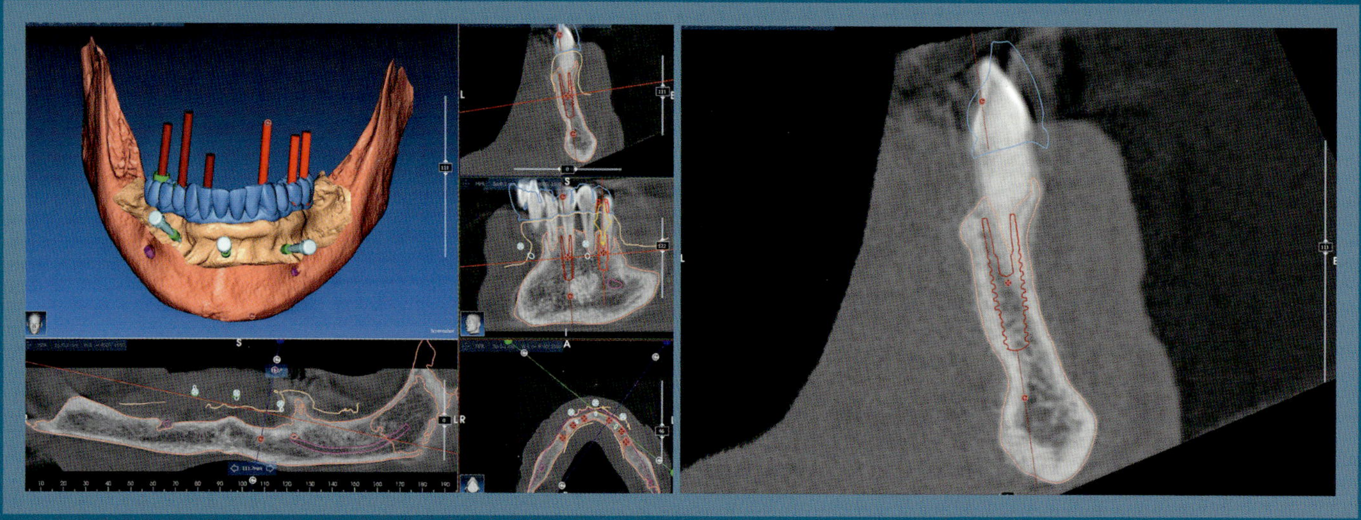

7.10 Planning the implant position based on the position of the prosthesis. Considering the reduced thickness of the crest, conical implants are chosen, in order to avoid fenestrations in the apical area of the implants.

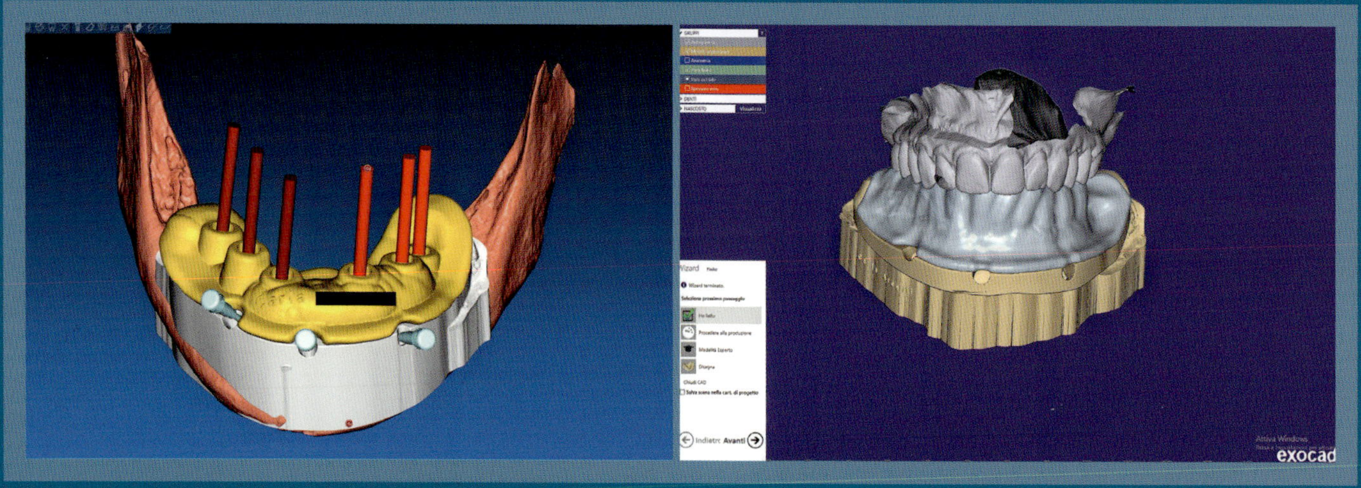

7.11 Design of the surgical guide and its components, i.e. the base with the sleeves for the intra-osseous pins (part B) and the resin bite (part A1), which will enable proper positioning in the patient's oral cavity thanks to occlusion with the upper arch and the teeth present in the lower arch. Tooth 38 is extracted to make proper housing of the surgical guide easier.

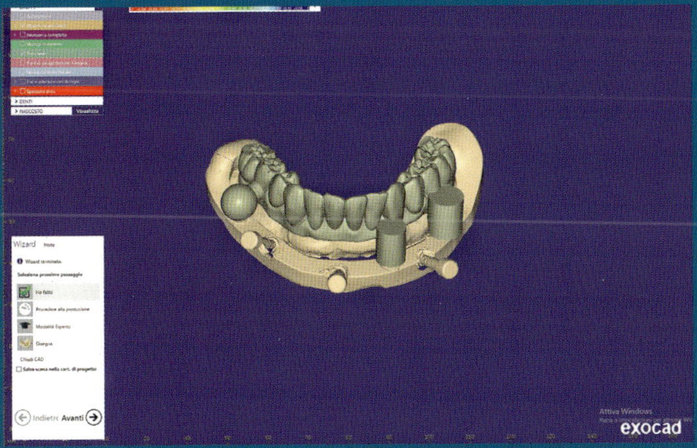

7.12 The prosthesis also has supports to be connected to the base of the index (part A5), thereby ensuring the utmost precision during the rebasing stage on the conometric copings.

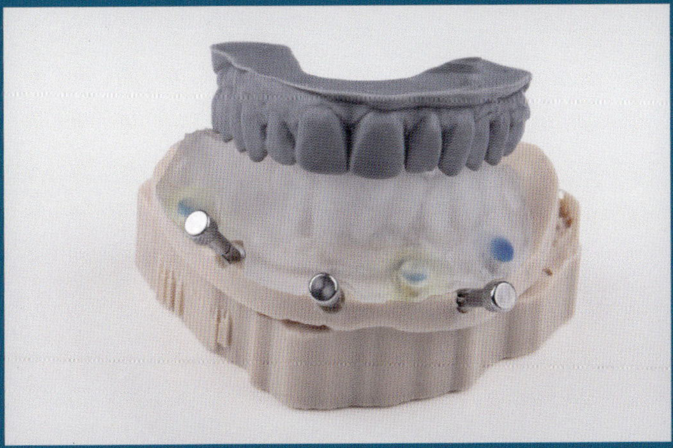

7.13 From top to bottom, antagonist model printed in resin, part A1 of the index according to the Digit protocol, part B with housing for the intra osseous pins, which must not interfere either with the position of the teeth to be extracted, or with that of the implants, initial model of the mandible with the teeth still present.

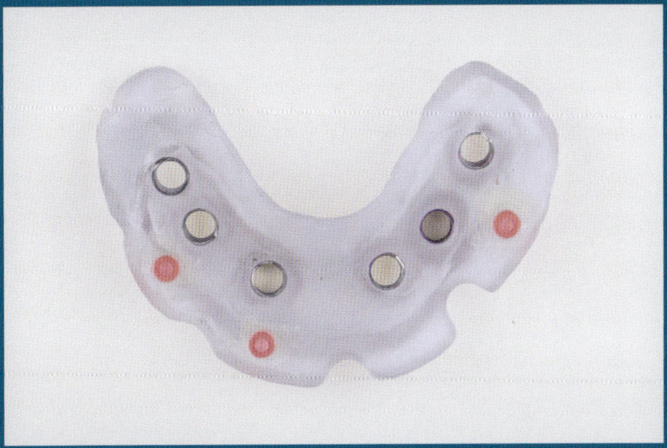

7.14 Part A3 of the index. In this case, part A2 (used for bone leveling) was not necessary as a flapless procedure was opted for.

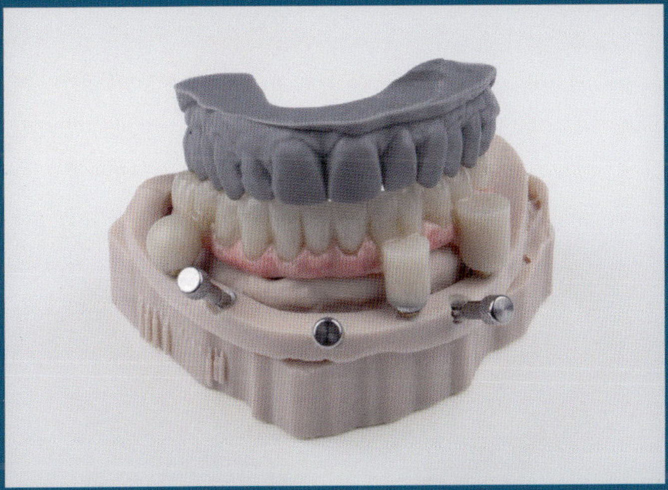

7.15 Compared to the situation shown in fig. 7.16, part A5 (Toronto prosthesis with attachment for proper placement) can be observed, supported on an edentulous model.

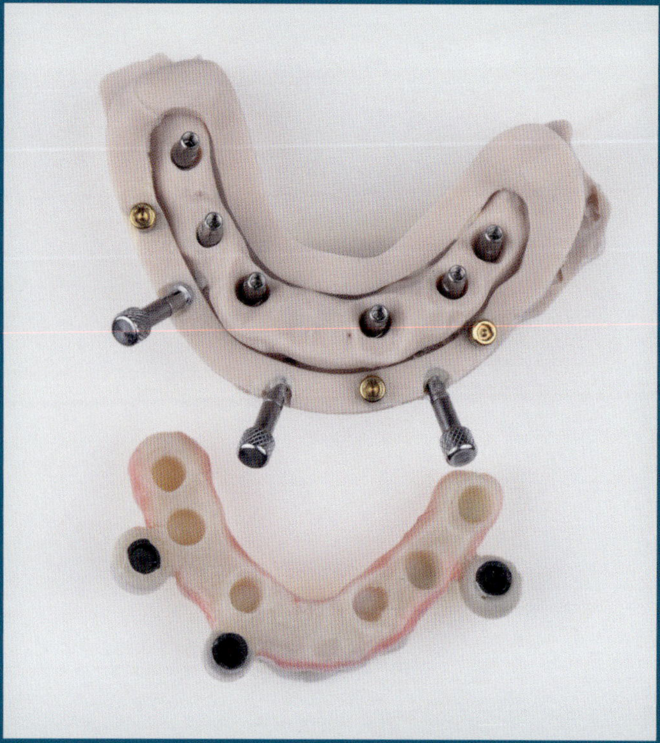

7.16 The edentulous model, with implant analogs (Myplant Bio) in position, can be observed. Implant abutments are inserted and the housings for the conometric copings are visible in the prosthesis. As all abutments are straight, part A4 (required to insert non-indexed angled abutments in the correct position) was not necessary.

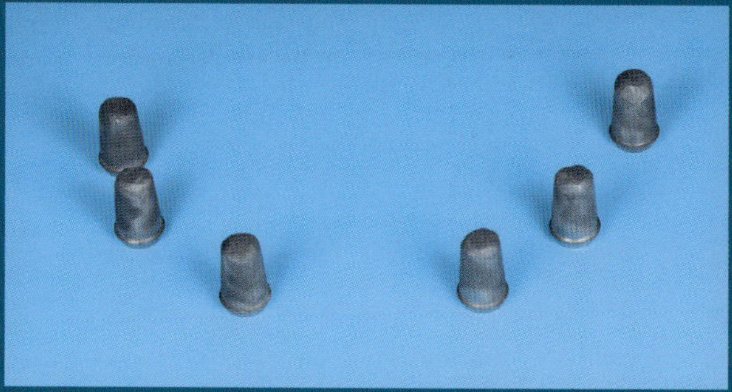

7.17 The copings are sandblasted prior to cementation with resin or composite in the appropriate housings.

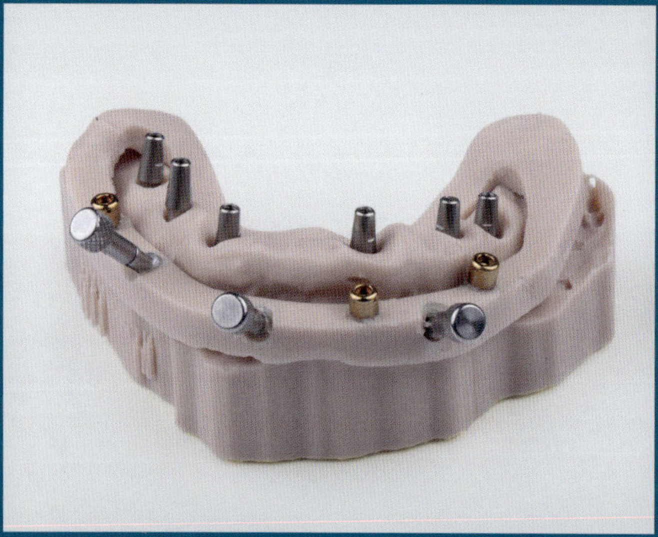

7.18 The model of the final patient situation, with part B of the index still in position.

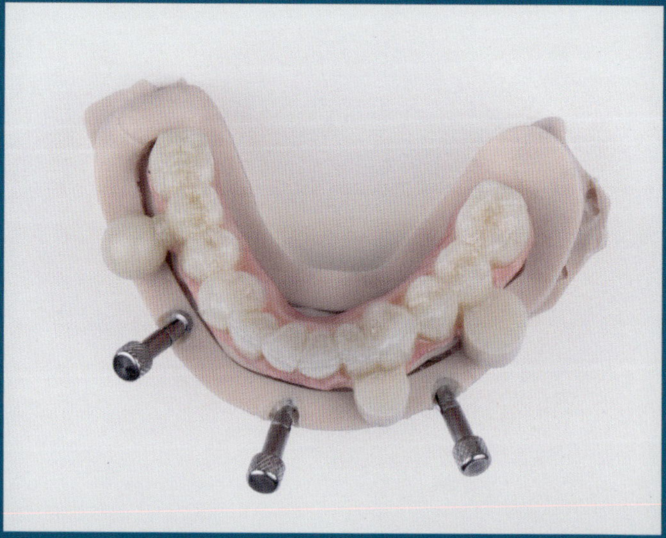

7.19 Occlusal view of the assembled parts.

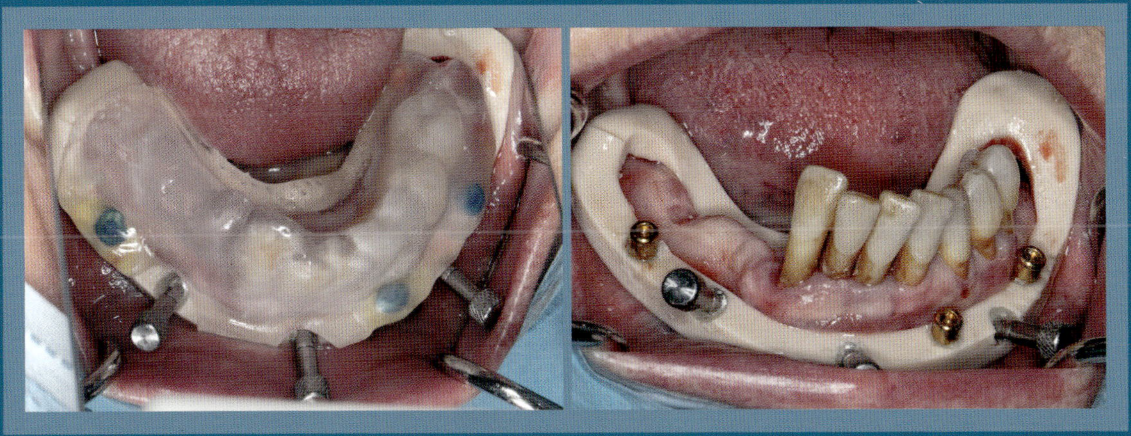

7.20 By using the resin bite, the guide is placed at the proper vertical position and secured with the pins.

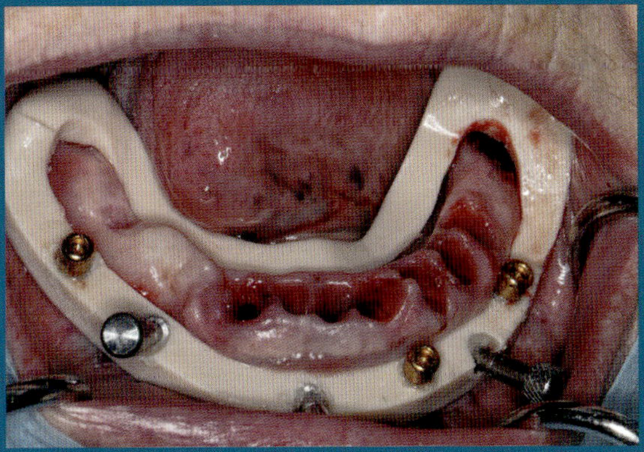

7.21 Teeth in the lower arch are extracted, while keeping the base of the guide in place.

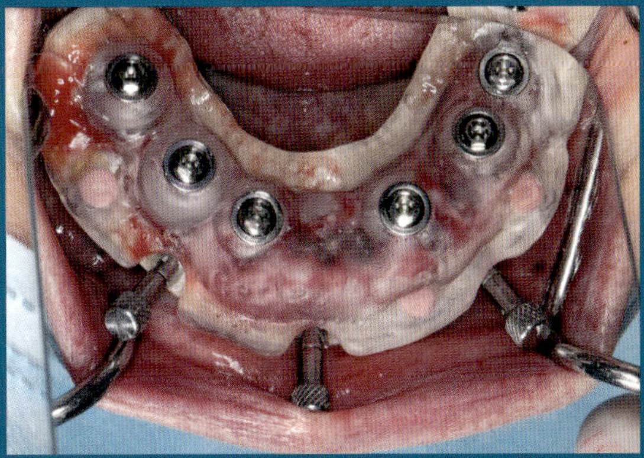

7.22 With the aid of the appropriate surgical guide, the six implants are inserted in the position previously decided and assessed on the basis of the designed prosthesis.

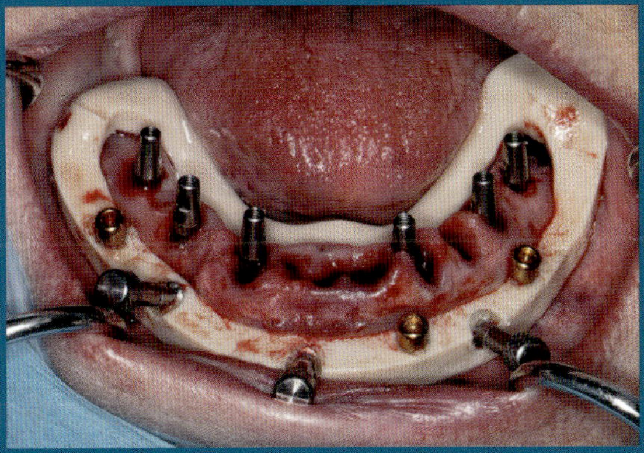

7.23 After removing part A3 of the surgical guide, the conometric abutments are inserted. At this stage, it is decided not to immediately load the implant in position 46, due to an insufficient insertion torque for immediate loading.

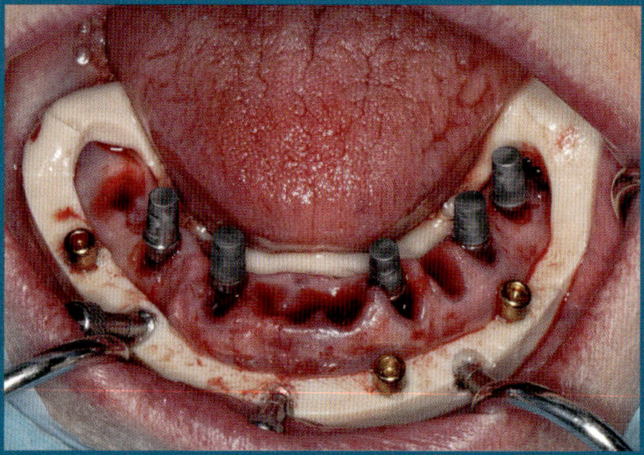

7.24 The conometric copings are inserted on the five implants to be loaded.

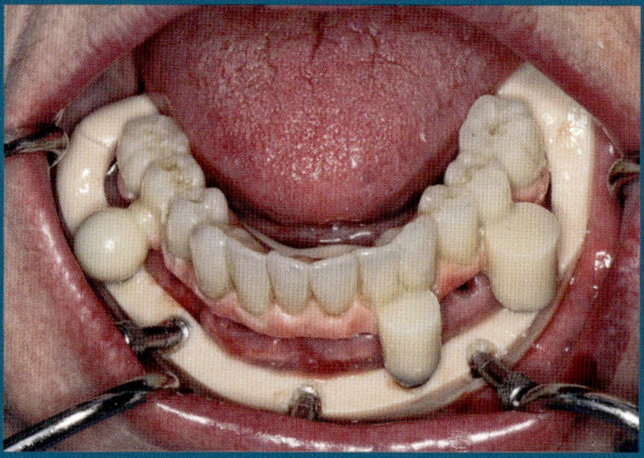

7.25 The provisional prosthesis is tested in position to assess its passivity.

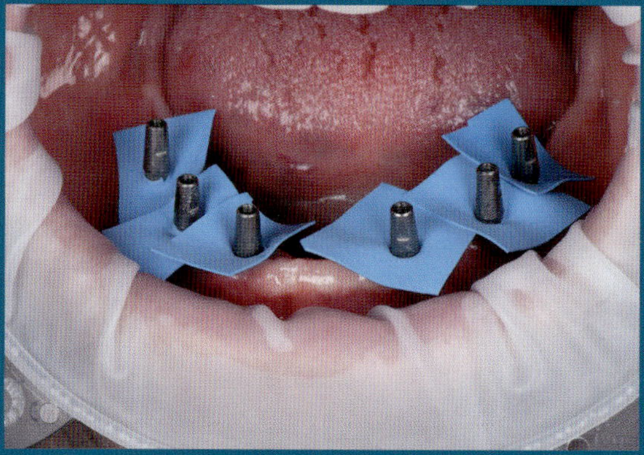

7.26 The underlying tissues are protected with rubber dam sheets before fixing the copings in the structure.

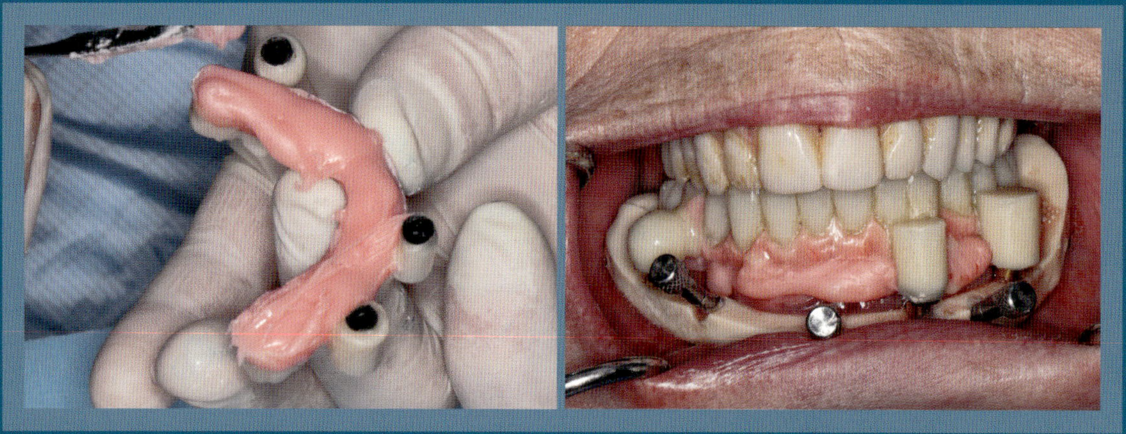

7.27 The copings are fixed in the prosthesis keeping as a reference the occlusion ensured by the ball attachments of the base index. In this case resin was used, but flowable composite may also be used.

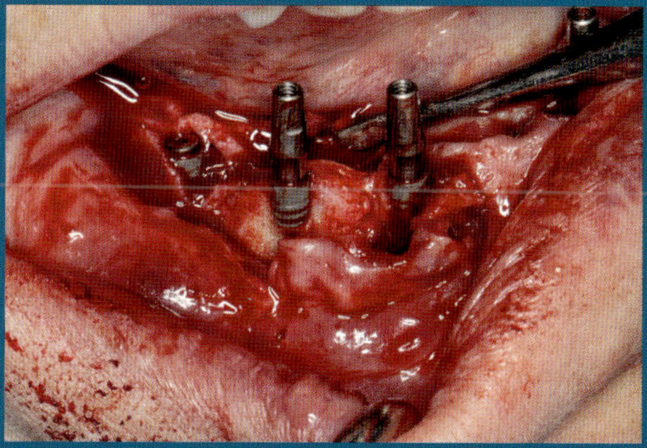

7.28 Bone defects: while waiting for the prosthesis to be completed by removal of the attachments and polishing, the residual bone defects around some implants in the fourth quadrant are treated with a regenerative technique.

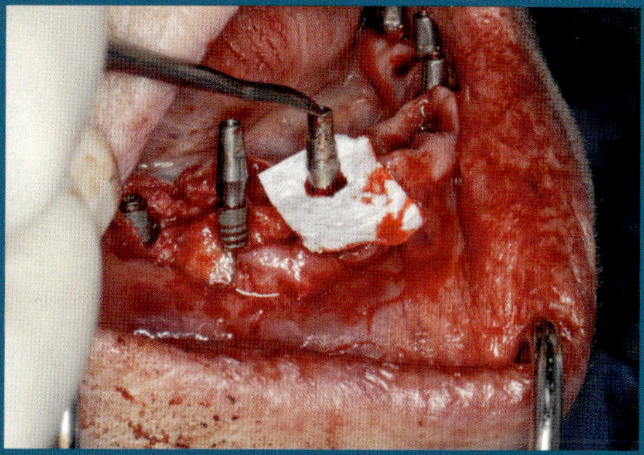

7.29 Resorbable membranes are positioned (Smartbrane Regedent) around the neck of the implants.

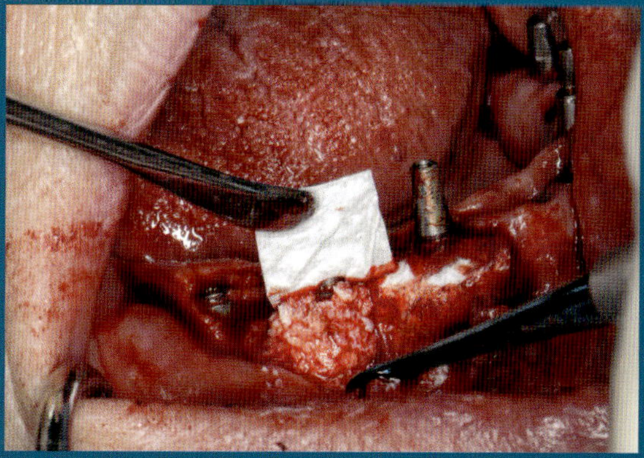

7.30 A mixture of de-proteinized bovine bone (Smartgraft Regedent) and autologous bone harvested during preparation of the implant sites is placed underneath the membranes.

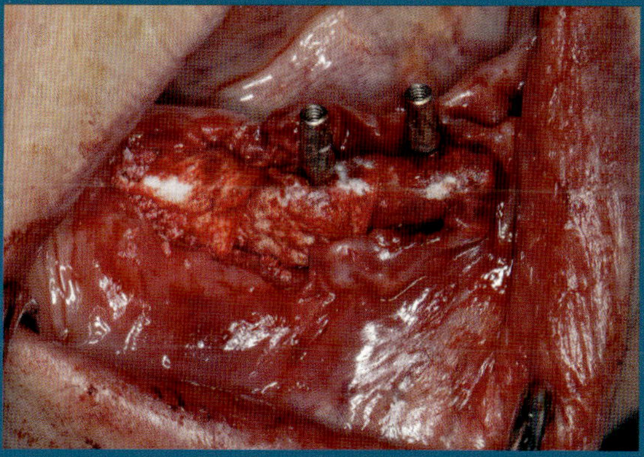

7.31 Membranes in the final position.

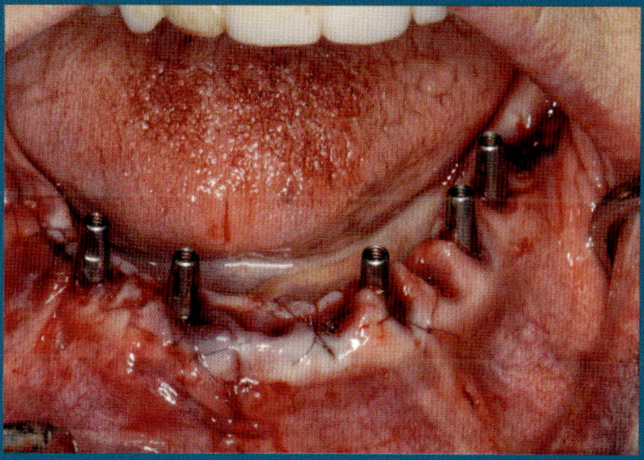

7.32 The flap is released and primary closure is obtained with an absorbable 6-0 suture.

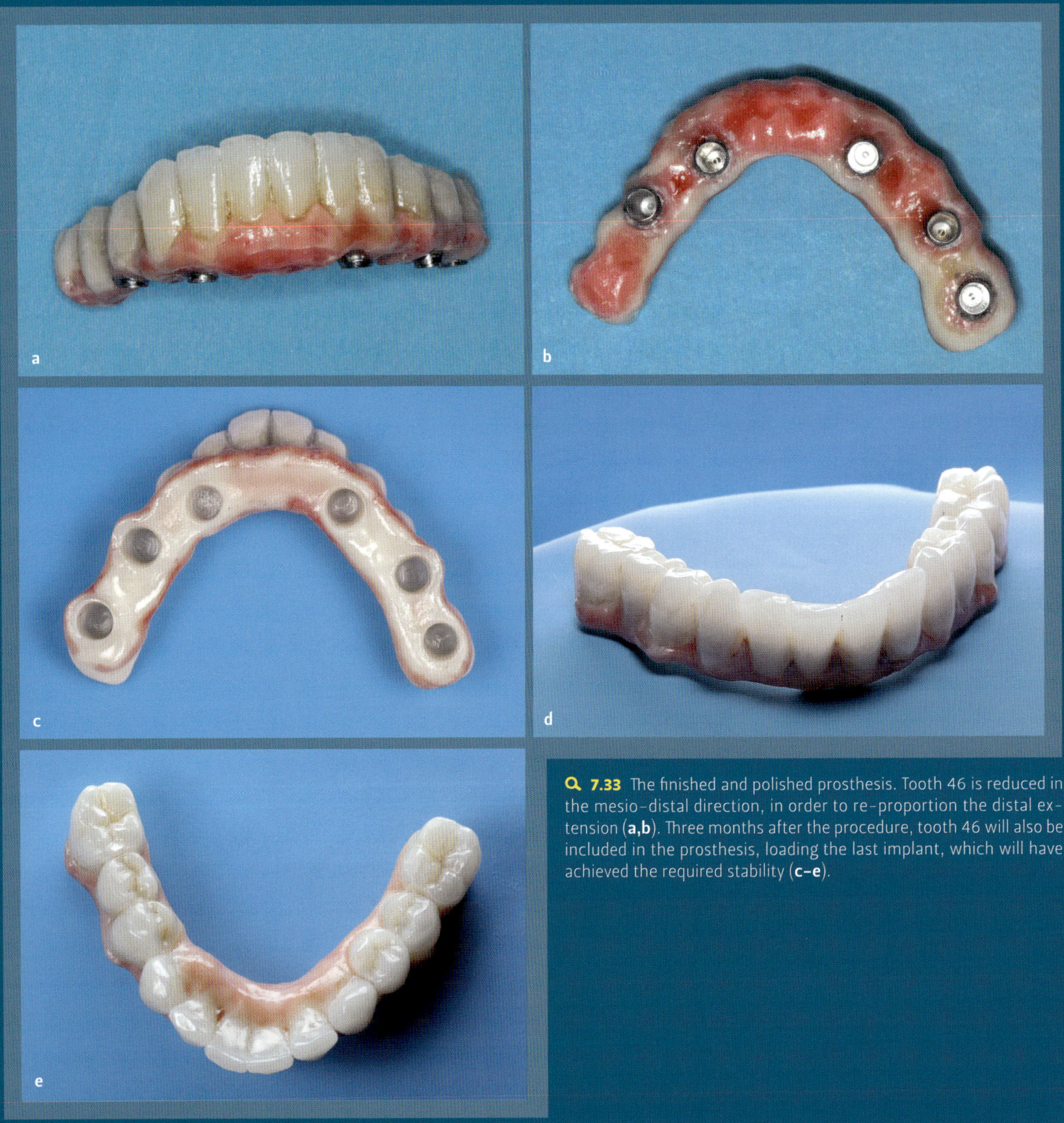

7.33 The finished and polished prosthesis. Tooth 46 is reduced in the mesio-distal direction, in order to re-proportion the distal extension (**a,b**). Three months after the procedure, tooth 46 will also be included in the prosthesis, loading the last implant, which will have achieved the required stability (**c–e**).

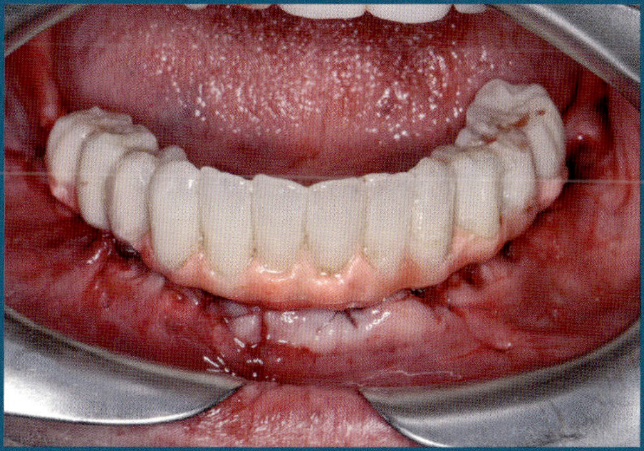

7.34 Prosthesis in place.

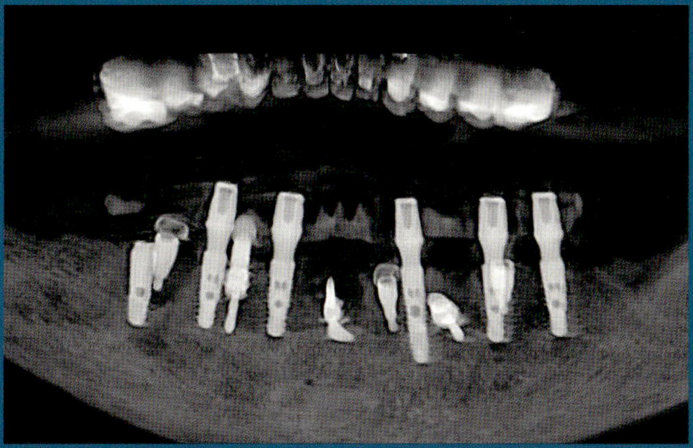

7.35 Control X-ray, where implants, pins and attachments of the prosthesis can be observed.

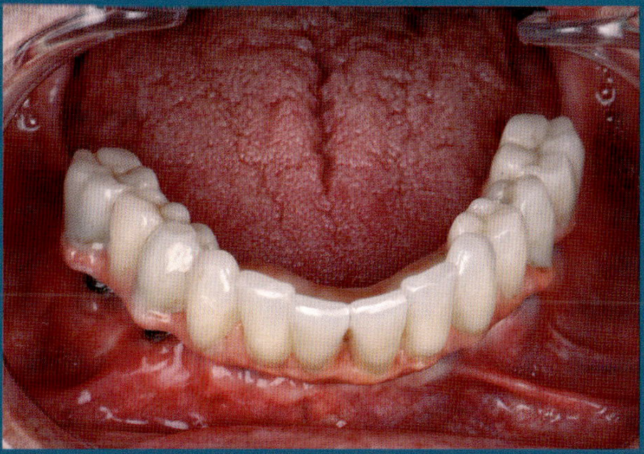

7.36 Situation after six months. It may observed that, in order to facilitate the patient's oral hygiene, a space was left between the prosthesis and the gums in the posterior regions.

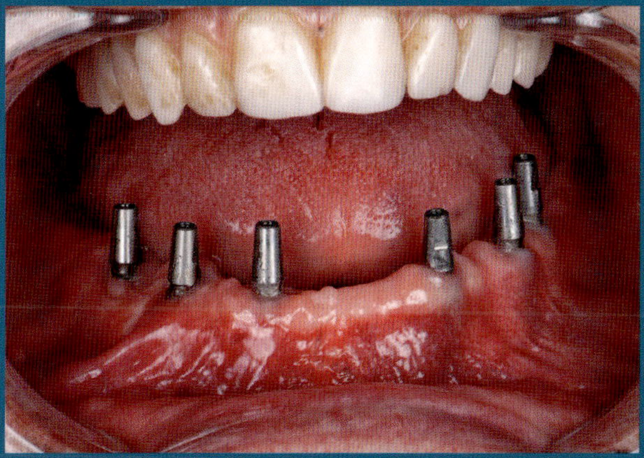

7.37 After prosthesis removal, healthy hard and soft tissues can be appreciated.

Clinical Case 2

Male patient, 59 years old

The patient complains of difficulty in chewing and unsatisfactory smile esthetics. No systemic issues are present. The objective examination shows no mucosal lesions. However, multiple inadequate restorations are observed in both arches. In quadrants I and II, two fixed bridgework with grade 3 mobility are present. An all ceramic bridge, from canine to canine, is also present but fractured. In the lower arch, teeth 36, 45, 46, 47 are missing. The remaining teeth show grade 2 or 3 mobility. On the first appointment, a PMMA bridge from 13 to 23 is placed, made with a chairside method to replace the previous fractured restoration in the anterior region (7.38).

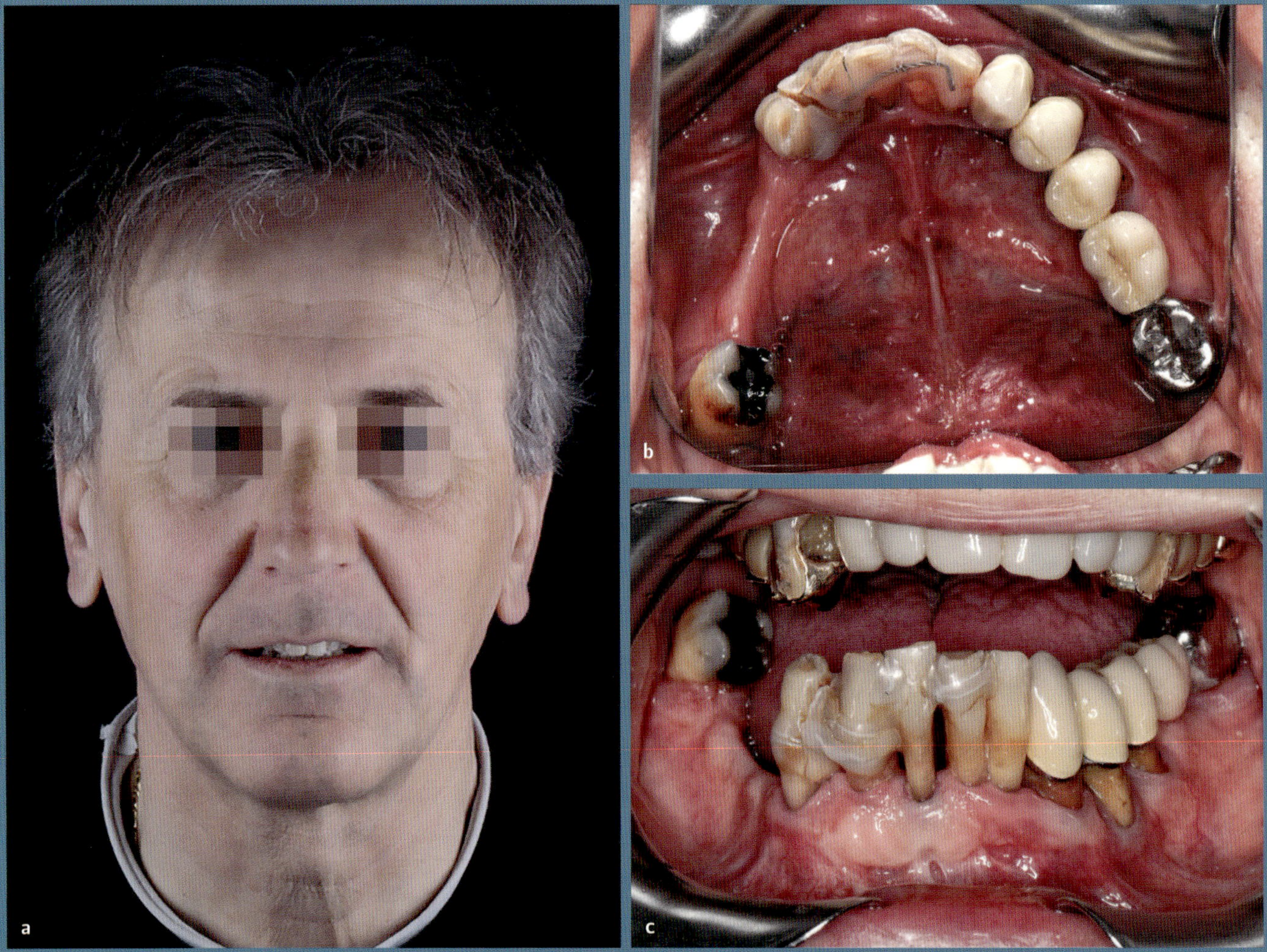

7.38 a) The patient complains of difficulty in chewing, widespread pain, bleeding. **b,c)** Occlusal and frontal view of the initial situation; note the unevenness of the periodontium.

The radiographic examination shows the marked resorption of the tooth supporting tissues in both arches, due to the quality of the restorations, incorrect distribution of the chewing load, but above all to an insufficient level of oral hygiene (7.39).

First of all, the lower arch is designed as shown in the steps (7.40). Once it is ascertained that the patient is able to achieve and maintain a satisfactory level of health of his gingival tissues, the guide is designed for the placement of six implants in the lower arch, in order to place a fixed total prosthesis (7.41a,b).

In the design, a space is also provided between the grid and the bone crest in the anterior area, in anticipation of horizontal regenerative surgery (7.41c).

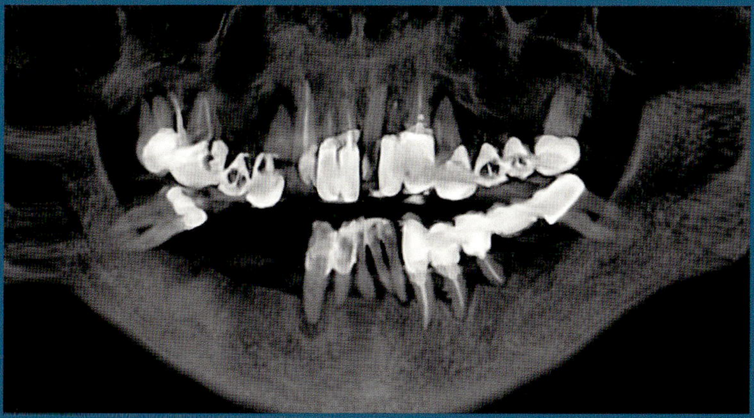

7.39 Panoramic X-ray showing marked lower as well as upper bone resorption. In the upper jaw, the treatment plan entails the retreatment of teeth 13,12, 11, 21,22, 23 and insertion of implants in the posterior sectors following bilateral sinus lift. At mandibular level, a Toronto-type prosthesis on six implants is planned.

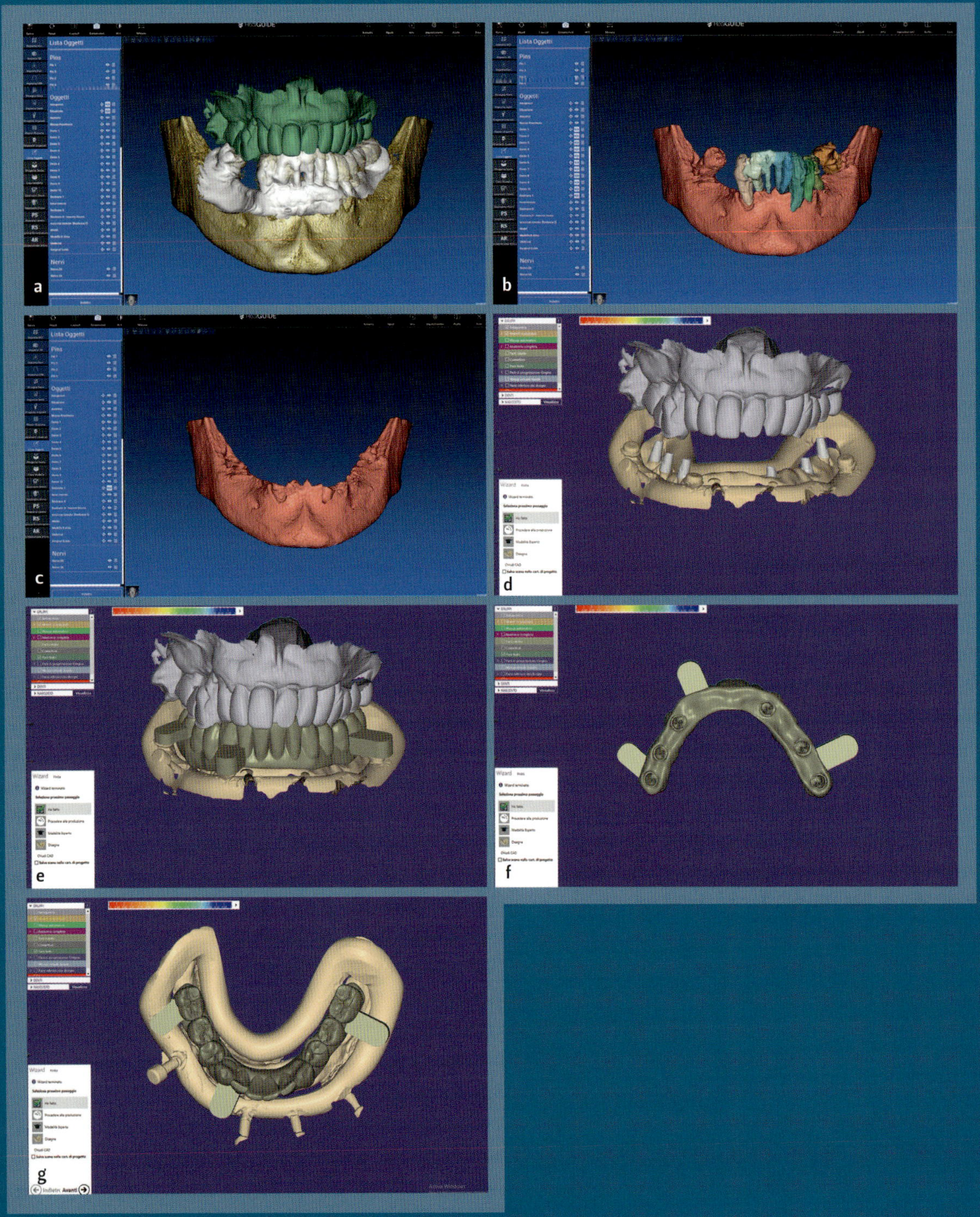

7.40 **a)** Matching CBCT and three-dimensional CAD rendering. **b)** The teeth to be removed with "virtual" extraction are highlighted and removed **(c)**, making the patient virtually edentulous. **d)** The implants and conometric abutments are inserted. **e)** The provisional prosthesis is fitted with the retentive attachments that will stabilize it on part B of the guide. **f)** The housings created for the retention copings - which will be cemented at the end of the surgical procedure - can be observed. **g)** Occlusal view of part B and of the provisional prosthesis (A5) assembled.

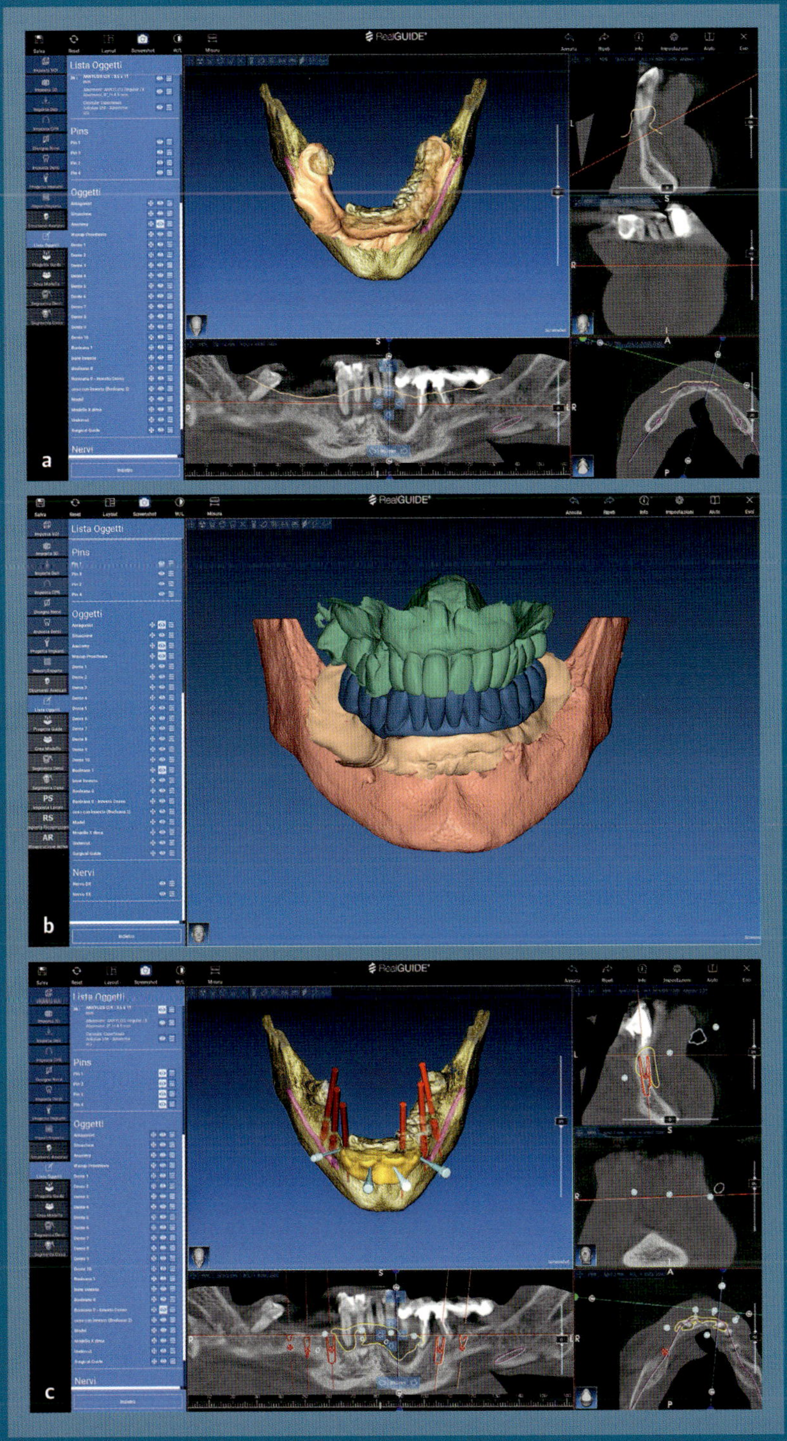

7.41 a) The CBCT examination is imported in the RealGuide design software (3Diemme) and matched to the intraoral scans. **b)** The Toronto prosthesis is designed. **c)** Surgical guide with insertion of the intra-osseous pins; the implants are inserted, despite the scant bone volume present.

The first step consists in fixing the base guide by means of a resin bite, held in position by the patient's occlusion (7.42).

After assembling the guide for implant insertion, the six implants are placed in the previously planned position (7.42 b-d).

After placing in the area of 32-33, a mixture of autologous and de-proteinized bovine bone, covered by resorbable membrane, a control X-ray is taken (7.43).

Finally, the provisional prosthesis is rebased on the conometric copings, based on the position determined by the ball attachments, and subsequently finished and polished. The provisional prosthesis is positioned again in the mouth and the copings are activated by means of the appropriate fixing instrument (7.44).

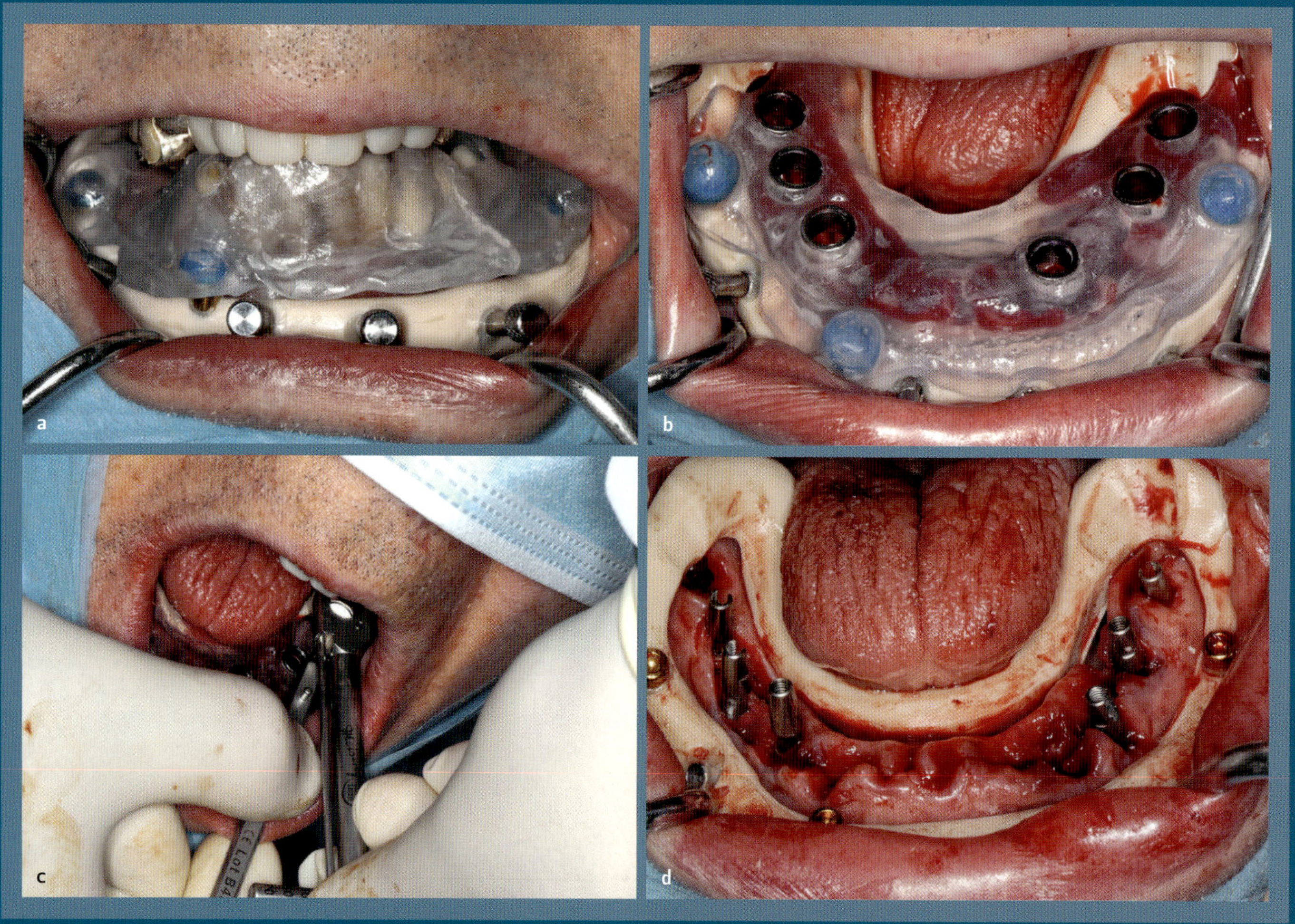

7.42 **a)** The bite in occlusion with the antagonist allows the exact positioning of part B of the surgical guide and consequently the insertion of the pins in the intended position. **b,c)** Part A3 of the guide in position for guided insertion of the six planned implants (Myplant bio). **d)** Implants and conometric abutments in position; part B of the index is still present.

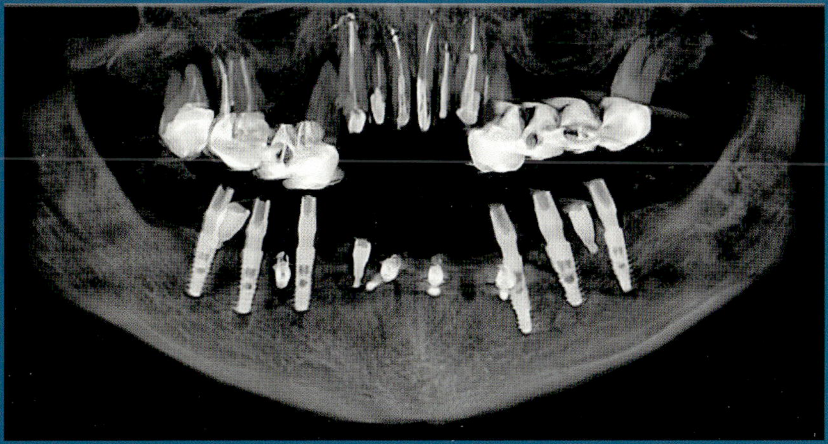

7.43 Control X-ray.

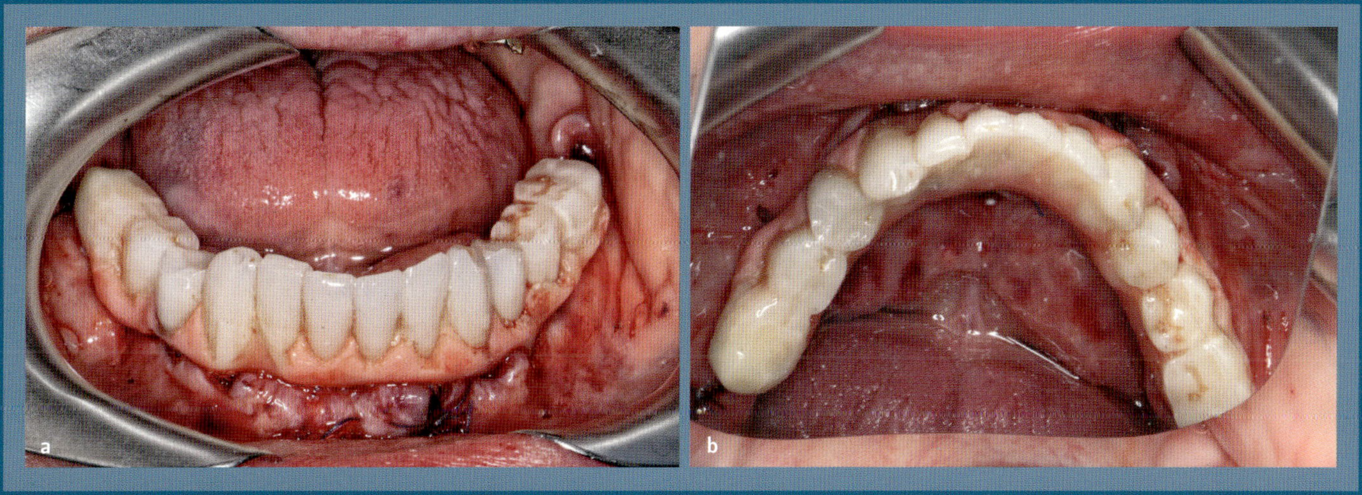

7.44 **a)** Prosthesis in composite material in position after attachments removal. **b)** Occlusal view.

Clinical Case 3

Male patient, 63 years old

The patient presents requesting a fixed rehabilitation for his lower arch. In the upper arch, a complete denture is present; in the lower one, the only surviving tooth is 33, however, it is compromised from a periodontal point of view, with grade 3 mobility. No systemic issues are reported (7.45- 7.46).

During the first appointment intraoral scans (7.47a) and CBCT are taken.

In order to make image matching easier, radiopaque markers were placed on the mucous tissue during CBCT acquisition. The radiographic examination shows marked crestal bone resorption. The analysis of the occlusion of the upper prosthesis highlights marked abrasion (7.47a).

A lower fixed prosthesis is then designed, supported by six implants (7.47b,c). The design of the prosthesis guides the implant position (7.47d).

An index is then fabricated which, placed in occlusion with the upper arch, can guide the placement of the grid for insertion of the pins, including the attachments for proper placement of the surgical guide and the provisional prosthesis. The prosthesis is designed on conometric abutments (7.47 e-h) as is consequently the surgical guide.

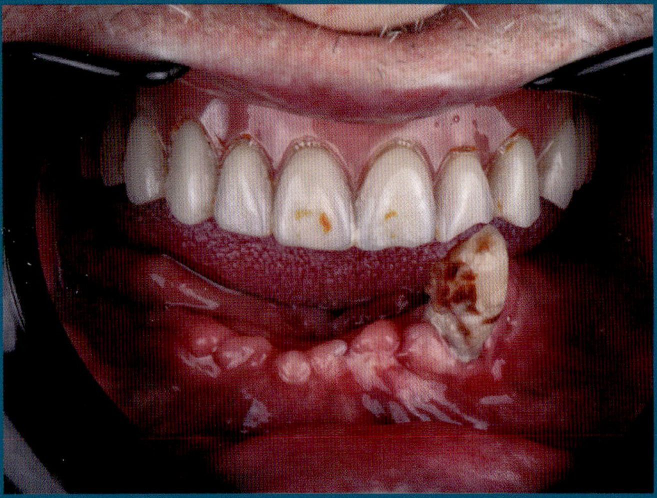

7.45 Initial situation.

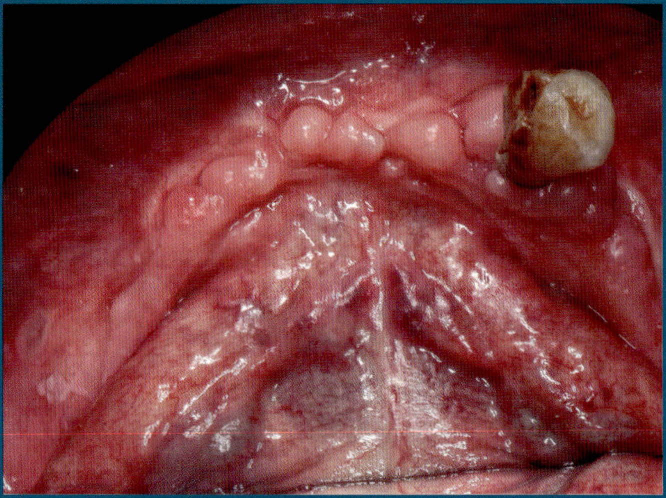

7.46 Occlusal view of the initial situation.

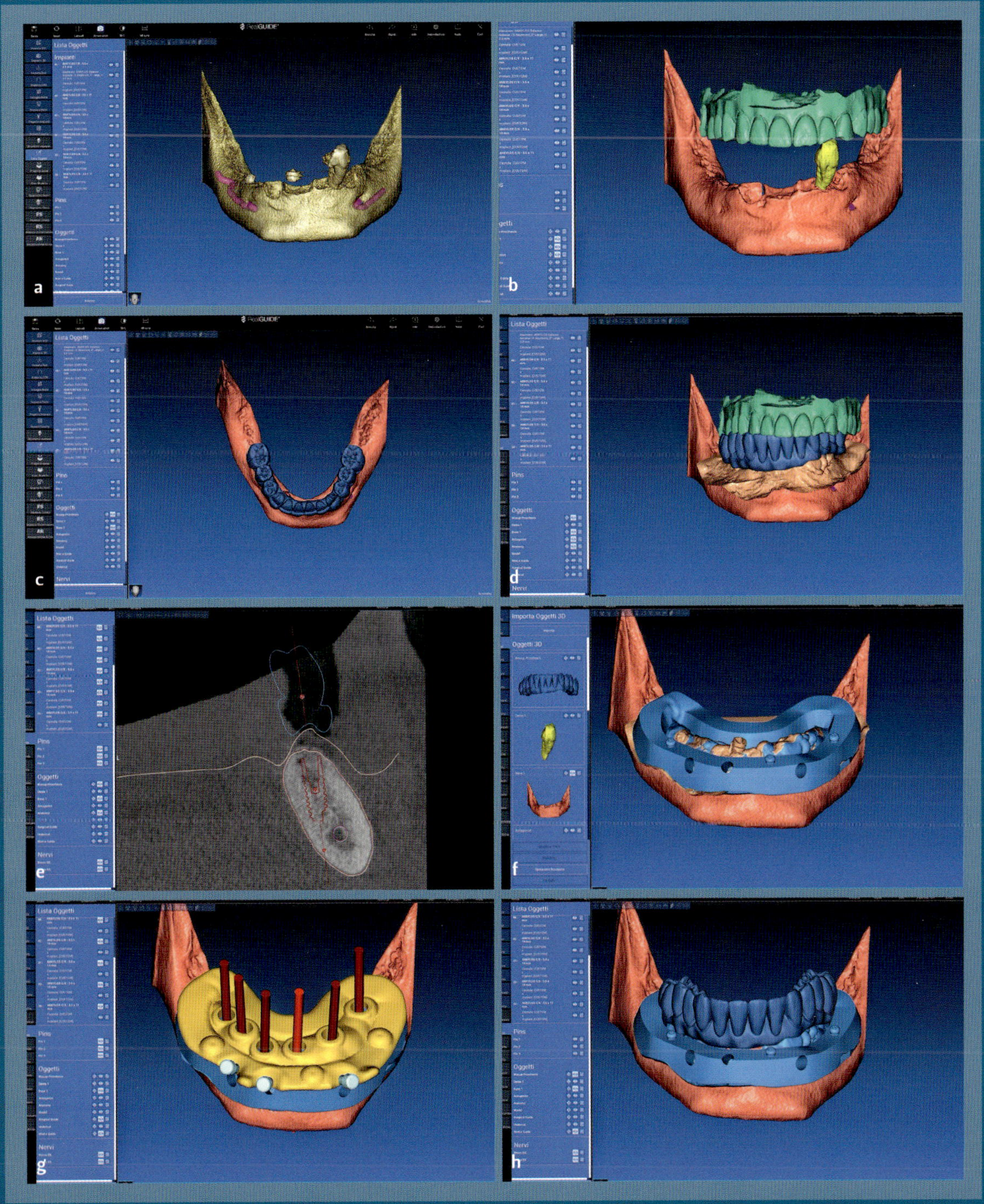

7.47 **a)** CBCT with highlighted layout of the mandibular nerves. **b)** Matched antagonist. **c)** Designed prosthesis, occlusal view and in relationship with the antagonist **(d,e)** The positions of the implants are identified on the basis of the prosthetic design. **f)** Design of part B of the guide. **g)** Part A3 of the guide. **h)** The same guide holding the prosthesis.

The components designed with the CAD software are fabricated with a milling machine (7.48a–d).

The provisional PMMA prosthesis is fabricated with posterior elements in composite, separately milled (7.48e).

The first surgical step was tooth 33 extraction (7.49).

The pins are then positioned through an index deriving from a diagnostic wax-up with mucous support, which replicates the provisional prosthe-

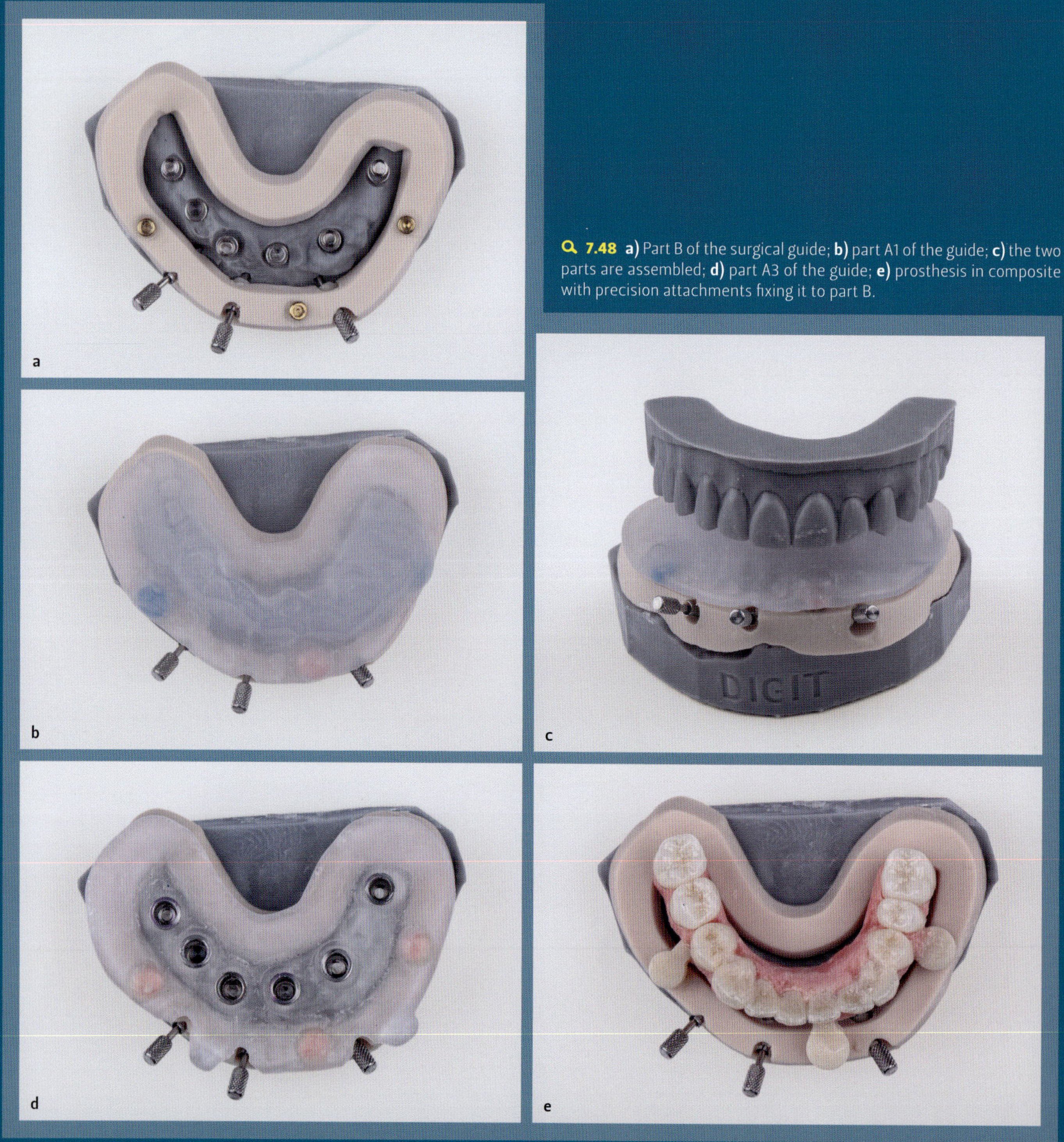

7.48 **a)** Part B of the surgical guide; **b)** part A1 of the guide; **c)** the two parts are assembled; **d)** part A3 of the guide; **e)** prosthesis in composite with precision attachments fixing it to part B.

sis in occlusion with the upper prosthesis (7.50). The surgical guide is applied for implant placement, then the implants are inserted (7.51).

The conometric abutments are positioned, with their copings, on which the prosthesis previously produced is placed (7.52).

The Toronto type prosthesis perfectly matches the attachments on the placement grid (7.53a), thus making it possible to fix the secondary copings with rebasing resin.

Finally, the situation with completed provisional prosthesis is shown (7.53b, 7.54).

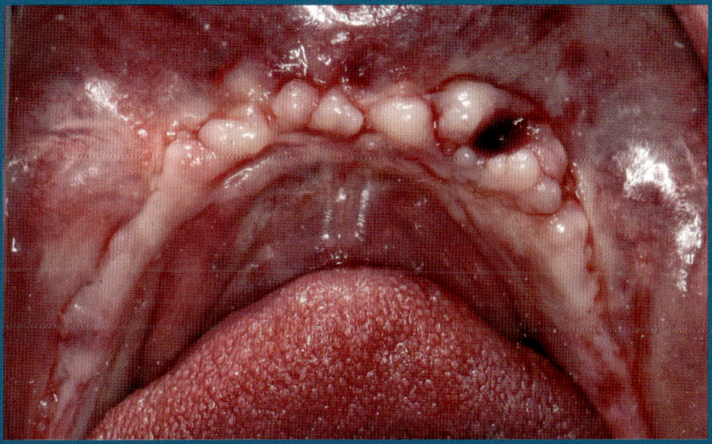

7.49 Occlusal view after tooth extraction.

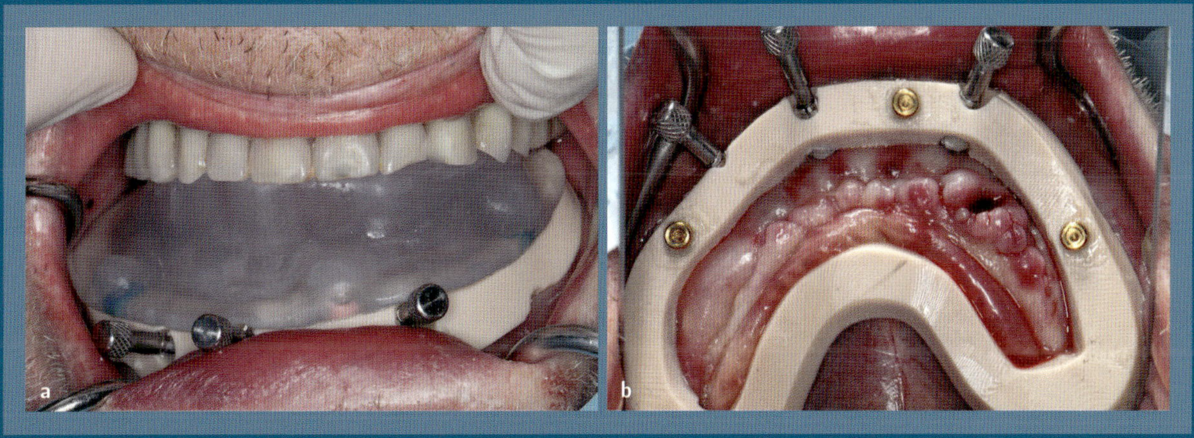

7.50 a) Part B of the guide locked in position thanks to part A1 in occlusion with the antagonist. **b)** Part B fixed with pins; the precision Locator attachments are visible.

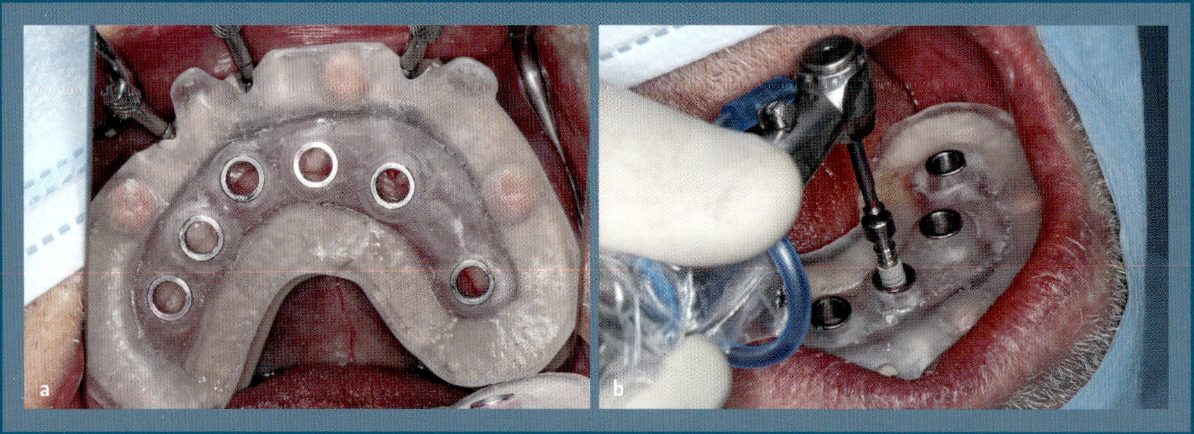

7.51 **a)** Part A3 assembled, required for guided implant insertion **(b)**.

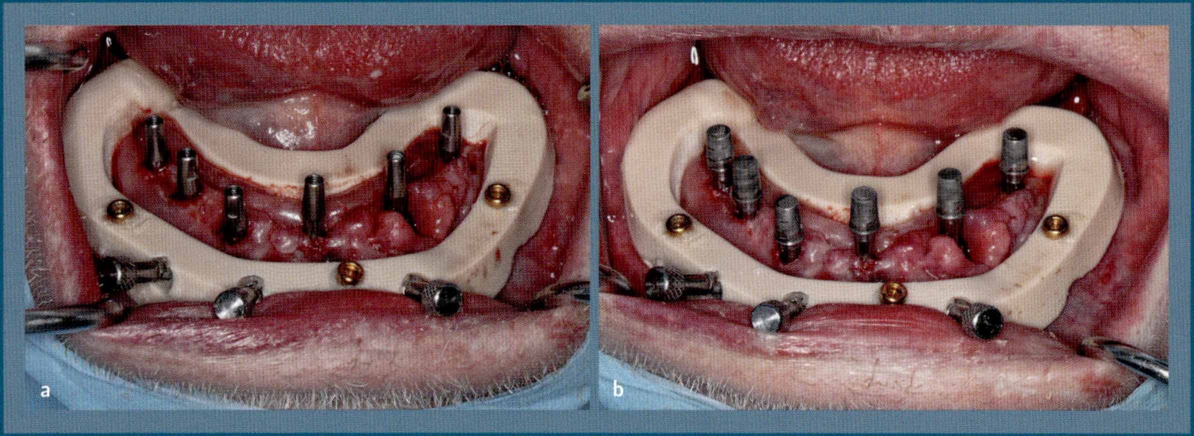

7.52 **a)** Inserted implants fitted with straight conometric abutment. **b)** Conometric copings application; these were sandblasted on the outside to ensure a more effective adhesion after cementation in the prosthesis housings.

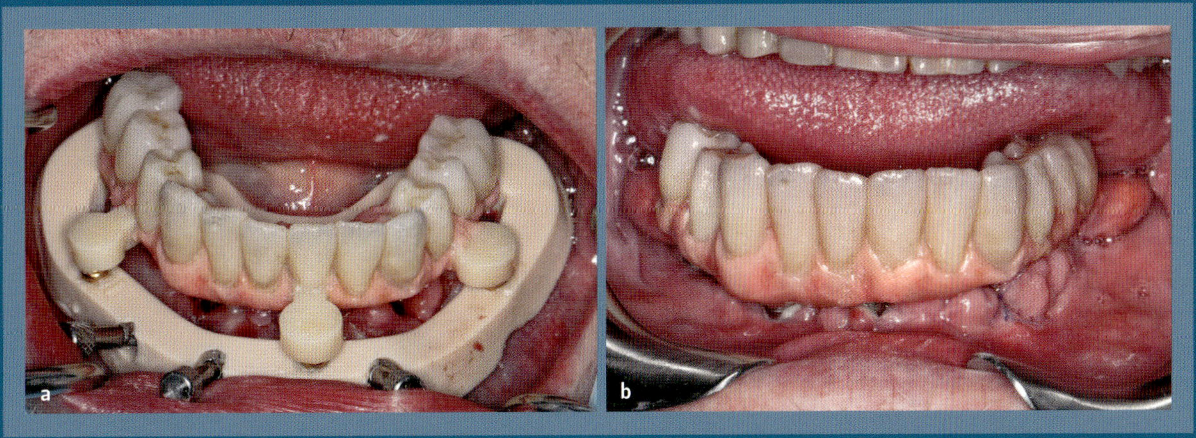

7.53 **a,b)** Prosthesis in position fixed to the attachments during rebasing: this system ensures its correct position with regards to the vertical dimension as well as to occlusion.

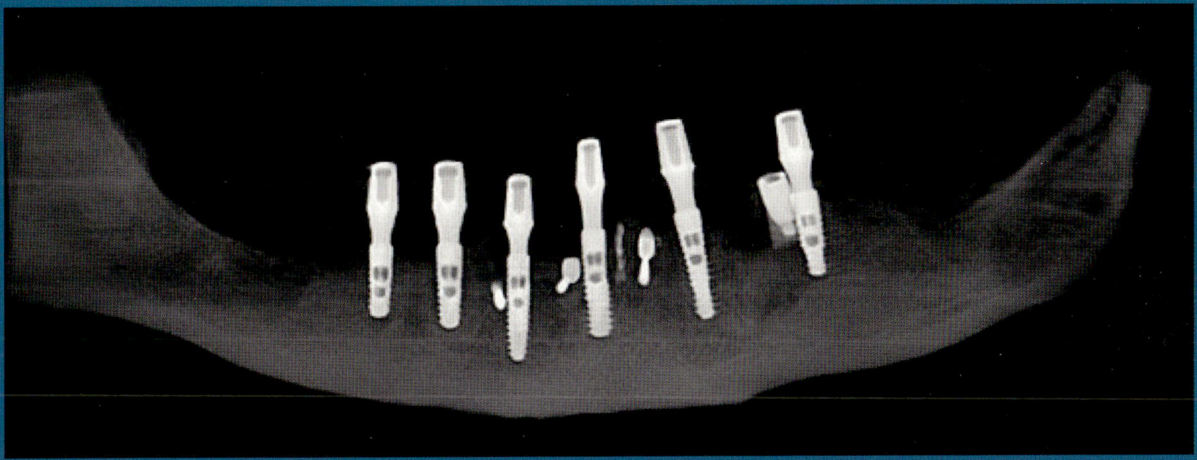

7.54 Control X-ray.